Practical intelligence

For many years, the study of intelligence has been dominated by the study of performance of intelligence tests. In recent years, psychologists, educators, and the lay public have become dissatisfied with tests that limit the measurement and conception of intelligence to performance on academic, and often obscure, kinds of tasks. The purpose of this book is to present a broader view of intelligence, to document the importance of intelligence not only in schools but in everyday life, including both job-related and domestic settings.

Practical Intelligence draws together fifteen chapters by distinguished experts in the field. It includes four main parts, plus introductory and concluding chapters. The first part deals with intelligence as it operates in job-related settings. The second part deals with intelligence as it operates in other everyday settings. The third part deals with the development of practical intelligence over the lifespan. The fourth part deals with the relations between practical intelligence, on the one hand, and culture and society, on the other. The chapters represent a diversity of theoretical and methodological perspectives. Together, they offer a comprehensive overview of the current state of thinking about practical intelligence. Psychologists, educators, and managers will all find *Practical Intelligence* an invaluable resource for themselves and their students, as will lay persons interested in conceptions of intelligence that are relevant to their everyday lives.

Practical intelligence
Nature and origins of
competence in the everyday world

Edited by

ROBERT J. STERNBERG *and* **RICHARD K. WAGNER**
Yale University   *Florida State University*

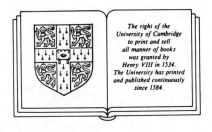

The right of the
University of Cambridge
to print and sell
all manner of books
was granted by
Henry VIII in 1534.
The University has printed
and published continuously
since 1584.

CAMBRIDGE UNIVERSITY PRESS

Cambridge
London   New York   New Rochelle
Melbourne   Sydney

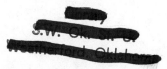

Essay Index

Published by the Press Syndicate of the University of Cambridge
The Pitt Building, Trumpington Street, Cambridge CB2 1RP
32 East 57th Street, New York, NY 10022, USA
10 Stamford Road, Oakleigh, Melbourne 3166, Australia

First published 1986

Printed in the United States of America

Library of Congress Cataloging-in-Publication Data
Main entry under title.
Practical intelligence.
Includes index.
1. Intellect.   I. Sternberg, Robert J.   II. Wagner,
Richard K.
BF431.P67   1986   153.9   85-28942

British Library Cataloguing in Publication Data
Practical intelligence: nature and origins of
competence in the everyday world.
1. Intellect.
I. Sternberg, Robert J.   II. Wagner, Richard K.
153.9   BF431

ISBN 0 521 30253 6 hard covers
ISBN 0 521 31797 5 paperback

Contents

260819

Contributors

Paul B. Baltes, Max Planck Institute for Human Development and Education, Berlin

J. W. Berry, Department of Psychology, Queen's University, Kingston, Ontario

Stephen J. Ceci, Human Development and Family Studies, Cornell University

Roger A. Dixon, Max Planck Institute for Human Development and Education, Berlin

Martin E. Ford, School of Education, Stanford University

Norman Frederiksen, Educational Testing Service, Princeton

Howard E. Gardner, Harvard Project Zero and Boston Veterans Administration Medical Center

Margarita Gomez-Palacio, Direccion General de Educacion Especial, Republic de Mexico

Jacqueline J. Goodnow, School of Behavioural Sciences, Macquarie University, Sydney, N.S.W.

S. H. Irvine, Department of Psychology, Plymouth Polytechnic

George O. Klemp, Jr., Charles River Consulting, Boston

Jeffrey Liker, Industrial and Operations Engineering, University of Michigan

David C. McClelland, Department of Psychology and Social Relations, Harvard University

Jane R. Mercer, Department of Sociology, University of California, Riverside

David R. Olson, Centre for Applied Cognitive Science, The Ontario Institute for Studies in Education and McLuhan Program in Culture and Technology, University of Toronto

Eligio Padilla, Department of Psychology, University of New Mexico

K. Warner Schaie, College of Human Development, Pennsylvania State University

Sylvia Scribner, Department of Psychology, City University of New York Graduate Center

Robert J. Sternberg, Department of Psychology, Yale University

Richard K. Wagner, Department of Psychology, Florida State University

Joseph M. Walters, Harvard Project Zero

Sherry L. Willis, College of Human Development, Pennsylvania State University

Preface

For many years, the study of intelligence was dominated by the study of intelligence tests. The domination of such tests in the study of intelligence had several unforeseen and unfortunate consequences. First, the study of tests tended to shift the focus of intelligence research away from theoretical issues and toward measurement issues. Although measurement issues are of interest in their own right, they can be studied more effectively when the research on testing is theoretically based. Second, creators and users of intelligence tests tended to be less than fully reflective about just what it was that the tests were measuring. The notion that intelligence is whatever it is that intelligence tests happen to measure has been a predominant one, whether or not this notion has been explicitly acknowledged. Third, intelligence tests were originally constructed for purposes of classification of students according to academic ability, with the result that theories and tests of intelligence tended to be focused on the academic domain. Behavior in everyday settings was seen as a possible criterion for validating intelligence tests as predictors, but everyday or practical intelligence received little attention in its own right.

During the last several years, a number of investigators have become increasingly dissatisfied with notions that restrict both the theory and measurement of intelligence to academic kinds of skills. Investigators have increasingly recognized the limited predictive value of conventional intelligence tests for everyday performance and, more importantly, have realized the theoretical limitations of academic conceptions of intelligence when the goal is to understand intelligence as it operates in the real world. As a result, increasing numbers of investigators of intelligence have turned their attention to the construct of practical, or everyday intelligence.

For the most part, research on practical intelligence is rather new. Relatively little work has been done in this area, and the existing research is scattered throughout the literature. This book attempts to bring together the theory and research of a number of leading investigators who have chosen to devote at least part of their research effort toward understanding and assessing the nature and origins of practical intelligence.

The book is divided into four main parts, preceded by an introductory chapter and concluding with a summary. The first part deals with intelligence as it operates in job-related settings, the second part deals with intelligence as it operates in everyday settings outside of occupational pursuits, the third part deals with the life-span development of practical intelligence, and the fourth part deals with the relationship between practical intelligence on the one hand, and culture and society on the other. Each contribution is by one or more leading investigators in the field of intelligence and represents an overview of a significant research program in the field. The chapters represent a diversity of theoretical and methodological perspectives and present a fairly complete overview of the current state of the field.

This book should be of interest to psychologists, educators, sociologists, and anthropologists interested in intelligence as it functions in the everyday world. Moreover, it can be used as a textbook in a variety of courses, such as those on intelligence, cognition, ecological psychology, individual differences, tests and measurements, and human abilities. The chapters have been written at a level that should be readable by beginning graduate students or even by advanced undergraduates with some background in the field of intelligence and human cognition. We believe that this book will be useful for instructional purposes and that it will set directions for research on intelligence in the coming years.

R. J. S.
R. K. W.

1   Introduction: The nature and scope of practical intelligence

Robert J. Sternberg

What is practical intelligence, and where is it found? This book contains thirteen responses to this question. These responses could be classified in any of a number of ways; indeed, the book is organized in terms of four parts that reflect four different orientations toward the problem of practical intelligence: practical intelligence as it is found in occupational settings (Part I), practical intelligence as it is found in daily life outside of occupational settings (Part II), the life-span development of practical intelligence (Part III), and the relationship between practical intelligence and culture and society (Part IV). The essays in this volume deal with many questions, but three seem preeminent: (1) What is practical intelligence? (2) In what ways is it similar to (or an extension of) academic intelligence, and in what ways is it distinctive from academic intelligence? (3) To what extent is practical intelligence domain-specific versus domain-general? In briefly summarizing each of the essays, we shall deal especially with these questions.

Chapter 1

This introductory chapter discusses some of the key questions that need to be answered about practical intelligence and summarizes the remaining chapters in terms of their answers to these questions.

Chapter 2

In her chapter, Thinking in Action: Some Characteristics of Practical Thought, Sylvia Scribner suggests that there are different kinds of thinking and that it is useful to distinguish between theoretical thinking, on the one hand, and practical thinking, on the other. She views practical thinking as the "mind in action," using the term to refer to thinking that is embedded in the larger scale purposive activities of daily life. Practical thinking serves to achieve the goals of the everyday activities in which one engages. Scribner and collaborators have studied practical thinking in a variety of settings, including the activities of workers in a milk-processing plant, of bartenders,

1

of sales engineers, and of waitresses. Using both ethnographic and experimental techniques, she observes how workers in these various settings use
fairly sophisticated methods of problem solving to accomplish their goals.
Although she and her colleagues have observed domain specificity in the
kinds of problems that practical thinkers must solve, they have found striking
resemblances in the kinds of practical reasoning that these workers bring to
their jobs to make the jobs easier. In particular, even mundane kinds of jobs
can involve an astonishing degree of complexity and show rather substantial
differences in functioning between experts and novices. Scribner presents
a rather detailed analysis of the kinds of practical reasoning that workers in
seemingly ordinary jobs bring to their tasks.

Chapter 3

In their discussion of What Characterizes Intelligent Functioning Among
Senior Managers?, George O. Klemp and David C. McClelland analyze the
generic competencies that distinguish between more and less successful
managers. Using a stunningly large data base accumulated over years of
experience in analyzing executive performance, Klemp and McClelland
identify eight generic competencies: planning/causal thinking, diagnostic
information seeking, conceptualization/synthetic thinking, concern for
influence (the need for power), directive influence (personalized power),
collaborative influence (socialized power), symbolic influence, and self-
confidence. Their list of competencies includes those that pertain to both
intellect and influence and, although these two kinds of competencies as
well as the additional competency of self-confidence can be separated from
each other, understanding the practical intelligence of managers requires
one to view how these various competencies interact. The authors show
how senior managers bring these competencies to bear upon their work.

Chapter 4

In their studies of Tacit Knowledge and Intelligence in the Everyday World,
Richard K. Wagner and Robert J. Sternberg study the influence of what they
call "tacit knowledge" upon practical intelligence among workers in two
occupations: business executives and college professors in the field of psychology. They argue that a key element of practical intelligence in occupational settings is the ability to learn and then apply information that is
never explicitly taught to workers but that is essential for success in their
jobs. This tacit knowledge, which is rarely verbalized, enables workers to
meet the often unwritten and unspoken demands of their jobs. Wagner and
Sternberg propose a framework for analyzing tacit knowledge. Within this
framework, tacit knowledge is divided by category and by orientation. The

categories deal with management of self, management of tasks, and management of others, and the orientations are local (short term) and global (long term). Although the specific contents of tacit knowledge may differ from one job to another, the basic framework does not differ. Moreover, there seems to be some generality in the learning of tacit knowledge: People who have acquired more of one kind of tacit knowledge generally have acquired more of other kinds as well. This generality should not be confused with the general factor in academic intelligence, however. The studies discussed by Wagner and Sternberg suggest that people who are high in academic intelligence do not necessarily fare well in acquired real-world tacit knowledge, and many of the people who are able to acquire this tacit knowledge are not particularly adept in performing on measures of academic intelligence.

Chapter 5

Norman Frederiksen, in striving Toward a Broader Conception of Human Intelligence, has taken psychometric testing paradigms well beyond the normal types of uses to which they are commonly applied. In particular, he has devised tests of practical intelligence that deal with a number of different aspects of the phenomenon. His goal has been to understand and then to measure quantitatively the kinds of skills that are needed for success in real-world thinking. For example, he has devised tests of scientific thinking that measure abilities such as those of formulating hypothesis, evaluating proposals, solving methodological problems, and measuring constructs. He has not only looked at these abilities, in general, but also in specific settings, such as solving medical diagnosis problems. In this research, for example, he has concentrated on how experts differ from novices in formulating hypotheses in rendering diagnoses. Frederiksen also reports on studies of interviewing behavior and of problem solving in business situations. In his studies of executives, Frederiksen has employed the "in-basket" technique that he originated, presenting to would-be executives simulations of the kinds of activities that business executives need to perform in accomplishing their jobs. Factor analysis has revealed eight factors of performances: acting in compliance with suggestions, preparing for action by becoming informed, concern with public relations, procrastination, concern with supervisors, informality, directing subordinates, and discussing. He has not only looked at the performance of business executives on an in-basket but also at the performance of school principals and others as they attempt to accomplish their jobs. Frederiksen's research represents what is probably the most sophisticated use of psychometric testing that has been accomplished in the practical domain. Although he finds overlap in the factors of competence across different occupations, it has become clear through recent research that the competencies needed for success in various fields differ somewhat as a function of the particular field and, moreover, that these competencies are not identical to those that are needed for academic success.

Chapter 6

In their essay Academic and Nonacademic Intelligence: An Experimental Separation, Stephen J. Ceci and Jeffrey Liker have proposed that practical intelligence represents a construct that is really quite distinct from any construct of academic intelligence. In order to study this distinction, Ceci and Liker have focused on racetrack handicapping. They have found that race track handicapping is an astonishingly complex task, and that experts incorporate a large number of variables in making their decisions about which horses will win races. They have been able to model the thinking of experts and of nonexperts in handicapping and have distinguished the weights the two groups of subjects give to various factors that affect which horses win and which lose. These investigators found that although handicapping ability is complex, it is quite distinct from the abilities involved in academic intelligence. Indeed, people with normal or even less than normal academic intelligence quotients can perform the tasks of race track handicapping in a highly effective and successful way. Their data require one to draw a rather firm line between academic intelligence, on the one hand, and practical intelligence, on the other.

Chapter 7

In her analysis of Some Lifelong Everyday Forms of Intelligent Behavior: Organizing and Reorganizing, Jacqueline Goodnow has studied intelligence as a judgment or attribution that can be made in both formal and informal situations. Her view of intelligence as an attribution reflects her extensive analysis of cross-cultural data, suggesting that people's notions of intelligence can differ substantially from one cultural setting to another. She is particularly interested in how people organize and reorganize information, and in how they use these organized forms of information in their planning and execution of the activities of everyday life. She shows that even the most mundane tasks involve complex forms of organization and reorganization, and that these forms of organization and reorganization are only minimally measured, if at all, by standard kinds of psychometric tests. She analyzes three components of organizational abilities: learning of physical constraints, social aspects, and facilitating conditions. Goodnow brings to bear both experimental and ethnographic literature and combines these literatures with her own observations of people organizing their information in their everyday lives.

Chapter 8

The Theory of Multiple Intelligences: Issues and Answers, by Joseph M. Walters and Howard Gardner, represents an attempt by these authors to specify the applicability of Gardner's theory of multiple intelligences as it applies to everyday life. The authors show how multiple intelligences are brought to bear upon everyday kinds of situations that people in a variety of different pursuits encounter. They argue that any unitary notion of intelligence fails to do justice both to the range of abilities people bring to bear on their everyday activities, and to the structure of intelligent cognition as it presumably exists in some form in their head. Like all new theories, the theory of multiple intelligences has now been subjected to a variety of critiques, and the authors spend some time rebutting the criticisms that have been raised against the theory, and showing how the theory can handle the arguments that have been raised against it. Walters and Gardner do not distinguish between academic and practical intelligence, per se, but rather argue that a good theory of intelligences would account for both academic and practical performance within the scope of a single theory. For them, the need is not for a separation of academic from practical intelligence, but rather for a separation of psychologically and functionally distinct intelligences from each other.

Chapter 9

In his essay, For All Practical Purposes: Criteria for Defining and Evaluating Practical Intelligence, Martin E. Ford proposes a taxonomy of human goals and a theory of the socially competent adult based on people's conceptions of the nature of social competence. The taxonomy of human goals represents an attempt to deal with one of the thorniest problems in the study of practical intelligence: What kinds of activities should serve as criteria for measuring the success of practical intelligence in life pursuits? Ford discusses eight main types of goals in his taxonomy: arousal goals, evaluation goals, experiential goals, physiological goals, safety goals, sex and reproduction goals, social relationship goals, and task goals. Criteria for evaluating practical intelligence should reflect a multiplicity of these goals. Ford seems to view practical intelligence largely in terms of social competence, and cites literature to support this point of view. His derived "implicit" theory of social competence includes four main clusters of skills: prosocial skills (e.g., is sensitive to the feelings of others, respects others and their viewpoints, is socially responsible), social-instrumental skills (e.g., knows how to get things done, has good communication skills, likes to set goals), social ease (e.g., is easy to be around, is socially adaptable, enjoys social activities and involvements), and self-efficacy (e.g., has own identity and own values, has a good self-concept, is open to new experiences). Ford's analysis of social competence is unique both in its sophisticated empirical derivation and in its provision of a new basis for measuring the various forms of social competence. Measurement issues have been predominant in the study of social competence because of the great difficulty investigators have experienced in measuring this construct, and Ford's work represents a new level of conceptual and methodological sophistication toward these measurement problems.

Chapter 10

In Toward Life-span Research on the Functions and Pragmatics of Intelligence, Roger A. Dixon and Paul B. Baltes present what they refer to as a neofunctional approach to understanding the "pragmatics" of intelligence. They distinguish these pragmatics from the "mechanics" of intelligence, the latter of which are measured by conventional psychometric intelligence tests. They show that although there can be certain declines in the mechanics of intelligence over the life-span, extending one's vision to include an analysis of the pragmatics of intelligence can result in the recognition of stability and even growth in practical intellectual performance. The authors review a wide range of literature, and especially philosophical literature, pertaining to their neo-functionalist orientation, and suggest that understanding changes in intellectual performance, both with respect to the mechanics and the pragmatics of intelligence, requires one to look at four essential aspects of life-span intellectual development: multidimensionality (the existence of multiple mental abilities, each with potentially distinct structural, functional, and developmental properties); multidirectionality (the existence of multiple distinct change patterns associated with these abilities); interindividual variability (the existence of large differences in the life-course change patterns of individuals); and intraindividual plasticity (the modifiability of intellectual behavioral patterns over the life course). The authors report on a series of theoretical and empirical analyses that suggest the importance of all four of these aspects of intellectual development to understanding both the mechanics and the pragmatics of intelligence. A key notion in their analysis of pragmatics is that of selective optimization with compensation. The idea here is that as people age, they need to make increasingly greater use of those mental abilities that remain strong and even that strengthen, at the same time that they need to figure out and implement ways of compensating for those intellectual abilities that may decline. As life goals and pursuits change, the pattern of selective optimization with compensation in adulthood begins to reflect the changing needs and desires of the individual in his or her adaptation to the everyday environment.

Chapter 11

In their study of Practical Intelligence in Later Adulthood, Sherry L. Willis and K. Warner Schaie analyze the relationship between psychometric abilities and practical intelligence in old age. These contributors report on two studies of the relationship of psychometric abilities to practical intelligence. In one study, they use a test of everyday competencies (e.g., reading maps, reading charts, filling out forms, and analyzing news text), relating these practical abilities to both fluid and crystallized abilities as measured by psychometric tests. They find strong relationships between traditional psychometric test performance and the ability of the elderly to perform on a variety of these practical tasks. However, the correlation is higher for younger than for older age groups. Both fluid and crystallized abilities proved to be important in practical task performance at all of the age levels they studied.

In the second study, Willis and Schaie examine age differences in perceived competence in everyday situations. Ability correlates of these age differences are examined. They find that with age, individuals perceive themselves as becoming more competent in certain respects and less competent in other respects. In particular, they find significant positive age/cohort differences in perceived competence for social, common, passive, and depriving situations, but negative age effects for the inverse dimensions of nonsocial, uncommon, active, and supportive situations. Thus, consistent with other investigators, perceived adeptness seems especially to increase in the social domain with increasing age. The authors also find the fluid abilities to be more powerful predictors than crystallized abilities of the various kinds of social competencies. High fluid abilities were found to be significant predictors of perceived competence in nonsocial, uncommon, and depriving situations, whereas low fluid abilities were found to be significant predictors in social, common, and passive situations. Their data show that although practical competencies can be distinguished from academic ones, academic competencies are surprisingly good predictors of the practical ones. In particular, fluid ability, which is often hypothesized as being less important than crystallized ability in later adulthood, actually proved in their studies to be the more important predictor.

Chapter 12

In Bricolage: Savages Do It Daily, J. W. Berry and S. H. Irvine center their analysis of practical intelligence around the concept of bricolage, which is work of an odd job sort. In studying bricolage in a variety of cultures, these contributors conclude that cognitive processes are very likely to be universal, but that they must be understood as they apply to the lower level, con-

crete, survival skills that can differ greatly from one culture and one occupation to another. Although many investigators studying practical
intelligence are concerned with the effects of context, Berry and Irvine are
fairly unique in presenting a taxonomy of levels of context. They discuss
four levels of context. Ecological context consists of the relatively permanent characteristics that provide the context for human action. Nested in
this ecological context are two levels: experiential context, or the pattern
of recurrent experiences that provides a basis for learning, and performance
context, or the limited set of environmental circumstances that may be observed to account for particular behaviors. The fourth context they discuss
is the experimental context, which represents those environmental characteristics that are designed by the psychologist to elicit a particular response
or test score. Berry and Irvine note that an experimental context may or
may not be nested in the first three contexts, and that the degree to which
it is nested represents the ecological validity of the task under investigation.

Paralleling the four contexts are four types of effects. The first, achievements, refers to the complex, long-standing and developed behavior pattern
that exists as an adaptive response to ecological context. Behaviors are
learned over time in the recurrent experiential context. Responses to performances appear in response to immediate stimulation or experience. Each
type of environment can be linked to a specific kind of effect, and understanding intelligence helps to make the link between the various kinds of
contexts and the effects they have. Berry and Irvine also distinguish between
specific abilities, cognitive styles, and general intelligence as they apply in
everyday life, and discuss the relations between these attributes and both
the ecocultural context in which they occur and the cognitive performances
to which they give rise.

Chapter 13

In their analysis of The Development of Practical Intelligence in Cross-cultural Perspective, Jane R. Mercer, Margarita Gomez-Palacio, and Eligio
Padilla discuss what they consider the two major approaches to conceptualizing the nature of intelligence: the academic approach and the social-
behavioral approach. They view the academic approach as concentrating on
the internal world of the individual and as devoted to the understanding and
measurement of cognitive processes and structures that are utilized to manipulate the symbolic systems of the culture and to solve various kinds of
problems encountered within the culture. A social-behavioral approach to
conceptualizing intelligence focuses on the individual's ability to deal with
the external world of social structures and interactions and to play a variety
of roles in various social systems. These authors discuss at length the dif-

ference between these two aspects of intelligence, and view them as relatively distinct, although with some degree of overlap. They discuss at some length their Adaptive Behavior Scales, which have been used to provide an operational definition of adaptive behavior as it occurs in real-world contexts. In particular, they define adaptive behavior in terms of the individual's social role performance in a variety of social systems as evaluated by others in those systems. They have identified six different kinds of roles that need to be taken into account in the analysis and measurement of adaptive behavior: family roles, community roles, peer roles, non-academic school roles, earner/consumer roles, and self-maintenance roles. They discuss various criticisms of the concept of social-behavioral intelligence, both in principle and as it is measured by their own scales, and provide data to support both the validity of their scales and the ability of the scales to counter criticisms that have been raised against social-adaptive intelligence. Their essay represents, in part, a sophisticated construct validation of the scales, as well as a demonstration that it is possible to measure practical intelligence in a way that is psychometrically sound as well as contextually relevant.

Chapter 14

In his essay on Intelligence and Literacy: The Relationships Between Intelligence and the Technologies of Representation and Communication, David R. Olson suggests that one of the greatest problems in existing conceptualizations of intelligence is the confusion of description with explanation. He argues that investigators of intelligence often reify descriptive behavior and, as a result, claim to provide explanation, whereas in fact they provide nothing more than hypothetical constructs that do not go beyond descriptions. Olson believes that intelligence tests simply sample behavior in the domain of linguistic competence as it is associated with literacy. The tests measure people's use of the categories of concepts upon which we construct and use systematic bodies of knowledge. It is important to emphasize that the tests do not measure the ability to do these things; rather, they measure people in actually doing the things. The tests are samples of competence, not measures of any underlying abilities. For Olson, then, intelligence is not an underlying quality of mind that explains why some people are better at some tasks than are other people. Rather, it is a descriptive concept that deals with the operations required for dealing with a human-made artifact, namely, written language. Olson does not believe that the cognitive operations measured by tests are universal, but he does believe that it is useful to measure these cognitive operations. His essay is thus not a critique of intelligence tests, per se, but rather a critique of the claims that have been made about the meanings of scores on intelligence tests.

Chapter 15

The final chapter of the book provides an organizing framework and comparative analysis of the various essays in this book, and it attempts to integrate them so as to provide an overall theoretical perspective on the field of practical intelligence.

To conclude, *Practical Intelligence: Nature and Origins of Competence in the Everyday World* provides an overview of the field of practical intelligence as it exists today. The field of practical intelligence is an evolving one, and we hope that this book will make some contribution toward furthering this evolution and toward directing it in constructive ways.

Part I

Intelligence on the job

2   Thinking in action: some characteristics of practical thought

Sylvia Scribner

If two and a half decades of AI research has done nothing else, it has given researchers a sense of awe in the face of the ordinary.

Waldrop (1984)

Is practical thinking a "kind" of thinking, and, if so, how does it compare to other "kinds"? Not many years ago, such a question, reflecting preoccupations of the naturalist rather than of the experimentalist, might not have found its way into discussions of human intellect. Yet today an increasing number of cognitive scientists are not only taking the question seriously but answering it in the affirmative. In constituting practical thinking as a kind, some set it up as a contrast class to a form of thinking considered instrumental for performance on intellectual tasks such as those encountered in school, on IQ tests, and in certain psychological experiments. This contrasting mode of thought is variously characterized as "academic," "formal," or, in my own usage (Scribner, 1977; Scribner & Fahrmeier, 1982) "theoretical."

Psychological archives, Neisser (1968) reminds us, are replete with other dichotomous schemes for organizing cognitive phenomena, from Freud's (1900) primary/secondary distinction to Levy-Bruhl's (1910) logical/alogical opposition and Vygotsky's (1962) comparison of spontaneous and scientific concepts. Why add another? As with any simple pair of dichotomous terms, the contrast is likely to be true in some respects (otherwise it would not be advanced as a serious proposition) and false or incomplete in other respects (it would otherwise displace competing categorical schemes and become the sole organizing framework for theory and research).

In spite of these well-remarked limitations of dichotomous schemes, several considerations suggest that a practical/theoretical distinction is a useful framework for thinking about thinking.[1] For one thing, a time-honored philosophical tradition, reaching back to old Aristotle (in McKeon, 1947) commends it as a distinction of substance. Contemporary interest is the outcome, not of faddism, but of sustained and serious efforts to make sense of accumulating evidence that people's intellectual accomplishments vary greatly

13

according to domain, task, and setting. Discrepancies between IQ levels and expertise in everyday affairs (see Chapter 6, this volume; Cole & Traupman, 1981; Wagner & Sternberg, in press) can no longer be ignored. More than a decade of research by anthropologists (Gladwin, 1970; Hutchins, 1980; Lave, 1877; Quinn, 1981) and cross-cultural psychologists (Cole, Gay, Glick & Sharp, 1971; Dube, 1982; Price-Williams, Gordon & Ramirez, 1969; Scribner, 1977) has documented sophisticated memory and reasoning abilities among traditional peoples who perform poorly on standard experimental tasks. In the laboratory, manipulations of task materials and demands (Donaldson, 1978; Hayes & Simon, 1977; Newman, Griffin & Cole, 1984) shift not only levels of performance but qualitative characteristics of the problem-solving process as well. We cannot review here the various theoretical responses to this unanticipated variability, except to note that some take the form of salvage operations designed to maintain unimodal theories of thought, while others abandon theoretical models altogether in favor of situationism and particularism. The construct "kinds of thinking" occupies middle ground between these positions, and, if empirically supported, would provide new possibilities for a coherent structure of explanation. The practical/theoretical distinction is one set of terms for a "kinds" taxonomy with special applicability to problem-solving systems. To proceed as if practical thinking were a natural variety requiring its own account has evident heuristic value.

Perhaps the most compelling argument for considering practical thinking as a definite mode of thought is that we now have on hand a small but growing body of research supporting such a conjecture. Formerly, attempts to claim *sui generis* characteristics for practical thinking foundered on inadequate evidence. Practical thinking was represented in the exchange primarily through anecdote, discursive description, or appeals to "what everyone knows." The imbalance in knowledge, although still great, is not nearly as one sided. In recent years, investigators from various disciplines have succeeded in extracting some specimens of practical thinking from the stream of naturally occurring behavior and studying them microscopically. A number of these specimens has been analyzed under conditions of control customary for laboratory tasks. Accordingly, we can begin to bring schematic ideas and hunches about the nature of practical thinking into confrontation with some acceptable, if still quite limited, evidence. We can ask: Do the specimens on hand exhibit common characteristics that justify us in considering them members of a natural kind rather than an accidental collection of singular tasks? If so, how do these characteristics compare with models of cognition representing formal or theoretical thought? Is practical thinking a "defective" version of "ideal" thought, as represented in these models, or is it qualitatively different but equal? Or – and the possibility should not be overlooked – do the characteristics of practical thought suggest that current cognitive models are defective for representing any mode of thought?

The project of this paper is to tackle only the first of these questions: do exemplars of well-analyzed practical thinking tasks exhibit common characteristics? On the basis of a selected set of studies, I propose to answer the question provisionally in the affirmative and to offer a description of salient characteristics of practical thinking. As will become clear, this descriptive model is based on research covering a limited range of practical activities, and thus it represents a speculative extrapolation from the evidence on hand. Its principal purpose is to open discussion on the characteristics of practical thinking and the usefulness of considering it a kind.

To provide a context for this portrait of practical thinking, I will first comment on the theoretical perspective I bring to the topic and then summarize the observational and experimental studies that constitute the core evidence for the model.

Starting points

My notion of practical thinking can be glossed as "mind in action." I use the term to refer to thinking that is embedded in the larger purposive activities of daily life and that functions to achieve the goals of those activities. Activity goals may involve mental accomplishments (deciding on the best buy in a supermarket) or manual accomplishments (repairing an engine) but, whatever their nature, practical thinking is instrumental to their achievement. So conceived – as embedded and instrumental – practical thinking stands in contrast to the type of thinking involved in performance of isolated mental tasks undertaken as ends in themselves.[2]

This orientation sets some parameters for the enterprise. Because it emphasizes dynamic processes – the functions of thinking – it entails no claims about the underlying abilities of individuals or structures of intelligence. Thus practical thinking in the present usage is not to be assimilated to notions of faculties or of factors of mind. Because this approach links thinking to action, it is also at variance with prevailing cognitive science approaches to thinking. The computer metaphor, dominant today, portrays mind as a system of symbolic representations and operations that can be understood in and of itself, in isolation from other systems of activity. Researchers adopting this metaphor seek either to model mental tasks undertaken for their own sake ("recall a narrative," "solve this arithmetic problem") or to analyze individual mental functions (e.g., inference, imagery) abstracted from tasks and separated from one another. Whatever may be said about the value of this framework and these research approaches (and their accomplishments are recognized), they offer little possibility for probing the nature of practical thought. This endeavor requires an analysis of the role of thought within a system of activity, not cut off from it. To achieve such an analysis, the investigator needs to select as her object of analysis not an isolated mental process or task in itself but an integral action directed toward some specifiable end and accomplished under specificable circumstances. Actions as units of analysis permit the researcher to tackle the what-for of thinking, to examine how thinking is related to doing, and to identify the factors in the world, as well as the representations in the head, that regulate its functioning.[3]

Consistent with this perspective, the research on practical thinking on which our model is based consists of studies of naturally occurring actions. Because I am most familiar with them, I rely primarily on studies of cognitive aspects of work which I carried out with colleagues in a milk-processing plant (Scribner, 1984a, 1984b; Scribner & Fahrmeier, 1982) and studies my students conducted, respectively, among bartenders (Beach, 1985), sales engineers (Laufer, 1985), and waitresses (Stevens, 1985). These studies take as their units of analysis job tasks ("goal-directed actions") that are a routine part of people's occupational activities. All employ a common methodology combining ethnographic and experimental techniques. This corpus is enlarged by other studies of problem solving at work, including research on tailors (Lave, in preparation), on magistrates (Lawrence, in press), on auto mechanics (McLaughlin, 1979), and on office workers (Suchman, 1985), which similarly take naturally occurring work tasks as their starting point and extend the analysis by simulation or test methods. Anthropological and sociological descriptions of occupational activities (among them, Applebaum, 1984a, 1984b; Chinoy, 1964; Gamst, 1980; Kusterer, 1978; Schrank, 1980; Zimbalist, 1979) contribute supplementary materials. The model of practical thinking we present is thus largely based on the study of well-defined and interdependent work tasks whose goals and conditions of accomplishment are socially determined and often highly structured. However, a crop of studies of quantitative problem solving in nonoccupational settings (de la Rocha, in press; Lave, Murtagh, de la Rocha, 1984; Carraher, Carraher & Schliemann, 1984) displays points of overlap and gives us some grounds for anticipating that the features we have singled out for attention may be attributes of intellectual activity in a wide variety of worldly pursuits.

Selected case studies from the dairy[4]

A modernized milk-processing plant was the scene of my early investigations of problem solving at work. The research program began with an ethnographic study (Jacob, 1979) that familiarized us with the dairy as a production system and social organization and highlighted the intellectual requirements of various jobs. We selected four for intensive study: product assemblers, wholesale delivery drivers, inventory men, and office clerks. After conducting systematic observations of principal work tasks in these occupations, we designed a series of job simulations and experiments to analyze the constituent operations and knowledge which these tasks involved. Participating in simulation studies was a panel of thirty-five workers with representation from each target occupation. Workers in the occupation from which the task was drawn served as experts; those from other occupations were novices. Ninth grade students were included in some studies for comparative purposes. Analyses of performance in both natural and simulated situations focused on modes of solution and features distinguishing the intellectual performance of novices from that of workers with on-the-job experience. Three job studies are summarized here.

Assembling products

Assemblers, classified as unskilled workers, are responsible for locating products stored in the warehouse and sending out to the loading platform the amount of each product ordered by drivers for their daily routes. Assemblers secure information about product orders from a computer-generated form that represents quantities according to a setting-specific system, using a dual metric of case and unit. Dairy products are stored and handled in standard size cases that hold a certain number of containers (units) of a given size (4 gallons, 9 half-gallons, 16 quarts, 32 pints, 48 half-pints). If a particular order involves a quantity not evenly divisible into cases, the order form represents it as a mixed number: x cases plus or minus (according to rule) 4 units. For example: 1–6 on the order form stands for one case minus 6 units. The numerical value of this expression depends on the container size it qualifies: 10 quarts, 26 pints, 4 half-pints. Whenever the assembler encounters a case-and-unit problem, he or she must interpret the symbolic representation on the form to determine the unit quantity needed, map this quantity onto the physical array, and collect as many units as will satisfy the order.

In our recorded observations of two product assemblers filling mixed case and unit orders on the job, we made several discoveries:

1. Assemblers often departed from the literal format of the orders.
2. They filled what looked like the identical order (e.g., 1 case − 6 quarts, or 10 quarts) in a variety of ways, depending on the availability of empty or partially filled cases in the vicinity. Observed solutions on this order included, for example, subtracting 4 from a partial case of 14 quarts and adding 2 quarts to a partial case of 8.
3. On all occasions, the mode of order filling, whether literal or nonliteral, was exactly that procedure that satisfied the order in the fewest moves – that is, of all alternatives, the solution the assembler selected required the transfer of a minimum number of units from one case to another. Assemblers

calculated these least physical effort solutions even when the "saving" in moves amounted to only one unit (in orders that might total 500 units).

4. Mental calculations for these least-effort solutions required the assembler to switch from one base number system to another. The mental effort involved in problem transformations was increased by the fact that assemblers typically went for a group of orders at one time, thus having to keep in mind quantities expressed in different base number systems.

5. Solutions representing least physical effort were accomplished with speed and accuracy; errors were virtually nonexistent.

6. In job simulations, only experienced assemblers consistently employed least physical effort strategies. Novice groups were literal problem solvers, filling orders only as indicated in the representations on the order form (always responding to the order "one case − 6 quarts," for example, by removing 6 quarts from a full case regardless of whether more efficient alternatives were available.

7. Over the course of many encounters with different types of problems in job simulations, novices acquired least physical effort strategies without instruction.

Pricing delivery tickets

Wholesale delivery drivers are responsible for determining the cost of their daily deliveries to customers. For this purpose they use standard delivery tickets, preprinted with the customer's name and products usually purchased. A driver who completes a delivery enters on the ticket the number of units of each product left with the customer (e.g., 24 gallons of homogenized milk; 428 half-pints of chocolate drink) and then computes its cost. For this chore, the driver has available a company price list displaying unit prices for each major product (e.g., price per quart or per half-pint of orange drink). Since the amount of each product is recorded on the ticket in units, and prices are in units, the computation task seems straightforward; that is, multiply number of units by unit price and enter the result in the appropriate column. School-taught multiplication algorithms, if executed properly, would always produce accurate delivery costs.

Recorded observations and interviews with drivers pricing out their tickets disclosed that algorithmic procedures could not account for all modes of solution, as demonstrated by the following instances:

1. Pricing problems with the identical structure (number units × unit price) were solved in a variety of ways, each exquisitely fine-tuned to the specific number properties of the problem at hand. One old-timer displayed twenty-three different solution procedures on his batch of eight delivery tickets.

2. Departures from the multiplication algorithm simplified the arithmetic required (were least-mental-effort solution procedures); as a result, drivers solved many problems mentally without the use of aids (paper and pencil, calculator, or adding machine).

3. A prominent problem-transformation procedure involved converting the unit amount of a product into an equivalent case amount, and computing cost through the application of case prices. In other words, drivers rep-

resented the case – a material object in the dairy – as a quantitative symbol. Since the case is not a fixed number but a variable (depending on the product container size) conversion of unit amounts to case amounts involved the driver's shifting back and forth in different base-number systems.

4. On all occasions, substitution of case for unit price reduced the work load of the arithmetic problem. Case conversion sometimes recast the multiplication problem in simpler form, as in the following example:

Problem on delivery ticket	*Problem reorganized by driver*
32 quarts skim milk @ .68 per quart	2 cases skim milk @ 10.88 per case

In other instances, combinations of case and unit quantities enabled drivers to reorganize multiplication problems into addition or subtraction problems:

17 quarts skim milk @ $.68 per quart	1 case skim milk @ $10.88 plus 1 quart @ .68
31 pints choc. milk @ .42 per pint	1 case choc. milk @ 13.44 minus 1 pint @ .42

5. In simulations in which problem parameters and computational resources were manipulated, drivers modulated their pricing techniques in accordance with the presence or absence of computational aids of a specific kind. Solution operations on the same problems changed under conditions of calculator use, paper-and-pencil arithmetic or mental arithmetic.

6. Computational techniques were dependent on each driver's personal knowledge of case and unit prices for particular products in particular amounts. Thus, solution procedures varied by individual as well as by problem and by calculating device.

7. Novices tended to solve all pricing problems by algorithmic procedures based on either unit prices or case prices.

8. On a paper and pencil arithmetic test such as those administered in school, drivers, whose on-the-job accuracy rate was near perfect, made many errors on decimal multiplication problems similar in format to their pricing problems.

Taking inventory

Taking warehouse inventory involves careful assessment of the quantities of some 100 products and accurate recording of these amounts on the paper forms. Counts for each product are recorded on the inventory form in case units and need to be accurate within a 1% or 2% margin of error. Typically, the entire quantity of one product is massed together in a single location in the form of stacks of dairy cases which are placed with sides touching and stacked six high, volume permitting. Large product arrays may contain as many as 1,000 cases. Because the warehouse is densely packed, inventory men have limited walk room for maneuvering around such arrays and for much of the time are taking counts of arrays containing invisible cases. Although clipboards and scratch paper were available, enumeration was primarily accomplished through mental arithmetic.

To learn the strategies used in counting these large masses of stock, we observed three men taking inventory and later simulated inventory counts in the laboratory with miniature arrays constructed of *lego* blocks. In a logical analysis of the inventory job, it would appear that the case is the countable and the product array is the set of countables. But empirical analyses disclosed that the "case" was rarely employed as a unit of count. Rather,

1. Inventory men had a wide variety of strategies for determining case number.
2. Strategies were closely fitted to properties of arrays. Quantities in large arrays (more than 300 cases) were arrived at by procedures building on multiplication. Men used known dimensions of the storage space (the depth of an area known to hold seventeen cases) and combined these with computed dimensions of the particular array to be enumerated (say, width of eight cases) and then multiplied again by fixed stack height (six cases). Combinatorial procedures, building on known and calculated dimensions and several arithmetic operations, varied with array configurations.
3. In the interest of using multiplication short-cut methods of enumeration, inventory men mentally transformed array configurations to make them amenable to these techniques. When a large array was not a solid rectangle, but had gaps, the men mentally squared off the array by visualizing phantom stacks and counting them. They then multiplied by rectangular dimensions and completed the solution by subtracting the phantoms from the product. In the instance of "add-ons" (protrusions), they mentally separated out a rectangular central core, multiplied and completed the solution by adding the "odd stuff" to the product.
4. Medium and small arrays were enumerated primarily by counting procedures. The unit of count varied, depending on the size of the array, its regularity and other physical properties. Counting strategies included jump counting by stacks, single counting of stacks, and jump counting by number of cases in each stack. At no time did we observe the single case used as the unit of count, although all counts were expressed on the completed inventory form in terms of case units.

A suggested model of practical thinking

Work tasks studied in the dairy present very simple instances of problem solving. Yet, even here, under the microscope, practical thinking emerges as an intricate and dynamic system organized by both factors in the world and subjective goals and knowledge. Its complexity, the "challenge of the ordinary," arises from this property – that it is simultaneously adaptive to ever-changing conditions in the world and to the purposes, values, and knowledge of the person and the social group.

Here we will consider some of the salient characteristics of skilled practical thinking, extrapolated from the dairy studies and other research. To stimulate thinking about kinds of thought, we will also draw contrasts where appropriate between these observed characteristics of workaday thinking and the properties of formal thinking offered by computer models of mind. We discuss each characteristic individually, but as attributes of a system they are interrelated and implicate each other.

Problem formation

Skilled practical thinking involves problem formation as well as problem solution. Models of formal problem solving suggest that problems are "given" and intellectual work consists of selecting and executing a series of steps that will lead to a solution; the initial problem may be decomposed into subproblems as part of the solution procedure, but its terms are fixed. By contrast, dairy studies suggest that expertise in practical problem solving frequently hinges on an apt formulation or redefinition of the initial problem. In commonplace everyday activities, Lave and associates discovered that problems do not necessarily control actions (Lave, Murtagh, & de la Rocha, 1984). Budget-conscious supermarket shoppers who claimed they were interested in figuring out best buys, rarely undertook the laborious arithmetic involved in unit price comparisons of bulk or packaged products and made their decision on other grounds, shifting the "problem space," as it were. Customers engaged in comparative arithmetic only when circumstances made it possible for them to reach an answer by simple computational or estimation procedures. Lave describes this process as the dialectical constitution of problem and solution.

In the world of work, people have fewer options for shifting problem terrain entirely. It is a peculiarity of occupational activities that many of the problems they pose are preset by social-institutional objectives and technological conditions. But even preset problems may be subjectively reconstituted. On many occasions, problems arise that have a general shape but not a definite formulation. One artful aspect of practical thinking is to construct or redefine a problem that experience or hunch suggests will facilitate a solution or enable the application of a preferred mode of problem solving (see discussion on effort-saving, below). This form of creativity is noticeable and has been well-remarked in professional activities, such as judicial decision-making (Lawrence, in press) and engineering and architecture (Schön, 1983) in which the capacity to devise problems that fit good solutions is highly prized. Dairy studies take us a step further. The dairy is a prototypical industrial system in which many occupational activities involve standardized and repetitive duties performed under highly constrained conditions. It would appear from job specifications that a great many problems are immutable. Yet closer scrutiny reveals that, on all jobs analyzed, experienced workers on some occasions (frequency varying by work task) departed from the literal format of problems and reformulated them in terms of new elements or operations. Drivers recast unit price problems into case price problems; product assemblers converted take-away problems (e.g., $16 - 6 = 10$) into add-to problems ($8 + 2 = 10$), and inventory men mentally squared off irregular areas to transform counting problems into multiplication problems. These examples indicate that if degrees of freedom are available, even in restricted activities, people find ways of redefining preset problems into "subjective" problems.

Flexible modes of solutions

Skilled practical thinking is marked by flexibility – solving the "same problem" now one way, now another, each way finely fitted to the occasion. Formal models of problem solving lead us to expect that repetitive problems or problems of the same logical class will be solved by the same sequence of operations (algorithms) on all occasions of their presentation. Variability sometimes enters the system in the guise of shifts in executive control from one higher-order strategy to another. These strategies, presumably, differ from each other in the modes of solution they regulate, but each generates consistent solutions to all instances of a given problem type.

Such models fail to account for the unexpected variability routinely displayed by dairy experts. Only novices used algorithmic procedures to solve problems. Comparisons of their performance with that of experts suggests that learning how to satisfy the intellectual requirements of a job is not so much a matter of becoming efficient in running off all-purpose algorithms as it is in building up a repertoire of solution modes fitted to properties of specific problems and particular circumstances. The variability experts displayed was exactly that type excluded from formal models: use of different component operations to solve recurring problems of the same kind.

What drives this variability? In the cases we studied, workers' proclivity to "do the same problem differently" on different occasions was unrelated to the objective outcome of performance. On well-practiced tasks of the skill level described, experts made few errors. In any event, available algorithms properly executed would always have yielded the right answer. Changing solution modes reflected experts' concern with the how of performance and were regulated by higher-order worker-evolved strategies for accomplishing the task in the least effortful ways (see description below). Here is an interesting example of a higher-order strategy generating inconsistency in modes of solution.

Flexibility in meeting changing conditions and ingenuity in devising "short cuts" are well-documented aspects of practical intellect across a broad spectrum of occupations. Schön (1983) considers "informal improvisation" the hallmark of professional expertise. Kusterer's (1978) exceptionally detailed studies of bank tellers and machine operators demonstrated that a good part of their working knowledge consisted of knowing how to handle conditions the "standard operating plan" did not cover. Suchman (1985) provides a striking example of the discrepancy between such plans and office-workers problem-solving procedures on the job. Secretaries learning how to use a new copying machine did not follow written instructions but collaboratively constructed effective methods for overcoming problem situations the instructions failed to anticipate. Suchman claims that these ad hoc procedures are unavoidable because they reflect the essence of how people use each other and their circumstances to "achieve intelligent action."

Incorporating the environment into the problem-solving system

Skilled practical thinking incorporates features of the task environment (people, things, information) into the problem-solving system. It is as valid to describe the environment as part of the problem-solving system as it is to observe that problem solving occurs "in" the environment.

This notion of the constitutive role of the environment in practical intellectual activities contrasts with prevailing conceptions of cognition–world relationships. In cognitive theories built on the computer metaphor, the world is a stage on which actors execute the outcomes of their mental operations. For others with a contextualist world view, the environment is a context, an external "envelope," as it were, affecting cognitive processes largely through interpretive procedures; the task in this view remains a unit (see Newman, Griffin & Cole, 1984, for a critique of the position that a "task" can be moved from "context" to "context" while remaining the "same" task). The characteristic we claim for practical thinking goes beyond the contextualist position. It emphasizes the inextricability of task from environment, and the continual interplay between internal representations and operations and external reality throughout the course of the problem-solving process – an interplay expressed in activity theory (Leont'ev, 1981) as the mutual constitution of subject and object. The thrust of the position has been captured by Neisser (1976, p. 183), who has argued that perception and action occur in continuous dependence on the environment and therefore cannot be understood without an understanding of the environment. We are extending this observation to the higher cognitive processes involved in practical problem-solving tasks, with a further critical elaboration. In problem solving, properties of the environment do not enter the problem-solving process deterministically or automatically; they assume a functional role only through the initiative and constructive activities of the problem solver.

Exploitation of the environment takes many forms. On some tasks in the dairy material objects in the environment functioned as terms in symbolic problems. Consider order filling on product assembly. A formal analysis would suggest that this task consisted of a written problem (the product order) that the assembler solved and later executed at the product array.

On the job, however, an experienced worker interpreted the written order, not as "the problem" but as input to an, as yet, unspecified problem. On arriving at the array, he used information from the physical configuration of containers in a case, in conjunction with symbolic information stored in memory, to define the form of the problem (addition or subtraction). A partial case functioned as one term in the equation and the assembler determined the number that needed to be combined with it to satisfy the order. Inventory provided a somewhat different example of experts' use of environmental properties to achieve an initial representation of the problem to be solved. Dimensions and configurations of product arrays were primary determinants of how the inventory person represented the generic problem of enumeration on different occasions, each time constructing a problem whose form best fitted properties of the object to be enumerated.

Skilled workers exploited the environment for problem-solution as well as problem formulation. The specific operations used to solve problems reflected the peculiar capacities and constraints of objects which social convention classifies as tools or aids for mental work. Recall how dairy drivers changed their arithmetic operations as they moved from paper and pencil to calculator arithmetic. Current research on computers, literacy, and culture-specific artifacts such as the abacus amply support the principle (Vygotsky, 1978) that modes of solution come into being around means of solution. But what is most revealing in current studies is the extent to which people, through cultural or individual invention, make mental "tools" of things in the environment the conventional functions of which are wholly unrelated to intellectual work. Lave (1977) draws attention to the ubiquity of specialized "environmental calculating devices": a piece of sheetrock is a metric unit for carpenters (Perin, undated) and a stack of dairy cases a unit of count for an inventory man; a cup is a canonical measure for a Liberian rice farmer (Gay & Cole, 1976), and the hull of a canoe establishes a scale for master boat builders in the Pulawat Islands (Gladwin, 1970). Nor is the role of objects in problem solving restricted to their quantitative properties. Bartenders learn to manage the memory load of their jobs by using glass shape and position as memory cues (Beach, 1985) and waitresses organize to-be-remembered customer orders by the location of food stations (Stevens, 1985). Most interestingly, things in settings may come to function as symbols, entirely separated from their material forms. An elegant example from the dairy is the drivers' use of "case" as a quantitative variable in arithmetic problems; what was initially a physical object takes on an instrumental role in problem solving in a purely symbolic mode.

These examples serve as accessible illustrations of the functional role of the environment in practical problem solving. They make the point, but do not limit it. The concept of the environment germane to practical problem solving is not a physicalist notion. Here "environment" includes all social, symbolic and material resources outside the head of the individual problem solver. In this sense, activities such as seeking information from other people, "putting heads together" to come to collaborative solutions, or searching documents and looking things up in files, may be understood as extended and complex procedures for intellectual use of the environment. Individual differences in abilities to use the environment in these ways may make a crucial difference to effective cognitive performance. In the dairy, experts displayed greater resourcefulness than novices in using things on hand in an effort to simplify and improve the accuracy of their solution procedures. Beach's (1985) experiments with bartenders also demonstrated that experience makes for greater rather than less reliance on environmental sources of information: Advanced bartending students used external memory cues to remember drink orders and recipes whereas beginners resorted more often to information retrieval from memory. If experts in a domain use the environment more (or more effectively) than novices, two implications follow: becoming skilled in a practical domain may move in a direction opposite to that posed by classic psychological learning theory, namely, from the abstract to the concrete. A second implication is that models of thinking that can only deal with the world as represented in the head may find analysis of many practical thinking problems quite intractable.

Effort saving as a higher-order solution strategy

Skilled practical thinking often seeks those modes of solution that are the most economical or that require the least effort. We have remarked that flexibility appears to be a defining characteristic of practical problem solving. Yet the kind of flexibility documented by the research implies more than random variation or variation for "its own sake" (although we certainly do not preclude these possibilities). As a hallmark of practical skill, flexibility requires that variation serve the purpose of "fitting means precisely to their occasions of use" (Welford, 1976). What is "fittingness" or "fine tuning to the occasion"? Analyses of dairy tasks suggested that fittingness was often indexed by a least-effort criterion: Workers chose just that mode of solution on a particular occasion that accomplished the required end with the fewest steps or the least complex procedures. Product assemblers reformulated "order problems" to save physical moves; inventory staff constructed mental representations for arrays that enabled substitution of short-cutting arithmetic procedures for lengthy processes of enumeration; drivers used case units to simplify multiplication problems on their delivery tickets. As these examples indicate, effort saving here is unrelated to an engineering concept of "efficiency" but refers rather to the psychological reorganization of practical tasks in the interests of economy or simplicity. Evidence on hand from other work settings (see Kusterer, 1978) indicates that effort-saving strategies are widespread and appear in clerical and technical occupations as well as those with manual components. And studies on everyday arithmetic (Lave et al., 1984; de la Rocha, 1985) indicate as well that procedures for simplifying and shortening solutions are common across a range of settings.

The principle of simplicity has been advanced as a criterion for good solutions in certain formal problem-solving domains. Although the concept is vague, Polya (1957) proposed that shortness of solution be considered one characteristic of what constitutes a good solution in mathematics. Empirical research indicates that math problem solvers often move spontaneously toward shorter solutions, even at a tender age (see Resnick & Ford, 1981). If these findings are subsumed under the rubric of effort saving, it would appear that the presence or absence of this higher-order strategy does not in itself set practical thinking apart from theoretical. But deeper probing suggests that certain regulative characteristics of the strategy may be quite different in the two domains. In practical tasks, least-effort strategies are commonly the basis for adoption of different solution modes for identical problems – a form of flexibility not yet documented, to my knowledge, for formal domains. What comes to the fore in this distinction is that practical problem solving tends to occur in task environments that have variable aspects. In a changing task environment, problems are often formally but not functionally the same. Thus, an understanding of least-effort strategies in practical thinking requires taking into account the environment and its conditions. Moreover, the analysis needs to be extended to the values and goals of the problem solver. Objective conditions in the task environment represent potential resources for problem solving, but people need to discover and take advantage of them. Numerous strands of evidence pointed to the fact that least-effort strategies in the dairy were the outcome of processes operating on a conscious level – workers wanted to make their jobs easier or otherwise more compatible with their needs. If least-effort strategies represent conscious constructions, their investigation requires going beyond the formal requirements of problems and the objective conditions of the environment to the larger institutional and cultural contexts in which individual tasks and purposes take shape.

Dependency on setting-specific knowledge

Practical thinking involves the acquisition and use of specific knowledge that is functionally important to the larger activities in which problem solving is embedded. In recent years the centrality of knowledge to intelligent performance has been widely recognized in cognitive theory. From earlier assumptions that problem solving can be understood in terms of "pure process," a consensus has arisen that problem-solving procedures are bound up with amount and organization of subject matter knowledge. Practical problem-solving research reinforces this view by disclosing the diverse forms of knowledge–strategy interactions and the complexity of the knowledge involved in even the simplest tasks. It also contributes some new insights into the specificity of practical knowledge and conditions influencing its acquisition, and our comments will concentrate on these.

The crucial role of setting and task-specific knowledge is well documented in practical problem-solving. The hallmark of expert problem solving in the dairy lay in the fact that experienced workers were able to use specific job-related knowledge to generate flexible and economic solution procedures. In every job examined, these procedures were constructed around, and relied on knowledge specific to the setting and relevant to the task at hand – case equivalencies, storage dimensions, numerical representation systems. What emerges unexpectedly from the research is the degree of specificity of the knowledge involved. From an analyst's bird's-eye point of view, the amount of even so-called specific knowledge required for task performance often appears vast and unbounded. But from the problem solver's point of view, what needs to be known may have quite definite boundaries, drawn in terms of the functional requirements of the task. A trivial example makes the point. Price knowledge was important to delivery drivers; it saved them time (pricing out was faster if they did not have to consult the company price list), and it reduced their risk of error. Yet drivers knew prices primarily for products they handled on their own routes – not prices in general as represented on the price list. Some were explicit about the functional bases of their knowledge. When questioned about prices in our interviews, they rarely said they did not *know* a price, but replied that they *did not handle* the product in question. A typical comment: "Gallons of chocolate drink, I don't even sell that. I don't even put that in my memory bank." Standard interviews conducted to assess workers' knowledge of a record-keeping form used by several occupations disclosed that members of a given occupation were able to explain only those portions of the form which they themselves had to read or fill in and were unfamiliar with the meaning of label headings to the right or left of the columns they used. Kusterer (1978), who conducted one of the most thorough studies of knowledge on the job, reaches similar conclusions about the extraordinary selectivity of some areas of working knowledge. More importantly, he suggests an underlying principle accounting for this selectivity – namely, that people acquire knowledge in the problem-solving mode: "unstudied phenomena remain unknown because they do not normally have any practical consequences affecting the worker's ability to carry out his assigned tasks" (1978, p. 131). Kusterer pointed out that knowledge acquisition varies greatly among individuals (some people have more or less intellectual curiosity) but general functional principles apply. Whether any individual's store of working knowledge is large or small is related to the diversity of functions she carries out and their degree of routinization. Less routinized activities pose more "problems" and thus require the aquisition of more information for overcoming problems. A group of machine operators in his study had to pack products as well as tend machine, but packing was a more routinized function. Kusterer found that, although most of the operators' physical activity involved the packing function, most of their working knowledge involved the machine-tending function.

Another possible functional factor is the saliency of knowledge for accomplishment of the activity goals. Dairy workers were found to organize their knowledge into hierarchical structures constructed along dimensions salient for their job functions. Thus, warehouse workers who had to locate products (the goal of their task) tended to use "location of the product in the warehouse" as a superordinate classification attribute, whereas office workers relied on "kind of dairy product" as the main taxonomic principle.

Knowledge–strategy relationships are so complex and so little explored in practical problem-solving research that generalizations are limited. What we know thus far, however, indicates that functional requirements have an important role in structuring these relationships.

Concluding remarks

The narrow evidentiary base of our description makes it likely that some characteristics selected for discussion may turn out to be particular to one or more practical pursuits rather than candidates for features of a general "kind." It is likely, too, that other aspects of practical thinking basic to its "kindness" have been overlooked. But whatever the limitations of the descriptive enterprise, studies of practical thinking under actual conditions clearly press against the restrictions of laboratory models. Unlike formal problem solving, practical problem solving cannot be understood solely in terms of problem structures and mental representations. Practical problem solving is an open system that includes components lying outside the formal problem – objects and information in the environment and goals and interests of the problem solver. Expertise in practical thinking involves the accomplishment of a fitting relationship among these elements, an accomplishment aptly characterized as functionally adaptive. Beneath the surface of adaptation, however, lie continuing acts of creativity – the invention of new ways of handling old and new problems. Since creativity is a term ordinarily reserved for exceptional individuals and extraordinary accomplishments, recognizing it in the practical problem-solving activities of ordinary people introduces a new perspective from which to grasp the challenge of the ordinary.

Notes

1 As we use the terms here, practical and theoretical thinking both refer to problem-solving activities; the scheme is not proposed as exclusive.
2 The classical antecedents of these distinctions are well-known. Compare Aristotle's descriptions of practical and theoretical thinking, which attributed a principal source of their qualitative differences to differences in their ends or purposes. He claimed that all practical processes of thinking go on for the sake of something outside the process, some end or good to be attained. Theoretical thinking, on the other hand, proceeds for its own sake; it is noninstrumental and "complete in itself." Accordingly, practical sciences have performance of actions as their end, while theoretical sciences are directed to the acquisition of knowledge.
3 Psychologists from several philosophical schools have advanced proposals for a psychology based on the analysis of action. Principles guiding our work are derived from Soviet activity theory; for a brief exposition, see Leont'ev (1979).
4 This research was supported by a grant from the Ford Foundation.
5 An earlier description of some of these characteristics may be found in Scribner (1984b).

References

Aristotle. (1947). *De anima* and *Introduction to metaphysics*. In R. McKeon (Ed.), *Introduction to Aristotle*. New York: Random House.

Beach, K. (1985, March). *Learning to become a bartender: The role of external memory cues at work*. Paper presented at Eastern Psychological Association, Boston, MA.

Carraher, T. N., Carraher, D. W., & Schliemann, A. D. (1985). Mathematics in the streets and in the schools. *British Journal of Developmental Psychology, 3*, 21–30.

Cole, M., Gay, J., Glick, J., & Sharp, D. W. (1971). *The cultural context of learning and thinking*. New York: Basic.

Cole, M., & Traupmann, K. (1981). Comparative cognitive research: Learning from a learning disabled child. In A. D. Pick (Ed.), *Minnesota/Symposia on child psychology* (Vol. 14). Hillsdale, NJ: Erlbaum.

de la Rocha, O. (1985). The reorganization of arithmetic practice in the kitchen. *Anthropology and Education Quarterly. 16*, 193–198.

Donaldson, M. (1978). *Children's minds*. New York: Norton.

Dube, E. F. (1982). Literacy, cultural familiarity, and "intelligence" as determinants of story recall. In U. Neisser (Ed.), *Memory observed* (pp. 274–292). San Francisco: Freeman.

Gay, J., & Cole, M. (1967). *The new mathematics and an old culture*. New York: Holt, Rinehart & Winston.

Gladwin, T. (1970). *East is a big bird*. Cambridge, MA: Harvard University Press.

Hayes, J. R., & Simon, H. A. (1977). Psychological differences among problem isomorphs. In N. J. Castellan, D. B. Pisoni, & G. R. Potts (Eds.), *Cognitive theory* (Vol. 2). Hillsdale, NJ: Erlbaum.

Hutchins, E. (1980). *Culture and inference*. Cambridge, MA: Harvard University Press.

Kusterer, K. C. (1978). *Know-how on the job: The important working knowledge of "unskilled" workers*. Boulder, CO: Westview.

Laufer, E. (1985, March). *Domain specific knowledge and memory performance in the work place*. Paper presented at Eastern Psychological Association, Boston, MA.

Lave, J. (1977). Cognitive consequences of traditional apprenticeship training in West Africa. *Anthropology and Education Quarterly, 8*(3), 177–180.

Lave, J. (1985). *Tailored learning: Education and cognitive skills among tribal craftsmen in West Africa*.

Lawrence, J. A. (1985). Expertise on the bench: Modelling magistrates' judicial decision-making. In M. T. H. Chi, R. Glaser, & M. Farr (Eds.), *The nature of expertise*. Hillsdale, N.J.: Erlbaum.

Leont'ev, A. N. (1979). The problem of activity in psychology. In J. V. Wertsch (Ed.), *The concept of activity in Soviet psychology* (pp. 37–71). White Plains, NY: Sharpe.

Levy-Bruhl, L. (1966). *How natives think* (Trans.). New York: Washington Square Press. (original work published 1910).

Murtagh, M. (1985). The practice of arithmetic by American grocery shoppers. *Anthropology and Education Quarterly, 16*, 186–192.

Neisser, U. (1968). The multiplicity of thought. In P. C. Wason & P. N. Johnson-Laird (Eds.), *Thinking and reasoning* (pp. 307–323). Baltimore: Penguin.

Newman, D., Griffin, P., & Cole, M. (1984). Social constraints in laboratory and classroom tasks. In B. Rogoff & J. Lave (Eds.), *Everyday cognition: Its development in social context*. Cambridge, MA: Harvard University Press.

Perin, D. (undated). Transcript of a carpenter at work. (Mimeo).

Quinn, N. (1981). A natural system used in Mfantse litigation settlement. In R. W. Casson (Ed.), *Language, culture and cognition* (pp. 413–436). New York: Macmillan.

Reckman, B. (1979). Carpentry: The craft and the trade. In A. Zimbalist (Ed.), *Case studies on the labor process* (pp. 73–102). New York: Monthly Review.

Resnick, L. B., & Ford, W. A. (1981). The psychology of mathematics for instruction. Hillsdale, NJ: Erlbaum.

Schön, D. A. (1983). *The reflective practitioner*. New York: Basic.

Scribner, S. (1977). Modes of thinking and ways of speaking. In P. N. Johnson-Laird & J. C. Wason (Eds.), *Thinking*. Cambridge: Cambridge University Press.

Scribner, S., & Fahrmeier, E. (1982). *Practical and theoretical arithmetic: Some preliminary findings*. Industrial Literary Project Working Paper No. 3. New York: The Graduate School and University Center, City University of New York.

Scribner, S. (1984a). Studying working intelligence. In B. Rogoff & Lave, J. (Eds.), *Everyday cognition*. Cambridge, MA: Harvard University Press.

Scribner, S. (1984b). Cognitive aspects of work. *Quarterly Newsletter of Laboratory of Comparative Human Cognition*. Univ. of Calif., San Diego.

Stevens, J. (1985, March). *An observational study of skilled memory in waitresses*. Paper presented at Eastern Psychological Association, Boston, MA.

Suchman, L. A. (1985). *Plans and situated actions: The problem of human-machine communication*. Palo Alto, CA: Xerox Corporation.

Vygotsky, L. S. (1962). *Thought and language*. Cambridge, MA: MIT Press.

Vygotsky, L. S. (1978). *Mind in society*. Cambridge, MA: Harvard University Press.

Wagner, R. K., & Sternberg, R. J. (1985). Practical intelligence in real-world pursuits: The role of tacit knowledge. *Journal of Personality and Social Psychology*.

Waldrop, M. W. (1984). Artificial intelligence (I): Into the world. *Science, 233*, 802–807.

Welford, A. T. (1976). *Skilled performance: Perceptual and motor skills*. Glenview, IL: Scott, Foresman.

Zimbalist, A. (Ed.). (1979). *Case studies in the labor process*. New York: Monthly Review.

3   What characterizes intelligent functioning among senior managers?

George O. Klemp, Jr., and David C. McClelland

As typically defined by psychologists, intelligence is whatever intelligence tests measure. These tests involve the manipulation of symbols to solve problems for which all the information is given. There is only one correct solution; the time allotted to reach the solution is short; and relevance to problems in real life is minimal (Neisser, 1976). But doing well on such tests cannot guarantee intelligent functioning in real life. For in real life, problems are rarely so clear cut: before figuring out a solution, one must first figure out the problem. Only then can one know what kind of information to seek out (it is not given) in order to solve it – and then choose a solution, usually from among several possible solutions. The process bears little relationship to the controlled one of an intelligence test.

Given this disparity in processes, psychologists who support intelligence tests are greatly concerned with trying to show the relationship between scores on such tests and functioning in real life. In general, there is a strong positive relationship between intelligence measured in symbol-manipulation tests and performance in school, where the task demands are similar to those in the tests. But the relationship between intelligence test scores and performance in other areas of life, such as work, is low if not nonexistent. For this reason, it has been argued that if we wish to learn more about intelligence, we must begin not with symbol-manipulation tests but with an analysis of intelligent functioning in the real world (McClelland, 1973; Sternberg, 1984).

In line with this orientation, Sternberg (1984) has defined intelligence very broadly, calling it purposive or successful adaptation in a real-world context. By this definition, intelligence includes whatever characteristics lead to such adaptation, if it is understood that "adaptation" covers changing the environment or selecting a new one if necessary. In this view, the way to advance knowledge of intelligent functioning is to compare persons who have had varying degrees of success in adapting to a given set of environmental demands, to see what characteristics differentiate them. For example, within a given occupation, what cognitive attributes distinguish the more successful people from the less successful ones?

31

The issue of intelligence is of great interest to most organizations. The leaders of an organization want to know what kind of intelligence, that is, what adaptive characteristics, are needed to do the organization's jobs well. Specifically, they want to know what qualities are needed for success as a senior manager, for it is on such managers that the success of the organization largely hinges.

Many experts, from Peter Drucker (1954) to Michael Maccoby (1981), have attempted to provide this information. On the basis of theory, experience, or clinical intuition, they have compiled lists of the characteristics of the successful executive. No one knows how accurate these lists are, however, as there is no way to test them – the characteristics are not concretely enough defined to be testable. For this reason, the generally accepted ideas about managerial intelligence in fact contribute little to our knowledge of intelligent functioning among managers.

For our clients in the worlds of business, education, government, and the armed services, it is important to be able not only to identify what the attributes of successful executive leaders and managers are, but to select people accurately on the basis of these attributes or to help persons acquire those attributes that they do not possess to the needed degree. Therefore, when we were asked about the issue of executive intelligence, we decided to investigate it scientifically, by applying an advanced type of behavioral technology. The technology is called *job competence assessment*. Job competence assessment employs systematic methods, first identifying top and average performers in a given occupation and then studying and analyzing them to uncover and measure the characteristics that distinguish the outstanding performers from the average ones. Upon their rigorous statistical validation, the results are both concrete and demonstrably applicable to numerous human-resource needs (Klemp, 1982).

For our purposes, we call these characteristics of outstanding performers *competencies* and define them more specifically as attributes of an individual that are necessary for effective performance in a job or life role. These attributes can include (1) general or specialized knowledge of use in an occupation; (2) abilities, both physical and intellectual; (3) traits, such as energy level and certain personality types; (4) motive or need states that direct individuals toward desired behavior patterns; and (5) self-images that reflect the roles people see themselves in and their concept of how effective they are in their roles. Further simplified, competencies can be classified into two broader types: (1) content competencies, or usable knowledge related to a role, and (2) process competencies, or attributes that bear on how knowledge is applied effectively. Thus, according to this definition, age and experience are not competencies themselves but may contribute to the acquisition of content and process competencies. The important thing to note is that competencies are defined within the context of a role, so that an attribute is a competency only if it contributes to effective performance in the role specified.

Since its development ten years ago, job competence assessment has been used to determine the competencies of more than eighty positions, ranging from those in human services and the foreign service to those of scientists, engineers, teachers, sales professionals, and various types of managers. The competencies, or combinations of competencies, are often specific to each occupation. But as we accumulated more and more information it became apparent that certain competencies are generic; that is, they appear in all the top performers of jobs of the same general type. This discovery is important because it enables us to compile a set of competencies that describe the outstanding senior manager in any type of organization.

In describing the competencies that distinguish outstanding senior managers, this chapter focuses on the intellectual competencies as they have been identified in various studies of senior managers, because the intellectual competencies are prominent in senior management positions, which require a high level of adaptive functioning. Moreover, because we and our colleagues have done numerous studies in this area, we have been able to cross-validate these competencies thoroughly – allowing us to ascertain statistically the senior manager competencies that are generic – those that apply to all jobs in this category.

But although we are focusing on the intellectual competencies, it should be remembered that competencies do not exist in isolation. The competency profile, or "model," that describes the high performer in a given job contains various competencies, all interacting. Thus, in order to explain how the intellectual competencies relate to adaptation in the occupational environment, we will also discuss the other competencies that must combine with intellectual functioning in order to yield managerial success.

Job competence assessment

Precisely how do we uncover, define, and measure the competencies needed to do a given job well? Job competence assessment has a series of specific steps that follow, as applied to the current subject, senior managers.

Step 1: Identifying the interview samples

The first step in job competence assessment is the identification of interview samples: a sample of outstanding performers in the job, and, for comparison, a sample of average performers in the job. (Poor performers are not studied because the focus of job competence assessment is exceptional performance as distinguished from adequate – not low – performance.) In the senior manager research, the interview samples were drawn from six diverse types

Table 1. *The interview samples in the studies of senior managers.*

Organization	Position	Number of outstanding interviewees	Number of average interviewees	Total number of interviewees
Diversified Fortune 100 company	General managers and division presidents	9	18	27
Volunteer organization	Executive directors	9	13	22
Fortune 100 company	General managers	6	9	15
Military hospitals	Commanding officers	11	11	22
Colleges	Presidents and deans	8	16[a]	24
Fortune 100 financial services organization	Senior executives	13	9	22
Totals		56	76	132

[a] See text for explanation of comparison-group composition.

of organization. Table 1 describes these samples, including the breakdown of outstanding and average performers studied in each type of organization.

The method of identifying the top performers within a job involve both objective performance measures and nomination by others in the organization. In addition to the application of the "hard" performance measures, superiors and peers in the target job specify the individuals in the job who are the "water walkers" – those whose performance, by every criterion, stands out as exceptional. The results are then combined to identify the performers who are consistently rated high.

The study of senior managers in the volunteer organization illustrates this process. First a selection was made, from among 150 executive directors of local units, of those whose units had shown the greatest financial growth. A list of all the executive directors was then distributed to each executive director; these people were asked to cross out the names of those peers whom they did not know and then to check, among the remaining names, those they considered outstanding. [Note that peer nominations are often found to be more valid than nominations by superiors, as people in the same job usually have a more precise knowledge of how well a person is doing that particular job (Kane & Lawler, 1978).] Finally, the chief executive officer (CEO) of the volunteer organization made his own list of the outstanding executive directors on the basis of his overall impression. When the results of these three identification processes were combined, only nine names were found on all three lists; these people would make up the interview sample of outstanding performers. Thirteen of the names did not appear on any list, so these employees were considered the average performers, making up the comparison interview sample. Although some outstanding performers can conceivably be missed in this process, this risk is acceptable in the effort to guarantee, through consensus, that only genuinely outstanding performers make up the first interview sample.

This process of identifying the interview samples was followed in all the studies of the senior managers except the study of college presidents and deans. Because a college has only one president and one dean per program, samples of both outstanding and average performers could not be drawn from within each institution; therefore, these people were compared with senior faculty and mid-level adminstrators in their institutions.

Step 2: The behavioral interviews

Once the outstanding job performers have been identified, the objective is to find out how they behave differently from the average performers in the job. To do this we would ideally be an invisible presence, following them around on the job and observing what they say and do, day in and day out. Kotter (1982) carried out an in-depth study of fifteen general managers from different organizations in which he had spent several weeks observing and taking notes on the behavior of these people as they sat in their offices, talked, attended conferences, and even flew on business to different cities. Such a procedure is far superior to the typical research interview or questionnaire, in which participants are asked to summarize how they spend their time, how they make decisions, and what characteristics they think are important in doing their work well.

From our point of view, this procedure has two limitations: (1) it is too expensive to use with the number of individuals that is needed in order to get statistically significant differences between the outstanding and average samples; and (2) it does not provide access to the thoughts and desires of the individual, that is, what a person thinks and what he or she says can be quite different yet equally important in the study of competence.

For these reasons, a behavioral interview was used as a primary source of information on how high-performing managers function. Adapted from Flanagan's critical-incident method (Flanagan, 1954), our behavioral interview was designed to uncover precise information on the actions and thoughts that make up competence in a given job. Following is a description of how the behavioral interviews were used in the study of senior managers.

First we asked managers to describe briefly their position and responsibilities, along with how they were prepared for the job and how they were selected for it. Next we asked participants to recall several key on-the-job situations in which they had felt particularly successful. They were then asked to choose one of these key situations to be described in complete detail. What led up to the event? Who else was involved? What did these other people say and do? What did the person want to accomplish? What was going on in the person's mind at every point during the event? Above all, what did the person say and do throughout the situation? In short, what we were trying to do was get a full report of a specific past occurrence, with a beginning, a middle, and an end, and with characters who wanted certain things, thought in certain ways, and acted in certain ways. What the interviewer is trained to avoid is getting generalizations about what the person usually does in typical situations. The reason is that everyone has ideas about what he or she does, and when and why, but these ideas are based partly on theories about the job, so they do not tell much about the person's actual behavior. By obtaining raw data on the person's behavior, the behavioral interview allowed us to get beneath the theories to the specific thoughts and actions that contribute to on-the-job success.

Throughout the interviews we avoided influencing the managers regarding their choice of situations to describe, for this choice itself is revealing: the kinds of situations that top performers and average performers recall often differ significantly. And although we asked for specific details of time, place, sequence, and words spoken, we did not "lead the witness" by asking yes-or-no questions; rather, we wanted the manager's ideas of what happened and might have happened, and we wanted these ideas described in full.

Each interview took two or three hours and covered four to six key situations. The interviews were tape-recorded, yielding sixty to eighty pages of double-spaced type when transcribed.

Step 3. Interview analysis

The next step in job competence assessment is to analyze the interview transcripts. First, all the transcripts are read for themes that seem to characterize the outstanding performers as a group, in contrast to the average performers. This is a major task, as a typical study may involve thirty-two transcripts, totaling more than 2,000 pages. The transcripts are read blind, without the readers' knowing which transcripts are from the outstanding performers, in order to maintain the readers' objectivity. Our general observation is that the better the criteria that were used to select the interview samples, the more accurately the transcript readers can identify the outstanding performers in the transcripts. When objective data have been used to sort individuals into outstanding and average performance groups, the readers' identification is accurate about 90% of the time.[1] When the criteria have been more subjective or in conflict, the readers' identification is accurate roughly 75% of the time.

Four to six members of the project team, usually including people from the client organization, perform this thematic analysis independently. They each read a set of transcripts, combing them for themes of outstanding performance and for the thoughts and behaviors of the interviewees that indicate the presence of those themes. They then meet in order to synthesize their analyses. The themes and critical behaviors each has identified are compared, discussed, and revised; these results are then combined to form a "codebook" of competencies and their indicators. With this codebook, the interview transcripts will be scored for the competencies, to see if these hypothesized competencies do indeed distinguish the outstanding performers from the average performers.

Typically, not all the interview transcripts are used in the preparation of the codebook, but only those that contain the richest, most complete material. A different set of readers then apply the codebook's behavioral definitions of the competencies – blind – to all the transcripts, to score for each appearance of a competency (this is called coding). If there is less than 80% agreement among the readers on any competency, the readers are retrained in coding. If the situation persists the indicators of the competency are redefined, and if the situation still persists the competency is dropped from the codebook. In addition, if the competency is scored in fewer than 20% of the transcripts, it is dropped.

After this blind coding is completed, the source of each interview, whether a top performer or an average performer, is revealed, to see whether the top performers do in fact score significantly higher than the average performers on the hypothesized competencies. The hypothesized competencies that pass this test are thus validated as the characteristics that distinguish the outstanding performers of the target job, and together they make up that job's competency model.

A comparison of competencies across managerial samples: what is generic?

For the present analysis, of senior managers in general, we examined the results of the application of the six codebooks that were prepared, by different teams, in the six studies listed in Table 1. These codebooks contained an average of sixteen competencies, with two to four indicators per competency. We performed a meta-analysis on this large body of information in order to identify competencies that appeared in most or all the codebooks, which would therefore differentiate the outstanding from the average performers in most senior management jobs. This task was thus a cross-validation of all the competencies. Although one might expect such an analysis to be difficult, given so many competencies, analysts, and types of managers involved, this was not the case. For in fact there were not so many competencies as it appeared: a few of the competencies proved to be specific to a particular type of manager, but many more – even if labeled differently – were found to be virtually the same.

Our focus will be the intellectual competencies of senior managers. These

competencies manifested themselves in the presence of other types of capabilities, such as interpersonal competencies (empathy and coaching) and
goal-attainment competencies (efficiency orientation and initiative). But the
context in which the intellectual competencies appeared most often was the
influencing of people regarding work-related objectives. For this reason, the
influence competencies will be treated along with the intellectual competencies in the discussion of our results. In addition, one competency seemed
to drive most of the others – self-confidence – so it too will be discussed.

Table 2 illustrates the nature of the raw material we worked with to find
the generic competencies, which cut across the six sets of samples of senior
managers. Most of the six codebooks included an intellectual competency
that involves planning or seeing the implications of events. It appeared in
the codebooks under various labels, as shown in column 2 of Table 2; sometimes it was called analytical thinking, other times anticipation, strategic
future orientation, or cause-and-effect reasoning. What demonstrates that
these different labels refer to the same competency is their indicators, which
are listed in the next column of Table 2: all of the indicators refer to a kind
of causal thinking, an "if X, then Y" mentality. The right-hand side of Table
2 shows that the senior managers who are outstanding performers displayed
this kind of thinking significantly more often than the average performers,
in three out of the four studies included in the exhibit. And in the fourth
study, of the commanding officers of military hospitals, there is a similar
distinction between the top and average performers, even though this difference does not reach a conventional level of significance. Moreover, the
fifth and sixth studies also supported these findings, although without the
statistical evidence needed for inclusion in Table 2. In the fifth study, of the
college presidents and deans, the competency appeared often enough to be
scored, but it did not differentiate significantly between these senior administrators and the senior faculty and mid-level administrators with whom
they were compared (had there been a comparison with average performers
in the same jobs, there might have been a significant differentiation). In the
sixth study, involving the senior executives of a Fortune 100 financial services organization, the competency was not identified on its own, but some
of its indicators occur as part of another competency, tactical flexibility,
which does differentiate between outstanding and average performers at the
.05 level of statistical significance. Thus, the case seems fairly strong for an
intellectual competency involving planning or causal thinking as a characteristic of outstanding senior managers in many types of organizations. This
competency enables them to see distant consequences of today's activities
and to design sound implementation strategies for their businesses or
operations.

Table 3 lists the eight generic competencies that we identified by comparing the results of the six individual studies. Some of the indicators, drawn

Table 2. *One generic competency ("planning/causal thinking") as it appeared in four studies.*

Study	Competency label	Competency indicators	Average frequencies of competency		Significance of difference (1-tailed p)
			In outstanding group	In average group	
General managers and division presidents of diversified Fortune 100 company	Analytical thinking	Anticipates problems or opportunities Identifies multiple implications of an action or event	7.78 ($n = 9$)	3.11 ($n = 18$)	.001
Executive directors of volunteer organization	Anticipation	Accurately predicts outcomes of activities or events Takes action to avoid problems that are foreseen	8.11 ($n = 9$)	3.92 ($n = 13$)	.01
General managers of Fortune 100 company	Analytical thinking and strategic future orientation	Identifies cause-and-effect relationships Anticipates future opportunities and requirements	5.83 ($n = 6$)	1.89 ($n = 9$)	.02
Commanding officers of military hospitals	Cause-and-effect reasoning	States implications of events and behavior States thoughts in a causal sequence ("If X, then Y")	1.45 ($n = 11$)	1.00 ($n = 11$)	.17

from different codebooks, of each competency are included. These competencies fall into three categories: (1) intellectual, (2) influence, and (3) other.

The intellectual competencies

Among the intellectual, or cognitive, competencies, the one described above is listed first: it is labeled planning/causal thinking. Next is diagnostic information seeking: pushing for concrete data in all sorts of ways, using a variety of sources. Then comes conceptualization/synthetic thinking, which involves seeing patterns in a series of events or identifying an idea that explains the essence of a situation. Planning/causal thinking is essentially hypothesis generation because it involves seeing either the potential implications of events or the likely consequences of a situation based on what has usually happened in the past. By contrast, conceptualization/synthetic thinking is essentially theory building to account for consistent patterns in recurring events or for connections between seemingly unrelated pieces of information; it is enhanced by diagnostic information seeking. The ability to conceptualize allows executives to create a strong sense of mission, and to mold the corporate culture to fit an adopted agenda (Deal & Kennedy, 1982).

As mentioned earlier, competencies always interact. Among the intellectual competencies, diagnostic information seeking is the natural outcome of planning/causal thinking, and it is the natural precursor of conceptualization/ synthetic thinking. Managers draw conclusions, from cause-and-effect reasoning and then seek information to check the accuracy of these conclusions. Once they have this information – particularly if it does not confirm their analyses – it forms the basis for the identification of patterns not recognized previously, which in turn lead the managers to more accurate analyses of implications. In the behavior of many senior managers, this process may express itself as an aggressively critical managerial style, marked by challenges to subordinates, making these managers appear both tough and incisive.

The influence competencies

The next group of competencies has to do with interpersonal influence. As indicated earlier, such influence is a key part of the managerial role. Four influence competencies appeared in our studies. The first is concern for influence – an alertness to the potentialities for influencing people. The indicators of this competency are essentially those that are used for scoring the need for power in Thematic Apperception Test (TAT) stories (Winter, 1973). Concern for influence appears in such statements as "When I walked

Table 3. *The eight generic senior manager competencies*

Competency	Competency indicators
The intellectual competencies	
Planning/causal thinking	Sees implications, consequences, alternatives, or if-then relationships
	Analyzes causal relationships
	Makes strategies, plans steps to reach a goal
Diagnostic information seeking	Pushes for concrete information in an ambiguous situation
	Seeks information from multiple sources to clarify a situation
	Uses questions to identify the specifics of a problem or other situation
Conceptualization/synthetic thinking	Understands how different parts, needs, or functions of the organization fit together
	Identifies patterns, interprets a series of events
	Identifies the most important issues in a complex situation
	Uses unusual analogies to understand or explain the essence of a situation
The influence competencies	
Concern for influence (the need for power)	States a desire to persuade people
	Anticipates the impact of actions on people
Directive influence (personalized power)	Confronts people directly when problems occur
	Tells people to do things the way he/she wants them done
Collaborative influence (socialized power)	Operates effectively with groups to influence outcomes and get cooperation
	Builds "ownership" of controversial decisions among key subordinates by involving them in decision making
Symbolic influence	Sets a personal example for an intended impact
	Uses symbols of group identity
Additional competency	
Self-confidence	Sees self as prime mover, leader, or energizer of the organization
	Mentions being stimulated by crises and other difficult problems
	Sees self as the most capable person to get the job done

into that meeting, I was trying to figure out how to persuade them to agree to my proposal.''

The next influence competency is directive influence: using one's personal authority or expert power to make sure that something gets done. The competency typically appears in a person's telling someone to do something, and it is particularly characteristic of first-line supervisors (Boyatzis, 1982). Directive influence is often referred to as personalized power, because it involves only the influencer's desire for power – as opposed to socialized power, which also involves the desires of the person being influenced (McClelland, 1975).

Socialized power in this study is labeled collaborative influence and is the third influence competency. In management language, this is selling rather than telling: it is building relationships for the benefit of both parites; and it is operating effectively with groups in order to get cooperation.

Fourth is the influence competency labeled symbolic influence. It is indicated by a use of symbols to influence how people act in the organization. A senior manager with this competency can, by personal example or a statement of mission, create a sense of purpose for the whole organization, which engenders individuals' loyalty and commitment to it.

An additional competency

In this category, at the bottom of Table 3, appears self-confidence. This important competency might well have been listed first, because we found it to be so prevalent among the outstanding senior managers. These people, although recognizing difficulties, never expressed any doubt that they would ultimately succeed. In the behavioral interviews, they displayed strong self-presentation skills and came across as very much in charge: they acted to make the interviewer feel comfortable, and they responded quickly and confidently to the request for key situations. By contrast, the average senior managers were more tentative, saying such things as, "To this day I don't know whether I made the right decision." Moreover, the outstanding managers expressed self-confidence by being stimulated by crises and other problems, rather than distressed or overwhelmed by them.

The frequency of the generic competencies – How big a role do they play?

Table 4 summarizes the frequency with which the eight generic competencies were present in the research results, as well as how often they distinguished outstanding from average performers at a statistically significant level. Consider self-confidence. This competency appeared in all six codebooks, which means that it occurred in at least 50% of all the participants (outstanding and average) in each of the six studies: each of these people showed one or more of the behaviors indicating this competency. Regarding this competency's importance, in five of the six studies the top performers showed evidence of self-confidence more often than the average performers at a statistically significant level: in one study at $p < .10$, in two studies at $p < .05$, and in two studies at $p < .01$.

Table 4. *The number of studies (out of six) in which each generic competency was present and significant*

Competency	Number of studies in which competency was present	Number of studies in which competency was significant	Levels of significance[a]
The intellectual competencies			
Planning/causal thinking	5	3	1 at $p < .05$
			2 at $p < .01$
Diagnostic information seeking	5	2	2 at $p < .10$
Conceptualization/synthetic thinking	5	4	1 at $p < .10$
			2 at $p < .05$
			1 at $p < .01$
The influence competencies			
Concern for influence	6	2	2 at $p < .05$
Directive influence	5	4	2 at $p < .05$
			2 at $p < .01$
Collaborative influence	5	4	3 at $p < .05$
			1 at $p < .01$
Symbolic influence	6	6	3 at $p < .05$
			3 at $p < .01$
Additional competency			
Self-confidence	6	5	1 at $p < .10$
			2 at $p < .05$
			2 at $p < .01$

[a] By a one-tailed t-test.

In noting the number of studies in which a competency was present, it is important to remember that the six competency analyses were carried out independently, at different times, by different teams of investigators – who proceeded purely inductively, without a priori hypotheses as to what competencies to look for. In other words, these results have a high level of validity. And even in the few cases in which an individual participated in more than one analysis and thus might have carried over expectations that influenced what was found, the strict statistical requirements for validation combatted this risk; a competency could not be included in a codebook unless concrete indicators of it could be located in at least half of that study's interview transcripts. Therefore, although the samples establishing the presence of a competency are small, together they provide solid evidence for the importance of the competency in senior managerial functioning.

Of the intellectual competencies, each appeared in five of the six studies of senior managers, and each study showed at least two of these three competencies. Conceptualization/synthetic thinking differentiated significantly between outstanding and average senior managers in four of the five studies in which this competency appeared. Planning/causal thinking differentiated similarly in three of the five studies in which it appeared, although this is a conservative statement, since in a fourth study the trend was in the same direction, and in a fifth study some of this competency's indicators were classified under another competency, which did differentiate significantly. By contrast, diagnostic information seeking differentiated less significantly between outstanding and average senior managers; the difference was significant in only two of the five studies in which the competency appeared, and at the level of $p < .10$. We interpret this finding to mean that diagnostic information seeking is a threshold competency; it is a minimum requirement for performing at the senior management level. That is, this characteristic is prevalent among senior managers (five of the six studies), but it does not differentiate between the top and average performers. In short, a job's threshold competencies must be possessed in order to perform the job at all.

In this connection, it is important to repeat that there were no poor performers in the research samples – no one who, for example, had been fired from senior management positions or had never even been considered for them. If such individuals had been included for comparison purposes, more threshold competencies would undoubtedly have appeared, as the differentiators between average performers and poor performers. But since the emphasis of the job competence assessment process is on the differentiators between average performers and outstanding performers, it does not usually uncover threshold competencies, which – because possessed by all who perform the job at least adequately – do not distinguish the outstanding from the average performers.

Regarding the frequency of the four influence competencies, each appeared in at least five of the six studies, and each study showed at least three of the four; three of these competencies differentiated significantly between outstanding and average senior managers. The competency that did not so differentiate is concern for influence; like diagnostic information seeking, it functions as a threshold competency, for it occurred in all six studies but differentiated significantly in only two of the studies. This finding is consistent with earlier results reported by McClelland (1975), who found that the need for power by itself does not distinguish outstanding from average managerial performance. What does differentiate is the need for power combined with two other elements – a lower need for affiliation and a high level of inhibition, or self-control – to form the "inhibited-power-motive syndrome." Stated in everyday language, the more successful managers have a concern for influence expressed in a controlled way and that is greater than the desire to be well liked. By contrast, a high need for power combined with a low level of inhibition leads to impulsive aggressiveness, which does

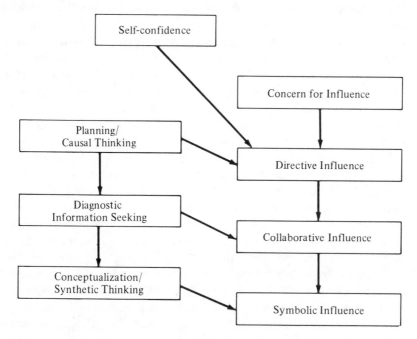

Figure 1. The interaction of the senior-manager competencies.

not normally characterize outstanding managerial performance (McClelland & Boyatzis, 1982).

The interaction of competencies

Simply listing the statistical significance of competencies, as in Table 4, does not convey very well how senior managers function to produce outstanding results; a depiction of how these competencies interact describes such functioning more clearly. Figure 1 is thus provided as a hypothetical model of the competencies' interaction that results in successful performance.

Figure 1 lists the competencies from top to bottom in roughly the order of how basic they are. Thus, self-confidence appears at the top of the model, for it acts as a prime mover of senior managerial performance, affecting the likelihood that the intellectual competencies will be expressed through a variety of influence strategies. Concern for influence appears next under self-confidence, for it activates the three other influence competencies; each of these three is associated with one of the three intellectual competencies.

The three competencies that appear under concern for influence are displayed according to the level of sophistication of their influence strategies.

Our research on managers has shown that these strategies tend to be associated with level in the managerial hierarchy: Directive influence strategies characterize effective first-line supervisors, collaborative influence strategies characterize effective mid-level managers, and symbolic influence strategies characterize effective senior managers. In functional terms, foremen must know how to tell people what to do, mid-level managers must know how to work with others, and senior managers must know how to make an impact on the whole organization through the use of mission statements and other symbolic activity.

Each of these influence strategies, in turn, appears to be dependent on a level of intellectual functioning, as represented by the three intellectual competencies. Thus, for managers to direct people successfully (directive influence), they must have a plan and see the implications of their plan (planning/ causal thinking). For managers to work with others (collaborative influence), they must be skilled at collecting feedback on their directive attempts so that they can diagnose where the organization needs adjusting and how and with whom they can work to bring about the adjustment (diagnostic information seeking). And for managers to develop mission statements and engage in symbolic activity (symbolic influence), they must be able to put the diverse pieces of information they have collected into a synthesized whole (conceptualization/synthetic thinking).

Kotter (1982) found in observing successful senior executives that they spent about 75% of their time talking to people; during these talks, they apparently did not make decisions, although if asked, most of them would say that they spend most of their time making decisions.[2] What, then, are they doing when they are talking? To borrow from the fields of linguistics and artificial intelligence, they are demonstrating surface behavior that links with the shared understanding, preconceptions, tacit assumptions, and informational history of others, so that while they seem to make no decisions, decisions "get made." In other words, they are exerting directive, collaborative, and symbolic influence: they are creating in those with whom they talk direction, a sense of ownership, and the feeling that there is a common agenda for the whole organization – that it has a mission to which all are contributing. In order to do all this, they must be good planners, diagnosticians, and conceptualizers – ultimately to produce a driving sense of purpose for the organization. In sum, the intellectual competencies inform and make possible the different influence competencies that are needed by the successful senior manager.

Intelligent functioning of senior managers

Figure 1 illustrates how the intellectual competencies combine with other competencies to produce intelligent behavior in a senior manager. Intelligence is here defined as Sternberg (1984) defines it: successful adaptation in the real world. Thus, as Sternberg points out, intelligence has only a contextual meaning. A given characteristic is indicative of intelligence – is a competency – only if it is adaptive: leading to success in a given situation. It may, therefore, be a competency in some situations and not in others. For example, directive influence is adaptive at the first-line supervisory level, but it may be quite disruptive, or maladaptive, at the mid-level management level. And analytic reasoning may be a handicap rather than a competency in certain military situations ("Yours is not to reason why. . . . "), because established procedures must be followed automatically for the unit to function effectively.

Another implication of seeing intelligence as successful adaptation is that its components include all the variables that influence behavior. According to the models developed by theorists such as Hull (1952) and Atkinson and Birch (1978), the components of intelligence include motivational, skill, or habit variables; knowledge or schema variables; and inhibitory variables. Figure 1 includes a motivational variable (the need for power, in concern for influence), several skill variables (collaborative influence and planning/ causal thinking), and a schema variable (a mission statement used in symbolic influence). But when intelligence is defined this broadly, it is necessary, for our description of intelligent senior managerial functioning, to specify the overt and covert behaviors – actions and thoughts – that signify the competencies relating to intellectual capability.

As far as this narrower intellectual area is concerned, what has been learned from our research? The identification of the three intellectual competencies is certainly not new. Nearly all theories of problem solving (Sternberg, 1984) include such performance components as the following:

> Causal thinking, or inductive reasoning, which involves seeing the implication of concepts or hypotheses
> Checking out the implications to see whether the facts fit the concepts or hypotheses (we call this diagnostic information seeking; Sternberg calls it selective encoding)
> Forming new concepts, which involves selectively combining diverse pieces of information to create a concept, which is then compared with other concepts in order to refine it

What is new about our findings is that we have observed these intellectual competencies in action and as operants in Skinner's sense (1938, 1953), rather than as responses to controlled situations or stimuli. Our data are clearly of a different order from what is obtained in an experimentally controlled situation, such as giving someone a problem to solve in an ability test. When we have administered such tests during the past three years to middle and senior managers as part of managerial-assessment programs that include complex business simulations, the tests tend to be uncorrelated with demonstration of complex problem-solving abilities in these simulations as well as with on-the-job performance. We would argue that this is to be expected, because many average managers are as adept in figuring out the solutions to narrowly focused problems as their outstanding counterparts. The major differences between outstanding and average managers in intellectual competence are that the former spend more time on the job exercising these capabilities than the latter and employ a greater repertoire of mental responses in doing so. In short, what we discovered is that the difference between capacity to act and disposition to act forms the distinction between average and outstanding senior managerial performance. Any theory of managerial intelligence must take this important difference into account.

What is also new about our findings is the behavioral detail they provide on how these intellectual competencies show themselves in the managerial context. Tables 2 and 3 illustrate some of this detail, which is displayed even more in the codebooks from which this material was taken. Traditionally, psychologists interested in theories of intelligence have focused on the behaviors involved in word games and puzzles invented as ability tests; such specific test behaviors are not necessarily how the intellectual competencies show themselves in the real world. Now, however, we have an extensive sampling of real-world intellectual behaviors on which to build more accurate theories of managerial intelligence.

The value of knowing such real-world intellectual behavior is much greater than that of knowing ability-test behavior. Consider training, for example. Training people in adaptive ability-test behavior will seldom prepare them for successful adaptation in the real world. Suppose it were found that performing well on a verbal analogies test is associated with successful managerial performance. Would anyone propose that training people to make verbal analogies will provide them with the skills to be better managers? In the first place, organizations would have great difficulty accepting such training as relevant but, more important, it is doubtful that training in this limited behavioral expression of an intellectual competency would generalize to the more complex expressions of the competency that characterize real-world adaptation. By contrast, the indicators documented through the job competence assessment process are highly generalizable. Because they are drawn from managerial performance in the real world, and because they are defined in concrete managerial terms, these indicators readily lend themselves to training designed to increase managerial competence. For example, training programs in leadership and management skills, based on competency research, have been carried out in the U.S. Navy and have resulted in improved operational effectiveness (U.S. Department of the Navy, 1984). Similarly, such indicators can be used in selection, to help identify the most promising candidates for senior management positions and, in performance appraisal, to help assess incumbents of those positions.

Does what we have found among managers relate to intelligent functioning in other occupations? The answer to this question is most certainly yes. In studies we have conducted on different kinds of jobs, we have found considerable consistency in the applicability of certain competencies. Outstanding performers in the helping professions – physicians, counselors, social workers, teachers – all rely on a high degree of planning/causal thinking and diagnostic information seeking in collecting and interpreting observations and data and making recommendations on the basis of their conclusions. Engineers and scientists depend on their ability to conceptualize problems in terms of their most important features, as well as to see connections between seemingly unrelated pieces of information. The best sales professionals are highly skilled both at diagnostic information seeking, which guides them in understanding their customers' true needs, and at all manners of influence. But what makes successful senior managers different from successful people in these other occupations is the specific combination of intellectual and other competencies that they require and the behavioral manifestations of these competencies in the appropriate context.

The particular combination of competencies described in this chapter, in fact, would be highly dysfunctional in nonmanagers from the occupations just noted. For example, scientists, engineers, and people in the helping professions who spend most of their time influencing others rather than solving their problems end up pleasing their superiors but not their clients, whereas sales professionals whose approach is too conceptual may confuse their customers by considering too many complex options rather than focusing on answering the customers' objections and making the sale. From our experience in studying people in these and other occupations, we conclude that individual competencies may be generic across occupations and situations, differing only in their behavioral manifestations and in how often they are required for effective performance. On the other hand, certain combinations of competencies tend to be specific and do not generalize well across occupations or situations.

The significance of our approach to research on job effectiveness is that it takes overall quality of performance and the situational context as the givens, from which emerge dimensions of difference between outstanding and average performers. This contrasts with an approach that begins with specific assumptions (e.g., on what constitutes "practical intelligence") and tests their validity in carefully contrived experimental situations. As our data spanning different studies begin to show consistent patterns and interpretations, and as these conclusions are matched by those derived from different approaches to assessing real-world performance, we expect that the value of job competence assessment will go beyond the practical need to select and train others more effectively. To the extent that it contributes to an empirical body of knowledge regarding how the mind functions effectively in the real world, it will enable us to develop increasingly accurate theories of intelligence.

Notes

1 Such accuracy can have interesting consequences. In one study, interviews had been conducted with eighteen supposedly outstanding employee relations managers; upon reading the transcripts, however, we had to report to the client organization that three of these people did not seem to be outstanding, at which point the client reported that these three average performers had been included in the outstanding sample to test us.
2 See, for example, Chester Barnard's classic book, *The functions of the executive* (1983), in which he pictures executives as decision makers.

References

Atkinson, J. W., & Birch, D. (1978). *Introduction to motivation* (2nd ed.). New York: Van Nostrand.

Barnard, C. I. (1938). *The functions of the executive.* Cambridge, MA: Harvard University Press.

Boyatzis, R. E. (1982). *The competent manager: A model for effective performance.* New York: Wiley.

Deal, T. E., & Kennedy, A. A. (1982). *Corporate cultures.* Reading, MA: Addison-Wesley.

Drucker, P. F. (1954). *The practice of management.* New York: Harper.

Flanagan, J. C. (1954). The critical incident technique. *Psychological Bulletin, 51,* 327–358.

Hull, C. L. (1952). *A behavior system.* New Haven: Yale University Press.

Kane, J. & Lawler, E. E. (1978). Methods of peer assessment. *Psychological Bulletin, 85*(3), 555–586.

Klemp, G. O., Jr. (1982). Job Competence Assessment: Defining the attributes of the top performer. In *The pig in the python and other tales* (collection of research papers presented before the 1981 ASTD National Conference). ASTD Research Series, Vol. 8.

Kotter, J. P. (1982). *The general managers.* New York: Free Press.

Maccoby, M. (1981). *The leader.* New York: Simon and Schuster.

McClelland, D. C. (1973). Testing for competence rather than for "intelligence." *American Psychologist, 28,* 1–14.

McClelland, D. C. (1975). *Power: The inner experience.* New York: Irvington.

McClelland, D. C., & Boyatzis, R. E. (1982). The leadership motive pattern and long-term success in management. *Journal of Applied Psychology, 67*(6), 737–743.

Neisser, U. (1976). General, academic, and artificial intelligence. In L. Resnick (Ed.), *The nature of intelligence.* Hillsdale, NJ: Erlbaum.

Skinner, B. F. (1938). *The behavior of organisms.* New York: Appleton-Century-Crofts.

Skinner, B. F. (1953). *Science and human behavior.* New York: Macmillan.

Sternberg, R. J. (1984). Toward a triarchic theory of human intelligence. *Behavioral and Brain Sciences, 7*(2), 269–315.

U.S. Department of the Navy. (1984). *A history of leadership and management education and training.* Washington, DC: Leadership and Management Education and Training Implementation Branch, Naval Military Personnel Command.

Winter, D. G. (1973). *The power motive.* New York: Free Press.

joint association of social class status should be minimized in such a comparison. That the tests predict training performance better than job performance suggests that the tests measure only a subset of the competencies required for real-world success.

Approaches to measuring real-world competencies

If traditional IQ and employment tests neglect competencies important to performance in real-world settings, how might remaining competencies be measured? A number of approaches to measuring aspects of real-world performance are ignored by traditional tests. We shall briefly consider three alternative approaches – the motivational, the critical incident, and the simulation – and then introduce the knowledge-based approach that we have taken.

The *motivational approach* has considered the role of motives that drive and are satisfied by intellectual behavior in real-world settings. The need to achieve (n-Ach), a motive that directs thought and behavior toward the goal of achieving excellence, has stimulated considerable research of both theoretical and practical importance (see, e.g., Atkinson, 1958; McClelland, Atkinson, Clark, & Lowell, 1953). One difficulty with this approach has been the somewhat low reliability of techniques, especially "projective" ones, that rely on subjects providing stories for pictures of the sort found on the Thematic Apperception Test (TAT) (McClelland, 1973). Helmreich, Spence, Beane, Lucker, and Matthews (1980) turned to "objective" measures, such as self-report, in an investigation of relations between success in the field of academic psychology and several personality attributes and motives, including achievement motivation. They reported small (.1–.2) but reliable correlations between several measures of success in academic psychology and the self-report measures of achievement motivation and personality attributes.

The *critical-incident technique* consists of asking people to describe several incidents they handled particularly well, as well as several incidents they handled particularly poorly (Flanagan, 1954; McClelland, 1976). These critical incidents are then analyzed qualitatively in an effort to determine the nature of the competencies that appear important to success in a given job. This approach is much more feasible than around-the-clock observation, but the approach assumes that people can and will provide incidents that are critical to success in their particular jobs and that qualitative analysis is sufficient for identification of underlying competencies.

The *simulation approach* consists of observing people in situations that have been set up to simulate job performance. The in-basket test (Frederiksen, 1966; Frederiksen, Saunders, & Wand, 1957) is a well-known example of this approach. A participant is presented with an "in-basket" that contains various memos, reports, and letters requiring action. Performance is evaluated in terms of how the items are handled. For example, are tasks delegated to subordinates when it is appropriate to do so? Another common example of the simulation approach is the Assessment Center, in which small groups of individuals are presented with a variety of simulation tasks including the in-basket test, simulated interviews, and simulated group discussions (Bray, 1982; Thorton & Byham, 1982). An advantage of the simulation approach is that it uses tasks similar to criterion performance. Disadvantages of this approach include (1) that it can be difficult to decide which parts of a job to simulate, and (2) that it is far from clear just how performance should be evaluated.

The approach we have taken is based on the *knowledge-based approach* used by cognitive psychologists and others in their study of the ways in which "experts" differ from "novices" in task performance relative to their domain of expertise (see, e.g., Chase & Simon, 1973; Chi, Feltovich & Glaser, 1981; de Groot, 1966; Jeffries, Turner, Polson, & Atwood, 1981; McKeithen, Reitman, Rueter, & Hirtle, 1981; Simon & Simon, 1978; Soloway, Erlich, Bonar, & Greenspan, 1982). Examples of tasks examined with this approach include chess, solving physics problems, and computer programming. The consistent finding has been that experts differ from novices primarily in the amount and organization of their knowledge about the task, rather than in underlying cognitive abilities.

Whereas the knowledge-based approach has been applied mostly to tasks of the "academic intelligence" variety, we sought to apply this approach in our study of practical tasks faced by individuals in several real-world pursuits.

An important claim we make is that much of the knowledge upon which competence in real-world settings depends is *tacit*, that is, not openly expressed or stated (*Oxford English Dictionary*, 1933). Tacit knowledge is considered (1) practical rather than academic, (2) informal rather than formal, and (3) usually not directly taught. Deciding which journal to submit a manuscript to is an example of a task that requires tacit knowledge. By our use of the word tacit we do not wish to imply that such knowledge is completely inaccessible to conscious awareness, unspeakable, or even unteachable, but merely that it usually is not taught directly to most of us. Although some tacit knowledge conceivably could be taught directly, much tacit knowledge may be disorganized and relatively inaccessible, making it potentially ill suited for direct instruction.

Consider how our approach relates to the other approaches to measuring real-world competence just presented.

Our approach shares with the motivational approach an interest in motivational aspects of real-world competence. But whereas the motivational approach has focused on the role of motives such as the need to achieve (n-Ach) in real-world accomplishment, our focus is on the "self-knowledge" an individual has about his or her individual motives and goals that might be useful in maximizing productive accomplishment. For example, whereas some individuals might find it difficult to work on a project unless it largely is of their own creation, others might prefer the diffusion of responsibility that comes with working on group projects initiated by others. Knowing which "kind" of person one is can be useful in selecting projects that best fit one's needs and preferences. We agree that motives such as n-Ach are important determinants of real-world competence; but we believe that real-world competence also is dependent upon one's knowledge about one's motivational "make-up," and one's knowledge about how to make best use of it.

Our approach differs from one based on the critical-incident technique in that rather than relying on persons to determine for themselves which incidents are in some way "critical," we ask subjects only to provide typical work-related situations and possible responses to them. We then identify "critical" items statistically using a variety of item-discrimination procedures. Thus, an advantage of our approach over one based on the critical incident technique is that we need not assume that people can and will provide incidents that are critical to success in their particular jobs and that a qualitative analysis of their responses is sufficient for identification of underlying competencies. A potential disadvantage of our approach is that critical areas of task performance might be overlooked in the initial stages of item development: Our item-discrimination procedures are only as good as the initial pool of items we apply them to.

Our approach shares with the simulation approach the view that eliciting practically important behavior in a test situation depends, in part, on the extent to which the test tasks resemble the tasks found in the everyday world. However, we rely on paper-and-pencil tasks that somewhat resemble simulations, rather than on actual simulations themselves, because it has been impractical to simulate the wide variety of tasks and situations that we have examined. There may be a tradeoff between the increased breadth of our inquiry and the decreased realism of our tasks. We now present our tacit knowledge framework and review findings from a number of experiments we carried out to examine various aspects of it.

Preliminary framework: three categories of tacit knowledge

We propose that practically intelligent behavior in professional and managerial careers depends in part on tacit knowledge, which we divided into three categories: tacit knowledge about managing self, managing others, and managing career (Wagner & Sternberg, 1985).

Tacit knowledge about *managing self* refers to knowledge about how to manage oneself on a daily basis so as to maximize one's productivity. Examples of tacit knowledge about managing self include knowledge about the relative importance of the tasks one faces, knowledge about more and less efficient ways of approaching tasks, and knowledge about how to motivate oneself so as to maximize accomplishment.

Tacit knowledge about *managing others* refers to knowledge about managing subordinates and one's social relationships. Examples include knowledge about how to assign and tailor tasks to take advantage of an individual's strengths and to minimize the effects of his or her weaknesses, how to reward in such a way as to maximize both performance and satisfaction, and how to get along with others in general.

Tacit knowledge about *managing career* refers to knowledge about how careers are established, how reputations can be enhanced, and how to convince superiors of the worth of one's ideas or products. A bad reputation can ruin a law career and can sidetrack the career of an advancing manager whether the reputation is well deserved or not. Examples of tacit knowledge about managing career include knowing to what extent one's priorities reflect what is valued by the organization or field, and how to convince others that your work is as good as it really is (or even better).

To limit the scope of our inquiry, our investigation has focused on two domains: academic psychology and business management. The domain of academic psychology was chosen because it is a domain with which we both have first-hand knowledge. Because our goal was to develop a framework that was not specific to any one domain, we conducted an investigation in a second domain that paralleled our study of academic psychologists. The domain of business management was chosen because it seemed somewhat far removed from the domain of academic psychology and, because business management is of interest to many people, a number of books have been written on success as a manager.

We turn now to a discussion of results from a series of experiments carried out to evaluate and further develop our tacit knowledge framework. The first three experiments examined the preliminary tacit knowledge framework that proposed three categories of tacit knowledge: tacit knowledge about oneself, tacit knowledge about managing others, and tacit knowledge about managing one's career. On the basis of the results of these experiments, the framework was expanded and this revised tacit knowledge framework was examined in two more experiments.

Experiment 1: Tacit knowledge in academic psychology

Method

We interviewed experienced and highly successful experts in the field of academic psychology, asking them to provide typical work-related situations and possible responses to them. On the basis of these interviews and the tacit-knowledge framework, we constructed a set of 12 work-related situations, each associated with alternative responses. A sample work-related situation and some of its associated response items follow. Additional examples of work-related situations are presented in Appendix A.

It is your second year as an assistant professor in a prestigious psychology department. This past year you published two unrelated empirical articles in established journals. You don't believe, however, that there is a research area that can be identified as your own. You believe yourself to be about as productive as others. The feedback about your first year of teaching has been generally good. You have yet to serve on a university committee. There is one graduate student who has chosen to work with you. You have no external source of funding, nor have you applied for funding.

Your goals are to become one of the top people in your field and to get tenure in your department. The following is a list of things you are considering doing in the next two months. You obviously cannot do them all. Rate the importance of each by its priority as a means of reaching your goals.

____a.   improve the quality of your teaching
____b.   write a grant proposal
____c.   begin long-term research that may lead to a major theoretical article
____d.   concentrate on recruiting more students
____e.   serve on a committee studying university–community relations
____f.   begin several related short-term research projects, each of which may lead to an empirical article
⋮
____o.   volunteer to be chairperson of the undergraduate curriculum committee

Performance on the tacit knowledge measure was then compared with performance on a number of external criterion reference measures appropriate to the domain of academic psychology.

There were three groups of subjects, totaling 187 participants in all. The *faculty group* consisted of fifty-four members of the faculty in twenty psychology departments, twenty-seven of whom were members of ten of the fifteen psychology departments rated highest in overall quality (Roose & Andersen, 1970), and twenty-one of whom were from ten other psychology departments. The *psychology graduate student group* consisted of 104 graduate students from twenty-one psychology departments, twenty of which were the same as were sampled for the faculty group, plus Yale University. The undergraduate group consisted of twenty-nine Yale undergraduates.

Results

Between-group analyses. Item ratings were correlated with a "dummy" variable that indicated whether the respondent was a member of the undergraduate, psychology graduate, or psychology faculty group. With a total of 160 response items in all, eight significant correlations between item ratings and the group membership variable would be expected on the basis of chance alone. In fact, significant correlations were found for fifty-eight items, with a binomial test of the probability of obtaining this many significant correlations on the basis of chance yielding $p < .001$. Percentages of subscale items yielding significant correlations with the group membership variable for the managing self, others, and career subscales were 25% ($p < .001$), 66% ($p < .01$), and 42% ($p < .001$), respectively. That items differentiated among groups whose members differed in level of professional advancement is consistent with the view that at least some items measured knowledge acquired as a result of experience and training in the field of academic psychology; but it was important to determine whether or not there existed within-group relations between tacit knowledge and criterion measures of performance.

Within-group analyses. Items for which ratings correlated significantly with the group membership variable were retained for this second phase of the analysis. Subscale scores for the three categories of tacit knowledge (managing self, others, and career) and a total score based on all the items were calculated by summing the ratings of response items associated with each category of tacit knowledge, after first reflecting the ratings for distractor items. Distractor items (i.e., item responses that novices believed to be important but experts knew to be unimportant) were identified by a negative correlation between the item rating and the group membership variable. (See Wagner & Sternberg, 1985, for details about scoring and for a full presentation of experiments 1–3.)

The within-group relations between tacit knowledge scores and criterion reference measures for the psychology faculty, psychology graduate student, and undergraduate groups suggested that (1) individual differences in tacit knowledge were related to various measures of career performance, and (2) the tacit knowledge measure was not just a proxy for a traditional IQ test. Correlations between tacit knowledge scores and criterion measures of performance are presented for the psychology faculty and graduate student groups in Table 1.

For the psychology faculty group, significant correlations in the range of .3 to .5 were found between the tacit knowledge scores and research-related criterion-reference measures such as number of publications, percentage of time spent in research, and whether or not an individual was a member of one of the top-rated departments. Significant negative correlations were found between the tacit knowledge scores and non-research-related criterion reference measures such as percentage of time spent in teaching and percentage of time spent in performing administrative duties.

For the psychology graduate student group, significant correlations in the .3 to .5 range were found between tacit knowledge scores and criterion reference measures such as number of years of graduate study completed,

Table 1. *Correlation coefficients between tacit-knowledge scores and criterion reference measures for faculty and psychology graduate student groups.*

| | Tacit-knowledge scores | | | |
Criterion reference measures	Total score	Self	Managing others	Career
Faculty				
# Publications	.33[a]	.16	.21	.35[a]
# Citations	.23	−.11	.53[b]	.30
# Conferences attended	.34[a]	.28[a]	.19	.37[b]
# Conference papers presented	.16	.16	.12	.24
Level of school	.40[b]	.34[a]	.43[b]	.39[b]
Academic rank	−.27	−.34[a]	.39[a]	−.11
Percentage of time spent in:				
Teaching	−.29[a]	−.24[a]	−.41[b]	−.31[a]
Research	.39[b]	.27	.27	.34[a]
Administrative duties	−.41[b]	−.37[b]	−.13	−.26
Advising students	.00	.07	.13	−.08
Editorial business	−.04	.19	.19	.00
Other	.14	.15	−.33[a]	.05
Year of Ph.D.	.04	.14	−.33[a]	.05
Psychology graduate students				
# Years completed	.39[b]	.15	.10	.43[b]
Level of school	.52[b]	.35[b]	.21[a]	.52[b]
# Research projects completed	.31[b]	.20[a]	.15	.41[b]
# Courses taught	.19	.08	.01	.23[a]
# Publications	.31[b]	.18	.08	.38[b]

[a] $p < .05$.
[b] $p < .01$.

whether or not the subject was a student in one of the top-rated departments, number of research projects completed, and number of publications.

For the undergraduate group, the only group for whom it was feasible to administer a traditional mental ability test, the correlation between total score on the tacit knowledge measure and performance on a standardized test of verbal reasoning was a nonsignificant −.04.

In summary, there are three important results. First, there were expert–novice differences in tacit knowledge across groups whose members differed in amounts of experience and training in the field of academic psychology. Second, there were strong relationships between performance on the tacit knowledge measure and various measures of career performance. Third, tacit knowledge scores of undergraduates were unrelated to scores on a verbal ability test.

Table 2. *Correlation coefficients between tacit-knowledge scores and criterion reference measures for business managers.*

	Tacit-knowledge scores			
Criterion reference measures	Total score	Self	Managing others	Career
Level of company	.34[a]	.00	.03	.40[b]
# Years formal schooling	.41[b]	.08	.05	.46[b]
Salary	.46[b]	.11	.05	.46[b]
# Years management experience	.21	.13	−.08	.20
Level of title	.14	−.11	.23	.16
Employees	.10	−.13	−.15	.25

[a] $p < .05$.
[b] $p < .01$.

Experiment 2. Tacit knowledge in business management

The purpose of experiment 2 was an attempt to generalized our findings to a second real-world pursuit, that of business management.

Method

There were three groups of subjects, totaling 127 subjects in all, whose members differed in amounts of experience and formal training in business management. The business professional group consisted of fifty-four managers, nineteen of whom were from among the top twenty companies in the Fortune 500 list, twenty-eight of whom were from companies not on the Fortune 500 list, and seven of whom did not choose to indicate their institutional affiliation. The business graduate student group consisted of fifty-one graduate students in five business schools that varied in level of prestige. The undergraduate group consisted of twenty-two Yale undergraduates.

Tacit knowledge in the field of business management was sampled by presenting subjects with twelve work-related situations, each of which was associated with from nine to twenty response items, for a total of 166 items. The work-related situations and response items were based on the tacit-knowledge framework and on interviews conducted with experienced and successful business executives. An example of a work-related situation and a sample of its associated response items follows, and other examples of work-related situations for business management are presented in Appendix B.

It is your second year as a mid-level manager in a company in the communications industry. You head a department of about thirty people. The evaluation of your first

year on the job has been generally favorable. Performance ratings for your department are at least as good as they were before you took over, and perhaps even a
little better. You have two assistants. One is quite capable. The other just seems to
go through the motions but to be of little real help.

You believe that although you are well liked, there is little that would distinguish
you in the eyes of your superiors from the nine other managers at a comparable level
in the company.

Your goal is rapid promotion to the top of the company. The following is a list of
things you are considering doing in the next two months. You obviously cannot do
them all. Rate the importance of each by its priority as a means of reaching your
goal.

_____a.   find a way to get rid of the "dead wood," e.g., the less helpful assistant
          and three or four others
_____b.   participate in a series of panel discussions to be shown on the local public
          television station
_____c.   find ways to make sure your superiors are aware of your important
          accomplishments
_____d.   make an effort to better match the work to be done with the strengths
          and weaknesses of individual employees
   ⋮
_____n.   write an article on productivity for the company newsletter

All scoring procedures were identical to those used in experiment 1.

Results

Between-group analyses. As was done in experiment 1, item ratings were
correlated with a "dummy" variable that indicated, in this case, whether
the respondent was a member of the undergraduate, business graduate, or
business manager group. Significant correlations were found between item
ratings and the group membership variable for thirty-nine of the original 166
response items, with a binomial test of the probability of obtaining this many
significant correlations due to chance alone yielding $p < .001$. Percentages
of subscale items yielding significant correlations with the group membership
variable for the managing self, others, and career subscales were 24% ($p <
.001$), 19% ($p < .05$), and 28% ($p < .001$), respectively. These results indicate
that performance on the tacit-knowledge measure differentiated groups varying in level of professional advancement in the domain of business
management.

Within-group analyses. Correlations between tacit-knowledge scores and
measures of criterion performance are presented for the business professional group in Table 2.

For business professionals, correlations in the .3 to .5 range were found
between tacit knowledge scores and criterion variables such as salary,
whether the individual's company was on the Fortune 500 list, and years of

schooling beyond high school. No reliable relations were found between tacit-knowledge scores and criterion variables for the business graduate student group. For the undergraduate group, the correlation between total score on the tacit-knowledge measure and performance on a standardized test of verbal reasoning was .16, $p > .05$.

In sum, with the exception of the lack of within-group relations between tacit knowledge and criterion performance for business graduate students, the results of experiment 2 replicated the results of experiment 1 in a new domain.

Experiment 3. Cross-validation study for business managers

Experiment 3 was carried out to cross-validate the results of experiment 2 on a group of bank managers for whom detailed performance evaluations were available.

Method

The subjects in this experiment were twenty-nine managers from offices of a local bank. The tacit-knowledge measure for business management used in experiment 2 was used without modification in this experiment. Scoring procedures were identical with those of experiment 2. Because the scoring system used in this experiment was that derived from and used in experiment 2, this experiment served to cross-validate the method of quantifying tacit knowledge used in the present experiments.

Results

The patterns and magnitudes of correlations between tacit-knowledge scores and criterion reference measures were similar to those obtained in the previous experiments. Correlations between tacit-knowledge scores and criterion measures of performance are presented for the bank manager group in Table 3.

Tacit-knowledge scores of bank managers were related to (1) average percentage of merit salary increase, (2) performance ratings for the area of "amount of new business generated for the bank," and (3) performance ratings for the area of "implementation of bank policy."

Summary: experiments 1, 2, and 3

The results of three experiments in two real-world settings support the relationship between tacit knowledge and competence in professional and man-

Table 3. *Correlation coefficients between tacit-knowledge scores and criterion reference measures for bank managers.*

| | Tacit-knowledge scores | | | |
Criterion reference measures	Total score	Self	Managing others	Career
Percentage salary increase[a]	.48[e]	.38[e]	.04	.33
Average performance rating[b]	.37	.15	.02	.31
Personnel management[c]	.29	.13	.15	.17
Generating new business[c]	.56[e]	.21	− .13	.53[e]
Following bank policy[d]	.39	.20	.01	.32

[a] $n = 22$.   [c] $n = 13$.   [e] $p < .05$.
[b] $n = 20$.   [d] $n = 21$.

agerial pursuits. Three major results were found across the three experiments:

1. Expert–novice differences in tacit knowledge about managing self, others, and career were found for groups of individuals whose members differed in amounts of experience and formal training. The set of response item ratings made to the work-related situations differentiated at better than chance levels among (1) psychology faculty, psychology graduate students, and undergraduates, in experiment 1; and (2) business professionals, business graduate students, and undergraduates, in experiment 2. However, because of the "between-group" item discrimination procedures used to score performance on the tacit-knowledge scale, it was not possible to compare performance levels directly across the various groups.

2. Differences in tacit knowledge were consequential for career performance in professional and managerial career pursuits. In each experiment, relationships were found between tacit-knowledge scores and a variety of performance measures in the domains of academic psychology and business management. The relations between overall tacit knowledge and career performance were surprisingly strong. Many of the obtained correlations between tacit-knowledge scores and various criterion measures of career performance were significant, and some were of a magnitude (.3–.5) of one and one-half to two and one-half times that of correlations typically found between performance on ability tests and job performance. Values of r^2 (proportion of variance accounted for) were from two to five times larger. However, convincing evidence of relationships between individual categories of tacit knowledge and career perfomance was available only for one of the three proposed categories of tacit knowledge, that of tacit knowledge about managing career.

3. Tacit knowledge was not related to verbal intelligence as measured by a standard verbal reasoning test. At least this was found for groups of participants who have previously been selected on the basis of academic or general aptitude, as is true for most people in managerial and professional careers.

We now turn our attention to some recent developments in our thinking about tacit knowledge.

Revised framework: categories and orientations of tacit knowledge

On the basis of the results just presented and further theorizing, the tacit-knowledge framework has recently been revised and extended in the senior author's dissertation, for which the junior author was dissertation advisor (Wagner, 1986). A new method for quantifying tacit knowledge has been developed, in which a person's performance is compared with a prototype derived from the responses of an expert group. A brief sketch of the revised framework will be provided and results from two experiments recently carried out to evaluate the revised framework will be presented.

The revised tacit-knowledge framework consists of three categories of tacit knowledge (managing self, tasks, and others) and two orientations (local and global). Orientation as used here refers to one's perspective in a given work-related situation.

Three categories of tacit knowledge

Three different categories of tacit knowledge were distinguished from each other.

Tacit knowledge about *managing self* refers to knowledge about self-motivational and self-organizational aspects of performance in work-related situations. An example of tacit knowledge about managing self is knowing how best to overcome the problem of procrastination.

Tacit knowledge about *managing tasks* refers to knowledge about how to do specific work-related tasks well. An example of tacit knowledge about managing tasks in the domain of academic psychology is knowing the value of beginning a manuscript by telling the reader what major points you plan to make.

Tacit knowledge about *managing others* refers to knowledge about managing one's subordinates and one's interactions with one's peers. An example of tacit knowledge about managing others is knowing how to reward subordinates so as to maximize both productivity and job satisfaction.

Two orientations of tacit knowledge

Two different orientations of tacit knowledge were distinguished from each other: (1) A *local orientation* refers to a focus on the short-term acomplishment of the specific task at hand, with no consideration given to one's reputation, one's career goals, or the "big picture"; and (2) a *global orientation* refers to a focus on one's long-range, career-related goals when making work-related judgments and decisions.

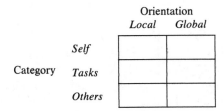

Figure 1. The revised tacit knowledge framework.

The revised tacit-knowledge framework, then, consists of three categories of tacit knowledge – managing self, tasks, and others – which are "crossed" with two orientations – local and global. This revised tacit-knowledge framework is portrayed in Figure 1. We will illustrate each cell in the diagram with a brief example.

Consider the previously mentioned problem of procrastination. Forcing oneself to spend at least ten minutes on a task is a strategy that works for some people – those who find that once they have begun, they will keep working at their task. According to the revised framework, knowledge that this strategy works for oneself is an example of tacit knowledge about managing self with a local orientation. However, if the task at hand were to write up several experiments to submit for possible publication, reminding oneself that getting tenure may hinge on finishing the manuscript soon also may help overcome procrastination. Knowing that this strategy works for you is an example of tacit knowledge about managing self with a global orientation. Such strategies are considered general across tasks, but possibly specific to individuals. Some persons may simply be unable to force themselves to spend even five minutes at a task and, others, reminding themselves that a future decision with important career implications may hinge on their timely completion of the task, may procrastinate even more!

Next, consider the previously mentioned task of how to begin one's manuscript. An example of tacit knowledge about managing tasks with a local orientation is knowing that it helps inform readers in advance about what one plans to say. Knowing where to submit which manuscrripts one has written so as to publicize one's work maximally is an example of tacit knowledge about managing tasks with a global orientation.

Recognizing that the time has come to let an employee go because of inadequate performance is an example of using tacit knowledge about managing others with a local orientation. Knowing that one should not let the employee go even though he or she deserves it because (1) one has terminated more employees than your colleagues, and (2) terminating employees is discouraged by one's company is an example of tacit knowledge about managing others with a global orientation.

Actualities and ideals

The comments of respondents in the Wagner and Sternberg (1985) experiments suggested the need to distinguish between two additional kinds of tacit knowledge: tacit knowledge about competence in the real world, that is, how good a given response alternative *actually is*, given the realities of one's situation; and tacit knowledge about competence in an ideal world, that is, how good a given response should be. Simply stated, the distinction is between what works and what's good or what should work, in some ideal sense. Use of the word "ideal" in the present context refers to a judgment about the quality of some course of action without regard to how practical or impractical it might be in one's actual job situation.

For example, an assistant professor attempting to get tenure in a prestigious department would probably be making a serious mistake by devoting most of her time to perfecting her introductory psychology class lecture (unless, of course, her teaching was so horrendous that she might have to be denied tenure on that basis alone). Given the realities of how tenure decisions are made, such a strategy would be less than optimal. But it is not inconceivable that oustanding introductory psychology classes might attract more and better students to major and go on to graduate school in psychology, thereby yielding a long-term, but perhaps dramatic, payoff to the field. The point is that whereas devoting most of one's time to teaching introductory psychology might well not be the best of strategies even in an ideal world, it is certainly possible that such a strategy would be better in an ideal world than it is in the actual world.

Two experiments were carried out to evaluate the revised framework. As was true for the previous experiments, the domains examined were those of academic psychology and business management. These experiments differed from the ones just presented in several important ways.

First, construction of the tacit-knowledge measures used in the present experiments was constrained by the tacit-knowledge framework: Every work-related situation and response item fit in one of the three categories and in one of the two orientations of tacit knowledge. Second, all response alternatives associated with a work-related situation sampled only one of the three categories and one of the two orientations of tacit knowledge. In other words, the response items associated with different categories of tacit knowledge and orientations were not intermixed within test item. Third, a new method of quantifying tacit knowledge based on deviation from an expert prototype was adopted (see Sternberg, Conway, Ketron, & Bernstein, 1981). Performance was scored in terms of squared deviations from a prototype derived from the mean ratings of an expert group. There were several important benefits associated with this new method of quantifying tacit knowledge: (1) all original items were retained on the final scales, yielding equal numbers of items (and, it was hoped, comparable reliability) across categories and orientations of tacit knowledge, and thus a more stringent test of the tacit-knowledge framework; and (2) direct tests of mean differences in performance across groups of different professional advancement, which were ruled out in Wagner and Sternberg (1985) because of the between-group item discrimination procedures used to construct the final scales.

The combined effect of the procedures was to facilitate more rigorous evaluation of the tacit-knowledge framework, including examination of the interrelations among the different kinds of tacit knowledge, and between the different kinds of tacit knowledge and career performance. These procedures were not possible in the earlier work because of differential reliabilities of the tacit-knowledge subscale scores.

Experiment 4: A prototype of tacit knowledge in academic psychology

Method

There were three groups of subjects, totaling 212 individuals in all, whose members differed in amounts of formal training and experience in the field of academic psychology. The *faculty group* consisted of ninety-one members of the faculty in twenty-six departments of psychology. Included in this group were fifty-one members of eleven departments that were highly rated in terms of the scholarly quality of the departmental faculty (Jones, Lindzey, & Coggeshall, 1982), thirty-nine members of fifteen departments less highly rated in terms of the scholarly quality of departmental faculty, and one person who did not choose to indicate his or her departmental affiliation. The psychology graduate student group consisted of sixty-one graduate students from the same departments sampled to obtain the faculty group. The undergraduate group consisted of sixty Yale undergraduates.

An academic psychology tacit-knowledge measure was constructed to sample tacit knowledge acquired as a result of training and experience in the field of academic psychology. The measure consisted of twelve work-related situations, each of which was associated with from nine to eleven response items. (Several of the work-related situations and response items were adapted from Wagner & Sternberg, 1985). Subjects read a given work-related situation and then rated each response alternative on a 1- to 7-point scale by either its quality (1 = "extremely bad," 4 = "neither good nor bad," and 7 = "extremely good,"), or its importance (1 = "extremely unimportant," 4 = "somewhat important," and 7 = "extremely important,"), depending on the particular response items. Subjects rated both the *actual* and *ideal* quality of each response item.

Of the twelve work-related situations, four were constructed to sample each of the three categories of tacit knowledge (managing self, tasks, and

Table 4. *Descriptive statistics for academic psychology tacit-knowledge scores (prototype method): actual and ideal scales.*

	Actual		Ideal	
	Mean	SD	Mean	SD
Psychology faculty (*N* = 80)				
Total score	215.9	59.1	195.1	56.6
Orientation				
Local	111.6	34.9	105.2	33.6
Global	104.3	31.0	90.1	28.1
Categories				
Self	71.9	23.2	63.1	19.7
Tasks	72.2	28.5	62.6	25.0
Others	71.5	23.3	69.5	22.9
Graduate students (*N* = 61)				
Total score	243.8	55.7	205.7	71.9
Orientation				
Local	123.5	29.2	113.3	46.5
Global	120.3	34.8	92.4	30.3
Categories				
Self	80.0	20.8	69.6	27.0
Tasks	82.4	28.2	67.3	31.1
Others	81.4	24.7	68.8	23.9
Undergraduates (*N* = 60)				
Total score	311.6	75.8	294.7	106.4
Orientation				
Local	157.7	47.0	166.7	65.0
Global	153.9	39.4	128.0	48.2
Categories				
Self	105.1	25.9	91.5	38.7
Tasks	98.2	30.2	95.0	35.7
Others	108.4	35.4	108.2	44.8

others). One-half of the twelve work-related situations were constructed to sample tacit knowledge with a local orientation, the other half to sample tacit knowledge with a global orientation. Thus, each work-related situation was constructed to sample one of three categories of tacit knowledge (managing self, tasks and others) with one of two orientations (local and global).

Results

Between-group analyses. Descriptive statistics for the tacit knowledge scores are presented in Table 4. Note that because the scores reflect deviation from an expert prototype, low scores signify better performance on the tacit-knowledge measure than do high scores.

Reliable differences in performance were found across the faculty, graduate student, and undergraduate groups. A significant decreasing trend was found in scores across groups with increasing levels of experience and training. These expert–novice differences were found (1) for each category of tacit knowledge, (2) for each orientation, and (3) for both the "actual" and the "ideal" ratings. (This conclusion was based on appropriate multivariate analyses of variance with correction of probabilities for follow-up analyses, rather than on multiple F tests.)

Within-group analyses. Correlations between tacit-knowledge scores based on the actual ratings and criterion measures of performance are presented separately for the faculty, graduate student, and undergraduate groups in Table 5.

For the actual scale, overall tacit knowledge was strongly related to research-related criterion measures. Total score, a measure of overall deviation from the expert prototype, was negatively correlated with criterion measures, including (1) rated scholarly quality of faculty in a person's department, (2) extent to which a person's work is cited in the literature, (3) quantity of publications, (4) percentage of time spent in research, and (5) number of conference papers presented. Total score was positively correlated with percentage of time spent in teaching and percentage of time spent in administrative duties, meaning that worse performance on the tacit-knowledge measure was associated with these patterns of behavior. Total score did not vary reliably as a linear function of academic rank, with means of 218.2, 224.1, and 204.3, for the assistant professor, associate professor, and full professor groups, respectively, yielding an $F(1, 74) = 0.59, p > .05$.

This pattern of strong negative correlations between measures of deviation from the expert prototype and research-related criterion measures, and positive correlations with several non-research-related criteria, was found for both local and global orientation, as well as for the tacit-knowledge categories of managing self, tasks, and others.

Results for the graduate student group were similar. Total deviation score was strongly and negatively related to criterion measures such as (1) rated scholarly quality of the student's department, (2) number of publications, (3) number of conference papers presented, (4) percentage of time spent in research, and (5) number of research projects completed. Correlations between total score with percentage of time spent in teaching and number of years of graduate study were not reliably different from zero, although most were in the appropriate direction.

For undergraduates, verbal aptitude was related to tacit knowledge about managing others, but not to tacit knowledge about managing self or tasks. The small but reliable correlations between verbal reasoning and both total score and score for the local orientation subscale derived from the strong

Table 5. *Correlation coefficients between tacit-knowledge scores (prototype method) and criterion performance in academic psychology: actual scale.*

| | | | Tacit-knowledge scores | | | | |
| | | | Orientation | | Categories | | |
Criterion reference measures	N	Total	Local	Global	Self	Tasks	Others
Faculty							
Rated scholarly quality of department faculty	77	$-.48^d$	$-.42^d$	$-.44^d$	$-.39^d$	$-.45^d$	$-.29^c$
No. of citations	59	$-.44^d$	$-.44^d$	$-.32^c$	$-.29^b$	$-.39^d$	$-.38^d$
No. of publications	59	$-.28^b$	$-.31^c$	$-.18$	$-.28^b$	$-.28^b$	$-.09$
Percentage of time spent							
Teaching	79	$.26^b$	$.24^b$	$.23^b$	$.29^c$	$.21^b$	$.11$
Research	79	$-.41^d$	$-.42^d$	$-.31^c$	$-.26^b$	$-.36^d$	$-.33^c$
Administrative duties	79	$.19^b$	$.22^b$	$.14$	$.15$	$.19^b$	$.13$
No. of papers presented	80	$-.21^b$	$-.24^b$	$-.14$	$-.15$	$-.19^b$	$-.15$
Age	80	$.22^a$	$.11$	$.29^a$	$.20$	$.16$	$.11$
Graduate students							
Rated scholarly quality of program faculty	61	$-.46^d$	$-.27^b$	$-.52^d$	$-.28^b$	$-.39^d$	$-.37^c$
No. of publications	59	$-.25^b$	$-.18$	$-.24^b$	$-.26^b$	$-.20$	$-.10$
No. of papers presented	80	$-.12$	$-.11$	$-.11$	$-.20$	$-.04$	$-.07$
Percentage of time spent							
Teaching	79	$.15$	$.20$	$.07$	$.19$	$-.07$	$.26^b$
Research	79	$-.48^d$	$-.43^d$	$-.41^d$	$-.35^c$	$-.30^c$	$-.46^d$
No. of research projects completed	61	$-.24^b$	$-.30^c$	$-.14$	$-.13$	$-.19$	$-.22^b$
No. of years completed	61	$-.07$	$.02$	$-.14$	$-.15$	$.07$	$-.12$
Undergraduates							
Verbal reasoning	60	$-.30^b$	$-.26^b$	$-.25$	$-.19$	$-.09$	$-.42^d$

^{a} $p < .05$, 2-tailed test. ^{c} $p < .01$.
^{b} $p < .05$. ^{d} $p < .001$.

relationship between tacit knowledge about managing others and verbal aptitude.

The pattern of results for the ideal scale was highly similar to that found for the actual scale. Total score did not vary reliably as a linear function of academic rank, with means of 212.9, 191.4, and 191.5, for the assistant professor, associate professor, and full professor groups, respectively, yielding an $F(1, 74)$ of 1.14, $p > .05$. One difference in results from that obtained for the actual scale concerned relations between tacit knowledge scores and verbal ability. In contrast to results obtained for the actual scale, performance of undergraduates on the ideal scale was more broadly related to performance on the reference measure of verbal reasoning ($r = .4$).

One final aspect of experiment 4 was to replicate directly the Wagner and Sternberg (1985) results and procedures. Performance on the tacit knowledge measure was re-evaluated using the Wagner and Sternberg item-discrimination procedures and scoring procedures. The results were highly similar to those reported for the prototype method, which both replicates the earlier work and demonstrates that the findings are not specific to one method of quantifying tacit knowledge.

Experiment 5: A prototype of tacit knowledge in business management

Method

There were three groups of subjects, totaling 149 individuals in all, whose members differed in amounts of formal training and experience in the field of business management. The business professional group consisted of sixty-four managers from a nationwide sample of thirty-one companies. Included in this group were twenty-six managers whose companies rank among the top forty on the Fortune 500 list, thirty-three managers whose companies are not among those on the Fotune 500 list, and five persons who did not choose to reveal their company affiliation. The business graduate student group consisted of twenty-five graduate students from seven business schools, including fifteen persons whose schools are among the highest ranked in the nation and ten individuals whose schools are not among the higher-ranked business schools. The undergraduate group consisted of the same sixty Yale undergraduates used in experiment 4. The undergraduates were given the tacit-knowledge measures for both business management and academic psychology in counterbalanced order.

The tacit-knowledge measure constructed was theoretically isomorphic to that used in experiment 4, but the content was appropriate for the domain of business management.

Between-group analyses. The pattern of results was identical to that found in experiment 4. A significant decreasing trend was noted in scores across the business professional, business graduate student, and undergraduate groups. Expert–novice differences were found (1) for each category of tacit knowledge, (2) for each orientation, and (3) for both the actual and ideal ratings.

Within-group analyses. Correlations between tacit-knowledge scores on the actual scale and criterion reference measures for the business professional, business graduate student, and undergraduate student groups are presented in Table 6.

Table 6. *Correlation coefficients between tacit-knowledge scores (prototype method) and criterion performance in business management: actual scale.*

| | | Tacit-knowledge scores | | | | |
| | | Orientation | | Categories | | |
Criterion reference measures	Total	Local	Global	Self	Tasks	Others
Business professionals						
Salary[c]	−.21	−.23	−.15	−.12	−.32[a]	−.11
Years management experience[d]	−.30[a]	−.40[b]	−.14	−.16	−.35[b]	−.18
Level of company[e]	−.05	.04	−.12	−.01	−.12	.01
Years schooling (post-H.S.)[f]	−.01	.03	−.05	.05	.02	−.10
Age[d]	−.12	−.28[a]	.05	−.12	−.13	−.05
Business graduate students[g]						
Level of school	−.34[a]	−.25	−.32	−.44[a]	−.36[a]	−.06
Years completed	.09	.02	.13	−.04	.13	.11
Years management experience	−.14	.06	−.27	−.06	−.05	−.27
Employed at present	−.24	−.02	−.35[a]	−.16	−.20	−.25
Undergraduates[h]						
Verbal reasoning	−.12	−.13	−.10	−.14	−.12	−.07

[a] $p < .05$.   [c] $n = 48$.   [e] $n = 46$.   [g] $n = 25$.
[b] $p < .01$.   [d] $n = 49$.   [f] $n = 50$.   [h] $n = 60$.

For the business professional group, overall tacit knowledge was related to years of management experience. Reliable relations were found between years of management experience and (1) tacit knowledge with a local orientation, and (2) tacit knowledge about managing tasks. No reliable relationships were found between tacit knowledge and level of company or years of schooling beyond high school. Salary was related reliably to tacit knowledge about managing tasks. Age was related reliably to tacit knowledge with a local orientation. For the business graduate student group, overall tacit knowledge was related to level of school. This relation was reliable for the categories of managing self and managing tasks. Years of schooling completed and years of management experience were unrelated to tacit knowledge. Whether or not the student was currently employed was related reliably to tacit knowledge with a global orientation. For the undergraduates, tacit knowledge was unrelated to verbal reasoning ability.

The pattern of correlations between tacit knowledge on the ideal scale and criterion reference measures was similar to that of the actual scale, although in general the relations appeared to be somewhat stronger for the ideal scale. For example, the correlations for business professionals between scores on the ideal scale and salary were in the range of .3 to .4. The point–biserial correlations for business graduate students between whether an individual's school was highly ranked or not and scores on the ideal scale were in the range of .4 to .5.

Generality of tacit knowledge. Members of the undergraduate group were given both the psychology and business tacit knowledge measures in counterbalanced order. Because there were no order effects on either the covariance structures or the mean scores for the tacit-knowledge questionnaires, it was possible to examine the generality of tacit knowledge, at least for the undergraduate group, by examining between-scale correlations. The correlations obtained between scores on the psychology and business tacit knowledge measures were moderate in size: total score ($r = .58, p < .001$); local orientation ($r = .54, p < .001$); global orientation ($r = .50, p <.001$); managing self ($r = .52, p < .001$); managing tasks ($r = .47, p < .001$); and managing others ($r = .52, p < .001$).

An attempt to replicate directly the Wagner and Sternberg (1985) results in the domain of business management proved partially, but not completely, successful.

First, expert–novice differences in tacit knowledge were found for groups of individuals whose members differed in amounts of training and experience in the field of business management. The set of item ratings differentiated at better than chance levels among the business professional, business graduate student, and undergraduate student groups. These expert–novice differences were found for (1) each category of tacit knowledge (managing self, tasks, and others); (2) each orientation (local and global); and (3) knowledge regarding competence in the actual business world (actual scale) and an ideal business world (ideal scale).

Second, results relating differences in tacit knowledge quantified using the Wagner and Sternberg (1985) item-discrimination procedures to differences in measures of career performance were mixed. Reliable relations were found between some, but not all, of the tacit-knowledge scores and measures of career performance for the business professional and business graduate student groups.

Third, with the exception of tacit knowledge about managing others in an ideal academic world, tacit knowledge did not appear to be related to verbal intelligence for members of the undergraduate group.

General discussion

The results of experiments 4 and 5 largely supported the value of the tacit-knowledge framework and measurement operations. Consider three sources of evidence.

First, it was possible to construct two theoretically isomorphic measures of tacit knowledge for two quite different domains, which indicates that the framework has considerable breadth. Further, the construction of the tacit-knowledge measures was completely constrained to the framework. In previous work (Wagner & Sternberg, 1985), instruments designed to sample tacit knowledge included items whose fit to the framework was Procrustean at best.

Second, in two experiments carried out in two domains, expert-novice differences were found for groups whose members differed in level of professional advancement. In contrast to the item-discrimination based scoring procedure of Wagner and Sternberg, the prototype method of quantifying tacit knowledge used in the present experiments permitted direct tests of between-group differences in tacit knowledge. The results supported the validity of the tacit-knowledge framework and measurement procedures. In both experiments, performance on the tacit-knowledge measures increased reliably across groups as a function of level of professional advancement. Follow-up analyses indicated that these expert–novice differences were present for each of the categories of tacit knowledge (managing self, tasks, and others) and for each of the orientations (local and global) proposed by the framework.

Third, in two experiments carried out in two domains, within-group differences in tacit knowledge were related to criterion measures of performance appropriate for each of the groups, with some correlations being of a magnitude (.3–.5) of one and one-half to two and one-half times that of correlations typically found between performance on ability tests and job performance. Values of r^2 (proportion of variance accounted for) were two to five times larger. For example, for psychology faculty, performance on the tacit-knowledge measure was related favorably to a variety of research-related criteria including, among others, number of citations, number of publications, rated scholarly quality of departmental faculty, and percentage of time spent in research. Performance on the tacit-knowledge measure was related unfavorably to non-research-related criteria such as percentage of the time spent in teaching and percentage of time spent performing administrative duties. For graduate students in psychology, performance on the tacit-knowledge measure was related favorably to research-related criteria such as number of publications. For business professionals, tacit knowledge was related favorably to performance criteria such as salary and years of management experience. For business graduate students, tacit knowledge was related favorably to whether their business school was one of the top rated in the country.

A pattern of results in the present experiments, consistent with a pattern observed in the earlier experiments, was that performance on the tacit-knowledge measure for academic psychology was more highly related to criterion performance than was performance on the tacit-knowledge measure for business management. The source of this pattern of results cannot be determined with certainty, but it may indicate that the tacit knowledge measure for academic psychology (a domain with which we have first-hand knowledge) is better constructed than the tacit-knowledge measure for business management (a domain with which we have no first-hand knowledge). Alternatively, the domain of business management may be a more differentiated domain than that of academic psychology, with needed competencies being somewhat specific to one's position, one's company, one's type of business, or all of these.

The earlier experiments found that tacit knowledge about "what works," that is, judgments about how good the response alternatives *actually* are, given the realities of the world as one knows it, is related to criterion measures of performance. The latter experiments showed that tacit knowledge about "what's good," that is, judgments about how good the response alternatives *ideally* are, also is related to criterion measures of performance. In addition, there was a strong relationship between individual differences in tacit knowledge about what works and tacit knowledge about what's good, with roughly one-third to one-half of the variance in total score on the actual and ideal scale being shared in the two experiments. Finding (1) relationships between criterion performance and performance on the ideal as well as the actual scale, and (2) strong relationships between individual differences on the actual and ideal scales, suggests that the kind of tacit knowledge acquired with experience in professional domains includes an awareness of both the quality and the practicality of alternative courses of action.

The results of comparing the performance of undergraduates across the academic psychology and business management tacit-knowledge measures yielded correlations between performance on the two measures in the .5 to .6 range. These results suggest that at least some tacit knowledge is general to the class of professions represented by the domains of academic psychology and business management. However, there is a need to replicate these results with those for persons who have more experience in the domains of study than do undergraduates.

Some concerns might understandably be raised about our principles and procedures for measuring tacit knowledge. Consider two such concerns:

1. *Can individuals "fake good" on our tacit knowledge measures?* One concern is whether respondents might have given "socially desirable" responses rather than responses that characterize what they actually would do. Because our focus has been on tacit knowledge about what to do rather than on actual performance, it is impossible for a person to "fake good" on the task, in any meaningful sense. Knowing what a good response is, regardless of whether it is something an individual actually would do, is precisely what we set out to measure! However, a limitation of our approach is that we do not measure a person's actual ability to do what he or she knows should be done. The strength of the correlations between tacit knowledge scores and criterion measures of performance does at least suggest that those who know what to do are capable of doing it.

2. *Whose values should be used to evaluate criterion performance?* Determining how good a person is as an academic psychologist or business manager is not easily done. For an academic psychologist, how much weight should be given to the quality of a person's research, to the quality of a person's teaching, or to some other aspect of the profession? Should the weighting be the same, regardless of the nature of one's position? Our strategy in handling this very difficult problem was, to the extent we were able, not to impose our own values, but to adopt the values of the field, as determined by selecting items on the basis of their ability to differentiate statistically among groups of individuals whose members differ in amounts of experience and formal training in a given domain. Not all individuals may share the dominant values of the field, however, and there certainly may be identifiable subgroups within a field that share different values. The strategy of adopting the dominant values of a field obviously limits the generalizability of the results to those who share these values, or who are judged by them.

Some conclusions about the nature of tacit knowledge in practically intelligent behavior

The results of five experiments carried out in two domains suggest five conclusions about tacit knowledge in practically intelligent behavior.

1. *Experts in real-world domains differ from novices in, among other things, having acquired domain-related tacit knowledge.* Furthermore, such tacit knowledge can be measured by presenting people with scenarios describing work-related situations and asking them to rate the quality of alternative responses. This conclusion is based on finding, in each of five experiments across two real-world domains, reliable expert–novice differences in tacit knowledge.
2. *Differences in tacit knowledge are related to differences in domain-related performance.* In each of five experiments, performance on measures of tacit knowledge was related to a wide variety of criterion measures of career performance. Many of these relationships were much stronger than those typically found between IQ or employment tests and job performance.
3. *Tacit knowledge of the sort examined in the present experiments is more than simple "careerism."* That is, knowing how to promote one's career appears to be just one aspect of the type of tacit knowledge acquired over the course of experience in such fields as academic psychology and business management. In experiments 4 and 5, differences in level of professional advancement were associated with differences in tacit knowledge useful in the short-term accomplishment of a wide variety of tasks, as well as in tacit knowledge useful in attaining one's long-range career-related objectives. These differences extended across work-related situations that required skill at managing oneself, tasks, and others, and they encompassed judgments about the quality (i.e., how good is this?) as well as the practicality (i.e., will this work?) of responses to various work-related situations.
4. *Acquisition of tacit knowledge does not appear to be closely related to performance on traditional measures of verbal intelligence.* In the four experiments for which scores on a standardized test of verbal intelligence were available, tacit-knowledge scores were related more to criterion measures of job performance than to scores on the standardized test of verbal intelligence and in most cases, the correlations between tacit-knowledge scores and verbal intelligence test scores were not reliably different from 0.

There are at least two possible explanations for the relative lack of relations between tacit-knowledge scores and verbal intelligence as measured by a standard psychometric test. First, people in professional pursuits represent a somewhat restricted range of verbal ability, having been selected on the basis of academic aptitude, either directly through selection based on test performance, or indirectly through selection based on school performance. Restricting the range of a variable tends to reduce its correlation with any other variable. Second, we agree with Neisser's (1976) contention that traditional IQ tests are better measures of intelligence of the "academic" rather than the "practical" variety.

5. *Individual differences in tacit knowledge appear to be general rather than specific in nature.* The magnitude of the intercorrelations among the categories and orientations of tacit knowledge and the highly similar patterns of relationships with a variety of external criterion measures observed in experiments 4 and 5 suggest that the categories and orientations proposed by the revised framework represent facets of a generalized fund of knowledge and skill, rather than specific psychological factors in their own right.

Similar findings of positive intercorrelations for academic tasks led Charles Spearman (1904, 1927), and later many others, to propose g, a construct representing a general ability that is measured to greater or lesser degree by most academic tasks. Might there be a comparable general ability for practical tasks?

Evidence in favor of a general ability for practical tasks from experiments 4 and 5 includes (1) the strong intercorrelations (.5–.8) among scales that were constructed to measure distinct categories and orientations of tacit knowledge; (2) the strong correlations (.7–.8) between performance on the actual and ideal scales; (3) the moderately strong correlation (.6) found for members of the undergraduate group between performance on the tacit-knowledge measures for academic psychology and business management; and (4) the highly similar patterns of correlations with external criterion measures for the tacit-knowledge measures for academic psychology and business management, for the actual and ideal scales, and for each of the subscales corresponding to the categories and orientations of tacit knowledge.

It is important to note, however, that the tacit-knowledge measures were limited in scope to two professional domains. The evidence in support of a general ability for practical tasks will be more convincing when generalized individual differences similar to those found in the two career pursuits examined here are found for other career pursuits, and for competence in out-of-school situations for younger people, such as school-aged children.

Although the fact that a generalized ability accounts for much of the variance in performance on academic type tasks might lead to the expectation of a similar finding for more practical tasks, it is important to note that the evidence for a general ability in the domain of social intelligence or competence has been mixed, at best (see, e.g., Ford & Tisak, 1983; Keating, 1978; Sternberg & Smith, 1985; Walker & Foley, 1973). The issue of a general ability in the domain of social intelligence is difficult to resolve because there are few valid instruments for measuring social intelligence. It will remain difficult to determine the generality of knowledge and skills in practical and social domains until instruments are available for these domains that share the psychometric sophistication of instruments used to assess performance in the academic domain.

A number of important issues must remain unresolved for the present. The first concerns the acquisition of tacit knowledge: How is tacit knowledge acquired over the course of experience in a real-world setting? Can its acquisition be accelerated? If so, for which kinds of tacit knowledge is accelerated acquisition possible, and what methods (e.g., direct teaching, a mentor model) enable accelerated acquisition? (See Sternberg & Caruso, 1985, for a discussion of possible methods of acquisition for practical knowledge.) The second issue concerns how tacit knowledge is actually used in performance in real-world settings, and whether some uses are consequential to performance, whereas others are not. For example, tacit knowledge might be primarily useful for deciding what one should be doing and a strategy for doing it, or its primary benefit might be in better "real-time" task performance itself, or perhaps some mixture of both. (See, e.g., Scribner, 1982, and Chapter 6, this volume, for recent examples of inquiries into cognitive tasks requiring the use of practical knowledge.)

The results of the work described indicate that the first step in understanding competence in real-world settings has been taken. Instruments derived from a theory of tacit knowledge show marked changes in performance levels as a function of level of expertise of the examinees, something that few, if any, traditional measures of mental abilities have shown. The second step – understanding the nature of tacit knowledge and its role in competent performance in real-world settings – has yet to be completed, although tentative progress has been made. Should progress continue, it is not unreasonable to expect that attempts to take the third step – acceleration of the acquisition of tacit knowledge and ultimately the attainment of competence – are in the foreseeable future.

Appendix A

Additional academic psychology work-related situations and a sample of response items

2. A new student has come to you for advice on how to be successful in graduate school. You don't know the person well enough to speak in anything but generalities. Rate the following statements of advice about working strategies by how important the strategies are to being successful as an academic psychologist:

____a.   regularly set priorities that reflect the importance of your tasks

____b.   keep in mind who will ultimately see or use the results of your labor when setting task priorities

:

____f.   do your best on everything you do

3.   You have been asked to serve on an admissions committee that will select students to be admitted to your psychology department. You have been thinking about what leads to later success in the field of psychology. Rate the importance of the following graduate student characteristics to later success in the field of academic psychology:

____a.   scholastic aptitude
____b.   ability to set priorities according to the importance of your tasks

:

____t.   knowledge of the relevant literature

4.   Rate each of the following according to their importance in leading to a successful career in academic psychology:

____a.   doing research that should be of interest to a diverse audience
____b.   avoiding criticism of others' theories without proposing alternatives

:

____i.   making a point to meet the prominent people in your area of the field

5.   A number of factors enter into the establishment of a good reputation among scholars in one's field. Consider the following factors and rate their importance:

____a.   teaching ability
____b.   writing ability

:

____p.   visibility (i.e., well known to the scientific community)

6.   Rate the importance of the following in deciding to which journal to submit an article for possible publication:

____a.   reputation of the journal to the field of psychology as a whole
____b.   reputation of the journal in your field of expertise

:

____k.   breadth of journal readership

7.   Rate the following strategies of working according to how important you believe them to be to doing well at the day-to-day work of an academic psychologist:

____a.   always have a variety of projects in progress; many "irons in the fire"
____b.   think in terms of tasks accomplished rather than hours spent working

:

____p.   find a way to make a game of quickly completing mundane tasks

8.   Rate the importance of the following considerations when selecting a research project:

____a.   the project is in an area with which I am familiar
____b.   the project will enable me to demonstrate my research talents

:

____k.   the paradigm is an established one

9.   An undergraduate student has asked for your advice in deciding to which graduate programs in psychology to apply. Consider the following dimensions for rating the overall quality of a graduate program in psychology and rate their importance:

____a.   breadth of the program
____b.   prestige of the faculty
       ⋮
____p.   quality of the graduate students in the department

10.   You have been asked to edit a new journal. You would like to have guidelines available to those who will review submitted manuscripts for the purpose of deciding whether to accept or reject them. Rate the importance of the following criteria for evaluating the quality of research articles:

____a.   fit of findings into some psychological theory
____b.   an abundance of tables and figures
       ⋮
____n.   how interesting the article is

11.   In many areas of psychology, three or four researchers are acknowledged to do extraordinary work. Rate the following characteristics by how important you believe them to be for the success of the best people in academic psychology:

____a.   unusually creative
____b.   highly self-motivated
       ⋮
____n.   socially adept

12.   Rate the following motivations in terms of their importance as incentives for pursuing a career in academic psychology:

____a.   I enjoy the subject matter of the areas I am pursuing
____b.   I enjoy doing research in my chosen areas
       ⋮
____l.   I like the near-total security of a tenured position

Appendix B

Additional business management work-related situations and a sample of response items

2.   A subordinate has come to you for advice on how to be more successful in the company. You don't know the person well enough to speak in anything but generalities. Rate the following pieces of advice by their importance to succeeding in the company:

____a.   regularly set priorities that reflect the importance of your tasks
____b.   try always to work at only what you are in the mood to do
       ⋮
____i.   do routine tasks early in the day so as to be sure you get them done

3.   Your company has sent you to a university to recruit and interview potential trainees for management positions. You have been considering characteristics of students that are important to later success in business. Rate the importance of the following student characteristics by the extent to which they lead to later success in business:

____a.   aptitude or intelligence
____b.   ability to set priorities according to the importance of your tasks
       ⋮
____t.   knowledge of the relevant areas of business (finance, production, etc.)

4. During one of your recruiting interviews at the university, a student asks you about things one can do to increase one's chances for success in business. Rate each of the following things one might do by its importance to a successful career in business:

____ a.   avoid criticism of others unless you have a better alternative to propose
____ b.   defend your views in the face of all criticism
       ⋮
____m.   take advantage of opportunities to get favorable attention from the local media

5. A number of factors enter into the establishment of a good reputation in a company as a manager. Consider the following factors and rate their importance:

____a.   critical thinking ability
____b.   visibility (i.e., well known throughout the company)
       ⋮
____q.   a keen sense of what superiors can be sold on

6. Rate the following characteristics of a job by their importance in leading to a successful career in a given company:

____a.   the job will bring your work to the attention of higher-level management personnel
____b.   the job is considered an important one by company personnel
       ⋮
____k.   You have your family's support on issues such as travel and working late or on weekends

7. Rate the following strategies of working according to how important you believe them to be for doing well at the day-to-day work of a business manager:

____a.   always have a variety of projects in progress; many "irons in the fire"
____b.   think in terms of tasks accomplished rather than hours spent working
       ⋮
____p.   find a way to make a game of quickly completing mundane tasks

8. You have just been promoted to head of an important department in the company. The previous head had been transferred to an equivalent position in a less important department. Your understanding of the reason for the move is that the performance of the department as a whole was mediocre. There were not any glaring deficiencies, just a perception of the department as so-so rather than as very good. Your charge was to shape up the department. Results are expected quickly. Rate the following pieces of advice colleagues have given you by their importance to succeeding in your new position:

____a.   always delegate to the most junior person who can be trusted with the task
____b.   give your superiors frequent progress reports
       ⋮
____ t.   promote open communication

9. You are looking for several new projects to tackle. You have a list of possible projects and desire to pick the best two or three among them. Rate the importance of the following considerations when selecting projects:

____a.   doing the project should prove to be fun
____b.   the project will enable me to demonstrate my talents
       ⋮
____ j.   the project will require working directly with several senior executives

10.   Rate the following kinds of experience by their importance to becoming a good manager:

_____a.   having completed an M.B.A. degree from a strong business department
_____b.   working for several years as a salesperson
    ⋮
_____i.   a strong background in the technology used by your company's production facilities

11.   In business, as in other fields, there are often several people who are acknowledged to do extraordinary work. Rate the following characteristics by how important you believe them to be for the success of these people:

_____a.   unusually creative
_____b.   highly self-motivated
    ⋮
_____p.   having virtually no outside interests – their job is their life

12.   Rate the following motivations in terms of their importance as incentives for pursuing a career in management:

_____a.   I think my abilities are a good match to this career choice
_____b.   I enjoy working with people
    ⋮
_____k.   I want to lead others but not be led by others

References

Atkinson, J. W. (Ed.). (1958). *Motives in fantasy, action, and society.* Princeton, NJ: Van Nostrand.

Bray, D. W. (1982). The Assessment Center and the study of lives. *American Psychologist, 37,* 180–189.

Charlesworth, W. R. (1976). Intelligence as adaptation: An ethological approach. In L. Resnick (Ed.), *The nature of intelligence* (pp. 147–168). Hillsdale, NJ: Erlbaum.

Chase, W. G., & Simon, H. A. (1973). Perception in chess. *Cognitive Psychology, 4,* 55–81.

Chi, M. T. H.,. Feltovich, P., & Glaser, R. (1981). Categorization and representation of physics problems by experts and novices. *Cognitive Science, 5,* 121–152.

de Groot, A. (1966). Perception and memory versus thought: Some old ideas and recent findings. In B. Kleinmuntz (Ed.), *Problem solving.* New York: Wiley.

Flanagan, J. C. (1954). The critical incident technique. *Psychological Bulletin, 51,* 327–358.

Ford, M. E., & Tisak, M. S. (1983). A further search for social intelligence. *Journal of Educational Psychology, 75,* 197–206.

Frederiksen, N. (1966). Validation of a simulation technique. *Organizational Behavior and Human Performance, 1,* 87–109.

Frederiksen, N., Saunders, D. R., & Wand, B. (1957). The in-basket test. *Psychological Monographs, 71* (9, Whole No. 438).

Ghiselli, E. (1966). *The validity of occupational aptitude tests.* New York: Wiley.

Helmreich, R. L., Spence, J. T., Beane, W. E., Lucker, G. W., & Matthews, K. A. (1980). Making it in academic psychology: Demographic and personality correlates of attainment. *Journal of Personality and Social Psychology, 39,* 896–908.

Jeffries, R., Turner, A. T., Polson, P. G., & Atwood, M. E. (1981). Processes involved in designing software. In J. Anderson (Ed.), *Cognitive skills and their acquisition* (pp. 255–283). Hillsdale, NJ: Erlbaum.

Jones, L. V., Lindzey, G., & Coggeshall, T. E. (Eds.) (1982). *An assessment of research-*

doctorate programs in the United States: Social and behavioral sciences. Washington, DC: National Academy Press.

Keating, D. P. (1978). A search for social intelligence. *Journal of Educational Psychology, 70,* 218–223.

McClelland, D. C. (1973). Testing for competence rather than for "intelligence." *American Psychologist, 38,* 1–14.

McClelland, D. C. (1976). *A guide to job competency assessment*. Boston: McBer.

McClelland, D. C., Atkinson, J. W., Clark, R. A., & Lowell, E. L. (1953). *The achievement motive*. New York: Appleton-Century-Crofts.

McKeithen, K. B., Reitman, J. S., Rueter, H. H., & Hirtle, S. (1981). Knowledge organization and skilled differences in computer programmers. *Cognitive Psychology, 13,* 307–325.

Neisser, U. (1976). General, academic, and artificial intelligence. In. L. Resnick (Ed.), *The nature of intelligence* (pp. 135–144). Hillsdale, NJ: Erlbaum.

Oxford English Dictionary. (1933). Oxford: Clarendon Press.

Roose, K. D., & Andersen, C. J. (1970). *A rating of graduate programs*. Washington, DC: American Council on Education.

Schmidt, F. L., & Hunter, J. E. (1977). Development of a general solution to the problem of validity generalization. *Journal of Applied Psychology, 62,* 529–540.

Schmidt, F. L., & Hunter, J. E. (1981). Employment testing: Old theories and new research findings. *American Psychologist, 36,* 1128–1137.

Scribner, S. (1982). Studying working intelligence. In Rogoff, B., & Lave, J. (Eds.), *Everyday cognition: Its development and social context*. Cambridge, MA: Harvard University Press.

Simon, D. P., & Simon, H. A. (1978). Individual differences in solving physics problems. In R. Siegler (Ed.), *Children's thinking: What develops?* (pp. 325–343). Hillsdale, NJ: Erlbaum.

Soloway, E., Ehrlich, K., Bonar, J., & Greenspan, J. (1982). What do novices know about programming? In B. Shneiderman & A. Badre (Eds.), *Directions in human–computer interactions* (pp. 27–54). Norwood, NJ: Ablex.

Spearman, C. (1904). "General Intelligence": Objectively determined and measured. *American Journal of Psychology, 15,* 201–292.

Spearman, C. (1927). *The abilities of man*. New York: Macmillan.

Sternberg, R. J., & Caruso, D. (1985). Practical modes of knowing. In E. Eisner (Ed.), *Learning the ways of knowing* (pp. 133–158). Chicago: University of Chicago Press.

Sternberg, R. J., Conway, B. E., Ketron, J. L., & Bernstein, M. (1981). People's conceptions of intelligence. *Journal of Personality and Social Psychology, 41,* 37–55.

Sternberg, R. J., & Smith, C. (1985). Social intelligence and decoding skills in nonverbal communication. *Social Cognition, 3,* 168–192.

Thorton, G. C., & Byham, W. C. (1982). *Assessment centers and managerial performance*. New York: Academic.

Wagner, R. K. (1986). *Tacit knowledge in everyday intelligent behavior*. Manuscript submitted for publication.

Wagner, R. K., & Sternberg, R. J. (1985). Practical intelligence in real-world pursuits: The role of tacit knowledge. *Journal of Personality and Social Psychology, 48,* 436–458.

Walker, R. E., & Foley, J. M. (1973). Social intelligence: Its history and measurement. *Psychological Reports, 33,* 839–864.

Wigdor, A. K., & Garner, W. R. (Eds.). (1982). *Ability testing: Uses, consequences, and controversies*. Washington, DC: National Academy Press.

5   Toward a broader conception of human intelligence

Norman Frederiksen

Aptitude or intelligence tests are typically printed tests containing items (usually in multiple-choice form) intended to measure such abilities as vocabulary, reading comprehension, arithmetic computation, inductive and other kinds of reasoning, spatial ability, and ideational fluency. In general, the skills are academic – they are those that are taught in school or are thought to predict success in school. The test items are well structured (Simon, 1973, 1978) in the sense that they are clearly stated, all the information needed is available (or, presumably, in the head of the examinee), and there is only one correct or "best" answer. The score is the number correct. Fluency or divergent-production tests (Guilford, 1967) are exceptions; by their nature they cannot be put in multiple-choice form, there is no single correct answer, and the score is usually the number, or number of unusual, responses given. Presumably they measure abilities involved in making broad searches of long-term memory in order to find words or ideas that satisfy some requirement.

"Practical" intelligence, on the other hand, may be thought of as what is reflected in one's cognitive responses to almost everything outside the school – the problem situations that arise naturally as one goes about his daily life. Such problems are often ill structured: they do not provide all the information needed to solve the problem, there are no definite criteria for determining when the problem is solved, they are often complex, and there is no "legal move generator" for finding all the possibilities at each step (Simon, 1978). The settings and the tasks generally do not resemble those encountered in school, and the problems rarely appear in multiple-choice form. Responses are not necessarily motivated by a need to get the right answer, and performance can be described in terms of many dimensions other than the number of correct answers. In view of such contrasts, it is not surprising that aptitude and intelligence tests often fail to predict very successfully evaluations of success in anything except educational accomplishment (Ghiselli, 1966; McClelland, 1973; Thorndike & Hagen, 1959). However, it should be stated that meta-analyses of studies involving clerical, industrial, and military jobs have shown that validity coefficients are substantially increased when corrections are made for sampling error, error of measurement, and restriction in range of ability (Hunter, 1980; Hunter & Hunter, 1983; Hunter, Schmidt, & Jackson, 1982; Schmidt & Hunter, 1977).

Our knowledge of the structure of abilities outside the realm of paper-and-pencil tests is extremely limited, probably because data collection by means of controlled observations of real-life behavior, or simulations of real-life behavior, is too inefficient and too costly for widespread use. But the economy and efficiency of conventional testing was achieved at the cost of introducing bias in regard to what is measured (Frederiksen, 1984).

There are two major ways in which paper-and-pencil tests fail to represent the whole domain of intelligent behavior. One has to do with the nature of the tests themselves. Most real-life problems cannot be posed in the form of conventional test items without seriously distorting the problem; even a "what would you do?" question about how to deal with, say, disruptive behavior in a classroom cannot possibly capture the complexity and immediacy of the real-life situation, even if posed in free-response form. Furthermore, the use of the multiple-choice format tends to limit the kinds of items that are written (Levine, McGuire, & Nattress, 1970) and in some instances the nature of the cognitive processes involved in taking a test (Ward, Frederiksen, & Carlson, 1980). And the restriction that scores be based only on the number of right answers limits the amount and kind of information that can be obtained.

The other major limitation of conventional testing is that there is very little variation in the situations in which data are collected. Tests are typically administered in academic settings where the expectation is that one should strive for as many "right" answers as possible, following specified time limits and procedures. Thus, the variety of options characteristic of real-life settings is not available. In real life one might decide to settle for an approximation or a probability that satisfies his or her needs rather than strive for an optimal solution; or one might postpone the problem until he or she can talk to someone or get a book off the shelf. And the strict, monitored setting might cause anxiety and interfere with one's efforts to solve a problem, in contrast with a relaxed or playful situation (Wallach & Kogan, 1965). As Lave, Murtaugh, and de la Roche (1984) put it, in life outside the school problems may present themselves in circumstances that encourage nonstandard methods of coping, in contexts that do not suggest a method of solution, or in guises that may not be recognized as problems.

Lave, Murtaugh, and de la Roche (1984) provide an example of a study of practical intelligence. They observed shoppers doing arithmetic in a supermarket. An observer with a tape recorder accompanied each shopper in the process of locating the items written on her shopping list and putting them in her cart. The shopper was encouraged to talk about her purchases and the reasons for her choices as she made her way along the shelves. Size, brand, and price were typically considered, in that order. Arithmetic problems arose particularly when comparing prices for packages that differed in size or weight. The shopper usually started with a probable or expected conclusion, which was to be verified. Numerical simplifications (e.g., changing ounces to pounds) characterized the calculations of most shoppers; but when a problem got too complicated, computations tended to be abandoned in favor of making a decision on some other basis. However, the actions based on the arithmetic of twenty-five shoppers was found to be virtually errorless, even though the hard problems were not completed. Shoppers were apparently able to select the "best buy" without an exact numerical solution. [See also a paper by Scribner (1984) and various papers by Tversky and Kahneman (e.g., 1973, 1974, 1983).]

Barker (1968) wrote that "It was one of the great achievements of psychology that

> . . . methods have been devised for identifying and measuring individual human constants. . . . It is unfortunate that these accomplishments have not been accompanied by progress in studying naturally occurring human behavior variation. But there is an incompatibility here: to achieve stable behavior measurements stable conditions must be imposed upon the person, and the same conditions must be reimposed each time the measurement is repeated. This method provides measures of individual constancies (under designated conditions), but it eliminates individual variations (under different conditions), and it destroys the naturally occurring contexts of behavior. (pp. 5–6)

This criticism applies particularly to psychometric psychologists; the standardization of testing conditions has eliminated the "naturally occurring contexts" of behavior and thus limited our conception of intelligence.

If it had been possible for psychologists to include in their test batteries measures of cognitive performance such as that exhibited by shoppers in supermarkets, and if the behaviors had been described more completely than in terms of number of correct answers, our conception of the structure of intellect might be quite different. We would no doubt have a larger and more varied set of cognitive abilities, and we perhaps would have been forced to pay more attention to the characteristics of the situations in which the observations were made. In building tests we have not followed the example of Bartlett (1932), who remarked in the Preface to his *Remembering* that

> I determined to try to retain the advantages of an experimental method . . . and also to keep my study as realistic as possible. I therefore built up, or selected, material which I hoped would prove interesting in itself, and would be of the type which every individual deals with constantly in his daily activities. . . . The book certainly claims to study that important group of mental processes which are usually included under the term 'remembering' in a realistic manner, just as they actually occur in any normal individual, both within and without the social group. (pp. v–vi)

Various methods in addition to intelligence tests have been used to assess intelligent behavior, including soliciting opinions (e.g., by means of questionnaires and rating scales), measuring knowledge (which is what most achievement tests do), eliciting "related" behavior (e.g., giving editing or rewriting exercises in lieu of tests that require writing), eliciting "what I would do" behavior (e.g., presenting a verbal description of a problem situation and asking the subject to write what he or she would do), eliciting lifelike behavior (e.g., interviewing simulated patients or using a flight simulator), and observing real-life behavior (Frederiksen, 1962a). Only the last two methods are based on direct observation of the behavior we wish to assess. Given a choice of the two, I would choose to elicit life-like behavior, using realistic simulations. My reasons have to do primarily with standardization and efficiency; one might have to wait a long time for opportunities to observe the desired real-life behavior under circumstances that make possible accurate interpretations of the data recorded. The simulation method seems particularly apt when we wish to understand intelligence as it operates in the worlds of home, work, and play as well as in the world of the classroom.

In the following sections I shall describe several attempts I have been involved in to develop tests that get closer to intelligent behaviors as they occur in real-life settings than do typical tests of intelligence. The use of such methods might lead to a more complete understanding of human intelligence and also to the role of situational factors in influencing responses to problems. More specifically, I shall attempt to show (1) that it is feasible to use simulations of real-life problems to elicit behaviors like those that occur outside the testing room, and to devise scoring methods that yield scores with adequate psychometric properties; (2) that different cognitive skills may be required when multiple-choice rather than free-response formats are used; (3) that many of the categories of intelligent behavior elicited by simulations do not match, and do not correlate appreciably with, the abilities measured by conventional tests of intelligence, while an appreciable proportion of the variance in scores may be accounted for by personal characteristics other than intelligence; and (4) that variation in the situations that elicit intelligent behaviors may significantly influence that performance.

Hypothetico-deductive thinking

The simulations to be described in this section permit the subject more freedom in responding than do typical psychological tests, but much less freedom than other simulations which will be described later. Here we shall be concerned with tests that constrain the subject to write hypotheses and, in some instances, to indicate what new information he or she needs in order to test the hypotheses or suggest others. These constraints may not be as limiting as one might suppose, however, since the problems posed are of the kind where hypothetico-deductive methods are commonly employed, as in scientific and medical problem solving. Such methods are also frequently used by laymen in attempting to deal with ill-structured problems, such as why the lights went out or why the blossoms fell off of the Christmas cactus.

Formulating hypotheses tests

I first became involved in studies involving hypothesis formulation when I was challenged to construct a "data-interpretation" test that really required interpretation, not just ability to read complicated graphs and tables (Frederiksen, 1959). The result was a test I called formulating hypotheses (FH), in which each problem consisted of a graph or table obtained from an actual investigation and a statement of a major finding based on that study. The task of the subject was to write "short statements of hypotheses (possible explanations) which you think might account for, or help to account for, the finding." One problem, for example, included a table showing by month the number of workers involved in work stoppages resulting from labor management disputes. The finding was that the number of workers involved in strikes was low in winter and high in summer. Some of the hypotheses suggested by subjects were, for example, that workers did not mind strikes in the summer because they could go fishing, that workers did not want to strike in the winter because fuel bills were high or because they didn't want to spoil the holidays for their families, and that union contracts typically terminated in the summer.

The development of a scoring system was an inductive procedure that first required making for each problem a classification of the ideas produced by a sample of subjects and then writing a generalized statement, or definition, of each category. A panel of judges then evaluated the categories in the light of the information available, and a quality value was assigned to each category. The coders' task, then, was merely to match each of a subject's responses to one of the hypothesis categories. Scores could then be generated by computer to represent, for example, the number of hypotheses suggested, their average quality, and the number of ideas that were of high quality.

Such items were used in two studies (Frederiksen & Evans, 1974; Klein, Frederiksen, & Evans, 1969) in which the effects of feedback on subsequent performance were investigated. In the first study, an experimental group of sixty-seven male college students was given feedback, after responding to each FH problem, in the form of a list of "acceptable" hypotheses – a list that was considerably longer than that typically written. A control group was given no feedback. The second experiment used the same problems in testing 395 college students (half male and half female). On completion of each problem, quantity feedback was given to one experimental group, quality feedback was given to the other, and a control group received no feedback. Quality feedback consisted of the six or seven hypothesis categories considered to be the best, each carefully worded. Reliabilities of the scores (based on tests of five or six problems) ranged from .60 to .95. Analyses of variance and covariance showed that the treatment effects were highly significant in both experiments, with performance changing in the direction of the feedback model. In view of the brevity of the treatments, the improvement was thought to be attributable to changes in subjective standards as to how good is "good enough," rather than to changes in ability.

From the standpoint of our concern about the nature of intelligence, the relationships of FH scores to other measures are of more interest. The first study showed that the number of hypotheses written was significantly related to both verbal ability (as measured by the SAT-V) and test anxiety, and that both relationships were *negative*. A significant interaction involving SAT-V and test anxiety was also found. In the case of test anxiety, the relationship was actually curvilinear, the middle level of anxiety being associated with the fewest hypotheses; a similar result was found in the second study, but only for male subjects. It appears from the data that the most productive subjects were in general those who were least able to evaluate their own ideas and least likely to be embarrassed by stupid answers. For whatever reason, in this experimental situation the relationships involving verbal ability are not what one would expect when tests are administered under ordinary testing procedures.

Tests of scientific thinking

In response to the Graduate Record Examinations Board's interest in research on creativity, four new tests, modelled after the FH test, were developed. These tests simulated several kinds of tasks required of research scientists, using problems that were thought to be of appropriate difficulty for senior psychology majors who planned to go to graduate school (Frederiksen & Ward, 1978). The four tests were named (1) Formulating Hypotheses (FH), (2) Evaluating Proposals (EP), (3) Solving Methodological Problems (SMP), and (4) Measuring Constructs (MC). Collectively they were called Tests of Scientific Thinking (TST). All made use of formats and scoring procedures similar to those just described. In the case of FH, a brief description of a psychological experiment or field study (based on an actual published study), a graph or table depicting the results, and a statement of the major finding were presented. The task was to write hypotheses that might explain or help to explain the finding. For EP the subject was asked to suppose that he or she was teaching a senior course in experimental design and methodology and had asked the students to write brief research proposals; the EP problems were the proposals supposedly submitted by the students. The task was to write critical comments regarding the methodology and design of the proposed study or the theoretical position taken. Each SMP problem was a brief statement of a methodological problem encountered by a student in planning a research study; the task was to write suggested solutions to the problem. And the MC test consisted of names or definitions of psychological constructs (e.g., bigotry, leadership, conservatism), and the task was to suggest methods for eliciting relevant behaviors that could be observed and measured without resorting to ratings or self-reports. Thus, the tests posed problems of a kind that are rarely encountered in an undergraduate program and that more closely resemble situations that might be encountered by research psychologists.

The time generally reserved for pretesting new items in a regular administration of the GRE Advanced Psychology Test was used to administer the four tests of scientific thinking, using an item-sampling procedure (Lord & Novick, 1968, Chapter 11). About 3,500 candidates for admission to graduate school participated, although of course no one person took all of the tests or even all of the problems from a single test.

The development of a scoring system again involved identifying categories of responses and assigning a quality value to each category. Six scores were generated that reflected in various ways the quality and number of ideas and the number that were both unusual and of high quality. Lower-bound estimates of the reliabilities of six-problem tests, calculated under the assumptions of the item-sampling procedure, ranged from .05 to .77; upper-bound estimates ranged from .21 to .88. The MC test yielded the most reliable scores, presumably because it elicited more responses, while SMP was least reliable. The least reliable of the six scores was the one based on the number of responses that were both unusual and of high quality.

The intercorrelations of scores for the four tests were factored, and three factors were identified. The first factor was clearly a number-score factor, with high loadings for the total number and the number of unusual responses. The other two factors were both quality factors, but they were differentiated by test, with one factor generally reflecting quality scores for FH and MC and the other quality scores for EP and SMP. The latter two tests tended to elicit responses concerned with technical matters of design and data analysis, while the other two allowed a wider range of responses.

The extension loadings of GRE scores on the TST factors were then computed. For factor II, a quality factor, the GRE-V and Q scores had the highest loadings (.39 and .44, respectively), and for factor III, the more technical quality factor, the loading for the Advanced Psychology Test was the highest (.47), presumably because factor III reflected applications of statistical and other technical knowledge to a greater extent than did factor II. But the loadings on factor I, the number score, were quite low; the loadings were .27, .22, and .23 for the GRE-V and Q scores and the Advanced Psychology

Test. Thus, the number of ideas generated was not well predicted by the conventional aptitude tests or even by a test of knowledge of psychology.

In April of the following year, when the subjects who had entered graduate school were near the completion of the first year of graduate study, the students were asked by mail to fill out a questionnaire dealing with such accomplishments as doing independent research, carrying out research as a collaborator, being an author or coauthor of a scientific paper, teaching, or designing laboratory equipment. Other items dealt with academic success, areas of interest, and self-appraisals of various skills. Correlations with GRE and TST were generally low but, because of a large N, standard errors were small.

It was found that the GRE tests were superior to the tests of scientific thinking for predicting the students' self-reported grades in graduate school, while the TST scores based on number and unusualness of ideas were more highly correlated with reported accomplishments. For example, the correlations of the GRE V, Q, and achievement tests were, respectively, .01, .02, and .13 with the total number of accomplishments reported, and the comparable correlations for the TST number scores (based on all four of the tests combined) were .18 for the number of responses, .24 for the number of unusual responses, and .16 for a less reliable score based on the number of unusual responses that were also of high quality. If one takes into account the crudity of the self-reported accomplishment measures and the fact that the students were enrolled in a wide variety of departments, the significance of these differences becomes more impressive.

Thus the scores reflecting number and number of unusual ideas appear to be related to real-life criteria that may have something to do with scientific productivity, while the GRE tests were related to grades, the conventional criteria for validating such tests. TST number scores have relatively low correlations with GRE aptitude tests, and they appear to be superior to the conventional tests in predicting scientific accomplishments during the first year of graduate school.

Another study (Ward, Frederiksen, & Carlson, 1980), also supported by the GRE Board, was concerned with the construct validity of just one of the tests of scientific thinking, the Formulating Hypotheses test. The idea was to investigate by correlational methods the cognitive processes involved in the formulation of hypotheses, using a battery of cognitive ability tests to measure skills that we thought would be involved in taking FH. On the basis of our theorizing about the cognitive processes involved in formulating hypotheses, we selected several tests to define each of five factors: verbal ability, reasoning, cognitive flexibility, ideational and expressional fluency, and knowledge of psychology.

We also wished to compare tests in free-response and multiple-choice formats with respect to the cognitive abilities involved in taking the FH test. We therefore converted some of our problems into multiple-choice form by replacing the answer spaces for each problem with a list of nine hypotheses, which were chosen to be representative of those we had obtained in free-response form with respect to quality and frequency of occurrence. Instructions were revised to allow selections from these lists; however, instead of choosing the one "best" answer, the subject could mark any of the options he or she thought might account for the finding. In all other respects, the multiple-choice problems were counterparts of the free-response form.

Six problems were in free response and eight in multiple-choice form. All the tests were administered to 174 paid volunteers from 11 colleges and universities; all were seniors majoring in psychology who claimed an intention to go to graduate school. Reliabilities of scores from the free-response problems ranged from .35 (for number of hypotheses that were both unusual and of high quality) to .79 (for mean quality). For the multiple-choice problems, reliabilities ranged from .32 to .90 (for number of hypotheses chosen).

Extension loadings of the FH scores on the cognitive factors were computed. It was found that the loadings of the quality scores from free-response and multiple-choice versions of FH had roughly similar loadings on verbal, reasoning, cognitive flexibility, and knowledge-of-psychology factors. The major difference had to do with the two fluency factors, where the loadings of the number and the number of unusual responses were substantial for the free-response form (ranging from .36 to .44) but almost zero for the multiple-choice version (ranging from .01 to .07). The major difference between the two formats with regard to skills involved is that fluency, or ability to search one's memory store for relevant words and ideas, is required when answers have to be conceived of and put into words by the subject rather than chosen from a list.

Several studies (Traub & Fisher, 1977; Vernon, 1962; Ward, 1982) have shown, by methods involving correlation, factor analyses, and multitrait–multimethod comparisons, that conventional multiple-choice tests measure essentially the same abilities as do free-response tests constructed by substituting answer spaces for the multiple-choice options. But if we begin with an existing free-response test, designed to measure complex problem-solving skills, and convert it to multiple-choice form, the result is different. Translation of FH problems into multiple-choice format nearly eliminated the need for making broad searches of long-term memory for relevant ideas.

Medical and nonmedical problem solving

The generation of hypotheses is, of course, only a small part of the process of problem solving. Elstein, Shulman, and Sprafka (1978) described the process of medical problem solving, for example, in terms of hypothesis generation and verification. According to their account, data are collected for the purpose of generating hypotheses, and additional data are obtained for the purpose of testing the old hypotheses and, if necesssary, generating new ones. Diagnostic accuracy is related to the thoroughness and accuracy of data collection. Errors may be due to faulty hypothesis formulation, misinterpretation, mistakes in combining evidence, or failure to collect the appropriate information. Thus, diagnostic problems are solved by a hypothetico-deductive method.

In the study here described, an attempt was made to extend the FH-test format by requiring subjects not only to generate an initial set of hypotheses but also to go through several cycles of requesting new information for evaluating the hypotheses and suggesting new ones, and revising the list in the light of the information obtained. The study was done in collaboration with the National Board of Medical Examiners and a consortium of medical schools (Frederiksen, Ward, Case, Carlson, & Samph, 1981). It was motivated by concern among medical educators that whereas conventional selection tests predict grades in the first years of medical school fairly well – the years when students are learning the scientific background for clinical practice – correlations with grades in the years of clinical training are near zero. From the present point of view, however, we shall be interested in how the protocols can be scored to reflect the cognitive processes involved in hypothesis generation and testing, the correlates of those scores, and how the processes differ when the problems are presented in multiple-choice rather than free-response form.

A set of medical problems was intended to provide criterion measures against which to evaluate the validity of an experimental nonmedical test that might be used in the selection process. In both sets the problems employed a format similar to that of the patient-management problems (PMP's) that are used in some medical schools for assessment and for training (McGuire & Babbott, 1967), except that a free-response as well as the multiple-choice format was used.

A medical problem began with a brief description of a situation (e.g., "you are a resident covering the out-patient clinic of a 400-bed hospital") and a small amount of information about a new patient ("a 45-year-old man has been brought into the clinic complaining of chest pains"). The subject first indicated the diagnostic possibilities that came to mind; then he or she was asked to decide what to do next (e.g., do a physical examination, interview the patient, or order X-rays). Then information compatible with that choice was presented, and the next task was to indicate what diagnostic possibilities were then being considered. (Thus the medical tests, unlike the nonmedical tests, allowed branching.) After several such cycles, the student decided on a diagnosis.

In the case of the patient complaining of chest pains, for example, thirteen hypothesis categories were identified in the protocols, including myocardial infarction/angina, pulmonary embolism, aneurysm, upper respiratory infection, myocarditis, and diabetes mellitus. Since nomenclature is well developed in medicine, it was possible to list almost all the possible terms that might be used to refer to each category, which made the coding process much easier than for the nonmedical problems. For example, any of the following terms were coded as myocarditis: myocarditis, Dressler's syndrome, pericardial tamponade, and pericarditis.

The nonmedical problem-solving tests necessarily differed from the medical tests in one important way. High proficiency in diagnostic problem solving requires a background of knowledge and experience that has been rehearsed so often that retrieval of needed information may be triggered automatically by the perception of a pattern of diagnostic findings (Anderson, 1982). Some degree of such proficiency may be expected even for fourth-year students. But there is no such common background of readily accessed information and expertise that can be assumed for candidates for admission to medical school (other than a general knowledge of biology). The prototype selection tests were therefore likely to differ in that they required a broad search of the memory store for relevant information rather than fast automatic retrieval based on much practice in the area of expertise.

The areas of knowledge involved in the nonmedical tests – education, sociology, ecology, and public health – were familiar in a very general way to any candidate for admission to medical school. The problems were posed in the incomplete form in which real-life problems are likely to occur, and the task was to write hypotheses that came to mind as possible solutions. Then the subject was given an opportunity to request new items of information, after which additional information was provided. The student then revised his or her list of hypotheses, and continued through a half-dozen cycles of requesting and receiving information and adding, retaining or discarding hypotheses until he or she was asked to write a solution to the problem.

One nonmedical problem, for example, required students to try to discover why certain trees in the middle of a hemlock hedge were dying. The hypotheses written by students could be classified into a number of major classes of hypotheses (e.g., soil, water, chemicals, insects, weather, animals) and subclasses (e.g., acid soil, too much water, used acid fertilizer, borers, hot dry weather, deer). A quality value for each category was determined on the basis of judgments made by a panel of judges in the light of the information available to the student at the time the response was written.

Other problems were concerned with why there were relatively fewer old people in Iron City than in the state as a whole, why there had been a decline in the crab population in a small inland bay, whether the police chief's request for additions to the force was justified, and why the absence rate was higher in the Central District than in other districts of a certain school system.

The problem-solving tests, like FH, were scored to yield information about quality, number, and unusualness of the ideas written (or chosen from a list). Additional scores were devised to throw light on some of the cognitive processes involved, such as the number of ideas that presumably were directly suggested by the items of information provided, the number presumably requiring a step of inference, and the number that must have come from a search of long-term memory since they had no apparent relation to any information provided. Still other scores were based on the number of hypotheses that were appropriately (or inappropriately) dropped, retained, or added as new information was acquired. Reliabilities of scores were lower than for the tests previously described, no doubt because the scores were based on only three problems.

A battery of cognitive tests similar to that used in the construct-validity study of FH was administered, and scores from the Medical College Admissions Test and the National Board examinations were obtained from files. The intercorrelations of all these measures were factored; the six factors obtained were called Reasoning, Verbal Comprehension, Medical Knowledge (based primarily on the National Board Examinations), Ideational Fluency, Cognitive Flexibility, and Science Knowledge. Extension loadings on these factors were obtained for all the scores obtained from the medical and nonmedical tests, including both free-response and multiple-choice forms.

First let us consider the loadings on the cognitive factors for the free-response form of the nonmedical test. A score called number of ideas was found to load on Reasoning and on Ideational Fluency factors, primarily the latter (the loadings were .19 and .33, respectively). When only the number of *good* ideas was considered, the loadings were higher (.25 and .36). Mean scores and extension loadings suggested that the three methods of searching for ideas were indeed used; for example, for a score called the number of ideas directly suggested (by information provided in the problem), the loadings on Reasoning and Fluency were both relatively low, while for number of ideas indirectly suggested (those that required a step of inference), the loading for reasoning increased. There were few appreciable loadings on Verbal Comprehension, and none on Medical Knowledge, Cognitive Flexibility, or Science Knowledge.

In the case of the multiple-choice version of the nonmedical test, the loadings were much lower, ranging from − .20 to .21, with only a slight tendency for loadings of scores on Ideational Fluency to be highest; fluency loadings ranged from .07 to 21. Thus the test when put into multiple-choice format is much less demanding of the skills represented in our cognitive test battery. One might suppose that reasoning would be involved in evaluating the options, but its median loading was only .02. It was suggested that the ability required for the multiple-choice form involves making narrow directed searches of long-term memory in search of information that matches each option, rather than the broad search that is required by the free-response form.

A similar comparison involving the medical test is simpler to describe. For the free-response form, the most important factor was clearly Medical Knowledge. The availability of a body of relevant knowledge whose retrieval has been rehearsed makes much less necessary the broad-search strategy identified with Ideational Fluency. The loadings on Reasoning were moderate; but the role of reasoning was greater for scores based on the latter part of the problem, when more information was available (the loadings for early middle, and late parts of the problem-solving are $-.12$, $.23$, and $.29$, respectively). The role of medical knowledge was even greater for the multiple-choice version, where the loading was .42 for a score comparable to the number of good ideas.

Once again, we find that for free-response problems, problem-solving procedures are different; in the absence of a store of knowledge specifically relevant to a problem area, or with lack of practice in relating the body of information to a kind of problem, one must more and more rely on ability to search broadly the long-term memory store for appropriate ideas.

Interviewing behavior

The task here described permitted a much wider variety of behaviors than those described so far. The subjects were the same medical students used in the study just described. In addition to all the problem-solving and test-taking activities, each of the students spent the greater part of a day interviewing five simulated patients and five simulated clients whose problems were nonmedical (Frederiksen, Carlson, & Ward, 1984; Ward, Carlson, Case, Frederiksen, & Samph, 1982). Interviews were conducted in a simulated clinic complete with a receptionist, a waiting room, and rooms for six interviewers. Students were instructed to conduct the interviews just as they would in a genuine medical setting. Interviews lasted up to 20 minutes and were recorded on audio tape for subsequent coding. Each simulated patient had been assigned a medical history and a set of complaints and symptoms based on an actual case, and was trained to give appropriate information when asked and to display affect as appropriate. Each client was similarly assigned a counseling problem, one that did not require medical knowledge (e.g., whether or not to attend medical school).

A coding sheet was developed that provided space for recording which of 33 categories of interview behavior occurred in each thirty-second interval. The categories were concerned with the doctor's performance in greeting the patient or client and putting him or her at ease, eliciting information, giving information and advice, recognizing and dealing with affect, and providing support. Because of wide variations in frequency of occurrence, reliabilities of the category scores also varied widely, from zero to as high as .85. At the end of each interview the coder made overall ratings concerned with the organization of the interview, the warmth of the interviewer, and the interviewer's control of the interview; reliabilities of the ratings ranged from .27 to .61, with ratings of warmth being the most reliable. Other information available from the problem-solving study included the aptitude and achievement test scores that had been used by the medical schools in admission and assessment of the students, the scores from the battery of cognitive-ability tests, scores based on the medical and nonmedical problems, and variables drawn from letters written by deans in support of applications for residency appointments.

The relationships between the measures based on interview behavior and those just listed were examined by correlational and factor-analytic methods. Little evidence of significant relationships was found. The most notable relationship was a negative one; there was some evidence that those students who had the greatest knowledge of science were rated *poorest* with regard to warmth in interviewing. No significant correlations were found with measures based on problem-solving performance, with deans'-letter variables, or with cognitive test scores.

A number of previous studies have reported substantial relationships between "social intelligence" and cognitive abilities, particularly verbal abilities (e.g., Ford, 1979; Keating, 1978). But our results differed, perhaps because the measures of social behavior were based on performance of subjects interacting with live interviewees, not on verbal representations of social situations. Individual differences in interviewing behavior appear to be quite independent of measures of academic intelligence.

In-basket tests

The simulations to be considered next, like interviewing, provide a good deal of freedom. The subject is introduced to a simulated organization which he or she is to serve as an administrator. Information about the organization is provided to the subject in realistic form, and the subject is asked to deal with the problems posed by the material that has collected in his or her in-basket. The tasks may be solved in whatever way the subject chooses, including putting a document in the wastebasket. Three major studies involving quite different kinds of organizations and subjects will be described. We shall be especially interested in inquiring about the influence of the situation and the subject's personal characteristics on administrative performance.

Air Force in-basket test

Not long after World War II, I was asked to direct a project that had to do with developing methods for evaluating instruction at the Command and Staff School (CSS) of the Air University. The students were mainly Air Force majors and lieutenant colonels who had been selected for training to prepare them for greater responsibilities.

In talking with Air Force officers about their duties, it was noted that inevitably there were two baskets on each desk marked "in" and "out" and that a large proportion of the work an officer did alone (as opposed to interpersonal situations) seemed to center on the contents of the IN basket. These observations led to the idea of an in-basket test for realistically presenting problems typical of those one might expect to encounter in his or her assignments (Frederiksen, Saunders, & Wand, 1957).

The result was a simulation of a "Pine City Air Force Base" which housed the 71st Composite Wing. A considerable body of information about the wing and its mission was assembled, in order to make it reasonable for subjects to take action on a majority of the problems, and thus avoid the criticism that the only sensible answer to a problem is "it depends." The contents of the in-basket itself were modeled after problems that Air Force officers had actually encountered. Pencils, memo pads, buck slips, paper clips, and other items were provided to facilitate responding to the items. Each subject was instructed to read his mail and take appropriate action as though he were actually on the job; he could, for example, write memoranda, letters, or directives for others; write notes or reminders to himself; call staff meetings; give instructions to subordinates, or change their duty assignments.

The in-basket items were targeted at the specific problem-solving skills that had been identified by the CSS staff (Findley, Frederiksen, & Saunders, 1954), such as ability to use standard operating procedure (SOP) effectively, to evaluate data, to be flexible, and to demonstrate foresight in management procedures. It turned out that the statements of the course objectives provided too limited a basis for describing the in-basket responses for the CSS students (Frederiksen, Saunders & Wand, 1957); but the experience gained in developing the Air Force in-basket test encouraged us to try again in a situation that permitted us to discover from the protocols what the major categories of performance might be, rather than trying to measure a preselected set of behaviors.

Bureau of business in-basket

The next in-basket was developed as the prototype of an instrument for possible use in the selection and placement of government administrators. It was based on an organization we called the Bureau of Business (BB) (modeled roughly after the Chamber of Commerce), an organization that did not require that its officers possess a body of highly specialized knowledge (Frederiksen, 1962b). Each subject assumed the role of the newly hired Executive Officer. He was given appropriate information about the BB for preliminary study and later reference, as well as pencils, writing pads, memo forms, and so on. The in-basket contained the material that had presumably collected in his predecessor's in-basket – letters, memos, and notes of incoming phone calls. The subject was instructed not to play a role but to be himself, not to say what he would do but to do it. Some examples of BB in-basket items: a letter from a filling station proprietor asking about the advantages of membership in the Bureau; a letter, prepared by a subordinate for signature, which confirmed arrangements for a speaker at a forthcoming meeting; a memorandum from a subordinate asking for advice about how to handle an attached letter which accused one of the field representatives of some shady practices; and a note about a phone call from a man in Poughkeepsie who asked about some printed programs that were supposed to have been shipped and which were needed for a meeting the next evening.

As a first step in setting up the categories for a scoring procedure, a number of judges were asked to read samples of the in-basket responses written by subjects and to write brief statements of the kinds of variation in behavior that they observed, such as "overly critical," "neat," or "seeks temporary solutions." Several hundred such statements were obtained, which were sorted into sixty-eight categories of behavior. Examples include the following: recognizes good work, socially insensitive, plans to discuss with subordinates, asks supervisors for advice, asks for further information, delays or postpones, makes plans only, takes terminal action, initiates a new organizational structure, delegates completely, and exhibits courtesy to subordinates. A coding sheet listed the 68 categories across the top, and the thirty-six in-basket problem numbers were placed in a column at the left. The coders' task was to read the response to each problem and record a 1 or 0 in each of the 68 columns to indicate whether or not the behavior described by the category was displayed. The column totals indicated the number of times each behavior occurred.

Another method of scoring was based on what specific action was taken in response to each problem. By examining the protocols, a list of up to ten courses of action that had been taken by one or more subjects was prepared for each problem (e.g., referring a letter to the membership officer or asking for more information). Ten columns on the score sheet were reserved for recording the action or actions taken by each subject on each problem. The column totals were of course meaningless, but the grand total of actions taken provided a measure of productivity. We also developed scoring keys based on classifications of the actions, which made it possible to get counts of the actions in each category. Such scores included number of unusual actions, number of actions judged to be imaginative, and the number of actions that involved making changes in the organization. An attempt to obtain a score representing quality of the actions failed because judges did not agree very well as to what were good and poor actions. Reliabilities of the scores were largely a function of the frequency of the behaviors; reliabilities ranged from zero to .87.

The test was administered to 335 subjects, mostly federal government administrators but also including business executives, army officers, and a few business students. A factor analysis of the forty most reliable scores was carried out; their median reliability was .52. Eight oblique factors were identified; they were easily interpreted in terms of meaningful dimensions of administrative performance. The eight factors were named as follows:

Acting in Compliance with Suggestions   Concern with Supervisors
Preparing for Action by Becoming   Informality
   Informed   Directing Subordinates
Concern with Public Relations   Discussing
Procrastination

All eight factors seem to reflect procedural, strategic, or stylistic aspects of problem solving.

A second-order analysis produced two easily interpretable factors. The first, Preparing for Action, was characterized by deferring final decision and action and instead making preparations for action by obtaining relevant information and advice. The second factor was called simply Amount of Work.

Of the total of 208 federal administrators who took the BB in-basket, 115 had complete data on a number of additional variables, including some biographical data, scores on four cognitive tests, the Strong Vocational Interest Blank (SVIB), and the Thurstone Temperament Schedule (TTS). Correlations between these variables and thirty-five selected in-basket scores were computed (Frederiksen, 1966).

The four cognitive tests were called Interpretation of Data, Matrices, Vocabulary, and Reading Comprehension. Of the 140 correlations computed, only nine were significantly different from zero at the 1 percent level, eight of which involved the Vocabulary Test. Vocabulary correlated moderately with imaginativeness ($r = .41$), the number of subordinates involved ($r = .32$), and the number of words written ($r = .30$), to cite the highest coefficients. No doubt the correlations are in part attributable to the fact that the in-basket tasks required considerable reading and writing. Otherwise in-basket performance had little resemblance to the kinds of ability measured by scores on the cognitive ability tests.

Five items of biographical data were available: age, GS (Government Service) level, educational level, whether or not the subject's duties involved supervision, and whether or not he had been chosen for advanced training. The highest r involved GS level, which correlated with giving directions or suggestions ($r = .38$) and the number of subordinates involved ($r = .36$). Experience in high-level administrative positions appeared to be associated with acting through one's subordinates.

The correlations with selected scores from the SVIB suggest that the extent to which one's interests and preferences resemble those in specific occupations may influence his or her performance in an administraive situation. For example, discussions with subordinates were less likely to occur if one's interests were like those of policemen ($r = -.24$) or forest service men ($r = -.34$), but were more likely if interests resembled those of managers ($r = .32$) or life insurance salesmen ($r = .37$). And two of the TTS scales – the active and dominant scales – were associated with many of the in-basket scores, with correlations ranging as high as .42.

The study demonstrates that it is feasible to discover from the protocols a wide variety of problem-solving behaviors, many of which can be reliably measured. Most of these behaviors represent procedural or strategic approaches to problem solving. The results suggest the need to go beyond the cognitive domain and into the domains of interests, personality, and previous history if we are to understand the complex patterns of intelligent behavior that are observable in lifelike, if not real-life, settings.

School principal's in-basket

The most elaborate of our in-basket simulations (Hemphill, Griffiths, & Frederiksen, 1962) involved 232 elementary school principals. The purpose of this study was to learn more about the dimensions of administrative performance, particularly for elementary school principals, and their potential for use in selection and instruction. Each principal spent nearly five consecutive days acting as principal of the hypothetical Jefferson School. The first day and a half were spent learning about the new school and community by simulated visits (using movies and film strips), studying documents (such as personnel records and school census reports), and listening to tape-recorded events (e.g., comments at a PTA meeting and a school board meeting). The simulation was based on a real school that provided material and assistance in developing the orientation materials.

The ideas for in-basket problems came from such sources as university case-study files and interviews with school people. Three in-baskets were prepared, representing situations spaced over an academic year. Some examples of in-basket items: a letter from a college professor requesting use of students in a psychological experiment; a note from a teacher protesting the method of teaching fractions used by a substitute teacher; a set of recommendations from a Committee on Education of the Gifted; a note from the janitor about finding doors unlocked; and an announcement of the availability of free copies of the Constitution from a distilling company.

In addition to taking in-basket tests, principals "visited" the classrooms of probationary teachers (by way of kinescopes) and filled out probationary report forms; listened to taped recordings of conferences and school board meetings, and wrote answers to questions related to the topics discussed; participated in live committee meetings; and prepared and delivered (to a tape recorder) a speech to the PTA. A large number of subjective evaluations of performances were based on these events.

Finally, when the simulation was over, the subjects were given tests of 16 cognitive abilities, four of the National Teacher Examination (NTE) tests, the Strong Vocational Interest Blank, Cattell's 16-Personality Factor Questionnaire, and a biographical questionnaire.

The in-basket scoring procedure was similar to that described earlier. The same list of sixty-eight categories of behavior was used in the scoring, forty of which were selected for use in a factor analysis on the basis of their frequency of occurrence and reliability. Eight oblique factors were identified; their names are as follows:

Exchanging Information	Maintaining Organizational Relationships
Discussing before Acting	Organizing Work
Complying with Suggestions	Responding to Outsiders
Analyzing Situations	Directing the Work of Others

Four of the factors appear to be identical to four found for the Bureau of Business – those involving compliance with suggestions, directing the work of others, concern with public relations, and discussing. Two second-order factors were found, one a bipolar factor that was called Preparation for Decision vs. Taking Final Action, and the other was called Amount of Work. These higher-order factors match very closely the two second-order factors found in the BB in-basket study.

Composite scores, based on those scores with the highest loadings on a factor and low loadings on other factors, were computed for use in investigating the relationships of factors to other variables. The reliabilities of these composites ranged from .70 (for Responding to Outsiders) to .93 (for Directing Others).

Generally speaking, the best measures for predicting in-basket performance turned out to be two NTE scores, one called Administration and Supervision and the other Elementary Education. Their correlations with composite scores representing Exchanging Information, Discussing Before

Acting, and Maintaining Organizational Relationships ranged from .41 to .50. Correlations were even higher for the Imaginativeness score (.65 and .63). At the other extreme, correlations with Complying with Suggestions were very low (.05 and .01). Knowledge of elementary education and school supervision apparently provided the content needed for activities involving communication with others about school problems and for taking imaginative actions.

Of the sixteen cognitive abilities, verbal knowledge, three fluency tests, and inductive reasoning were most closely related to performance, primarily with Exchanging Information. And the verbal and fluency tests were also the best predictors of the Imaginativeness score.

The relationship of measures of in-basket performance to all the measures of interest and personality and all the evaluations of performance (in other tasks and in their real jobs) obviously cannot be discussed in detail here. But a few brief summaries may provide some insight into the nature of the relationships of performance on the simulated job to other variables (see Figure 5, pp. 328–329, of Hemphill, Griffiths, & Frederiksen, 1962).

Preparation for action. Those at the Preparation end of the scale for the second-order factor Preparation for Action vs. Taking Final Action were found to be fluent, facile with symbolic material, good at reasoning, and knowledgeable about school administration, elementary education, science, and the general culture. Their interests were like those of psychologists and lawyers, and they cared about fulfilling the educational needs of students. They were judged to be active and effective in group discussions and likely to suggest new procedures. Their superiors (in their real jobs) made positive evaluations of their work, as did the research staff members and the in-basket coders. The factor scores were unrelated to any of the biographical items.

Amount of work. The other second-order factor was Amount of Work Expended. Those who expended much work were generally of high ability, fluent with words and ideas, and knowledgeable about elementary education, school administration, and cultural and scientific material. But amount of work was unrelated to personality, interest, and value variables. High producers were effective in social interaction, talked a lot, and tried to influence others. Their superiors were only slightly positive in their evaluations, although staff members and in-basket coders were more positive. Performance was unrelated to biographical data.

Organizing work. One of the first-order factors, called Organizing Work, was characterized by scheduling one's work and following preestablished procedures. The composite scores were unrelated to measures of knowledge and ability or to biographical data, but were associated with being easily frustrated, inflexible, shy, insecure, unstable, and tense. Interests were unlike those of school superintendents, administrators, and psychologists. In discussions, the highly organized principals emphasized positive information, but they were judged ineffective. Evaluations by superiors were generally negative, but teachers who served under them in their real jobs regarded them positively from the standpoint of initiating structure.

Responding to outsiders. Another first-order factor was called Responding to Outsiders. Those who were high on this factor were low in cognitive abilities and in knowledge of science, mathematics, school administration, and general culture. They tended to be submissive, shy, naive, stable, and relaxed, and to have interests unlike those of public administrators and lawyers. In situations involving social interaction they tended not to participate and were regarded as ineffective. They tended to be older females with a large amount of teaching experience, and they were regarded somewhat negatively by their superiors and by other staff members.

Knowledge of elementary education and administration is clearly the best predictor of performance in the simulated job, although performance in the simulated job is also influenced by a wide variety of personality, interest, motivational and social factors, and cognitive abilities. Knowledge about elementary school teaching and supervision appears to be useful in suggesting the nature of one's actions and communications, and verbal ability and ideational fluency are the cognitive skills most involved in responding to the school in-basket problems.

We find that a set of in-basket scoring categories are applicable to the behaviors of two quite different administrative situations and different subject groups, suggesting that the categories may be sufficiently general to apply to a variety of situations. In contrast with the BB in-basket study, we find higher correlations with academic ability tests. Correlations are especially high for tests of the relevant professional knowledge, and an important role for interest and personality measures as predictors of performance is again found. But some of the major categories of performance, especially Discussing Before Acting, are essentially unrelated to any of the conventional measures of intelligence.

California Department of Commerce in-basket

One purpose of another in-basket study was to test the feasibility of carrying out experimental research in simulated situations. More specifically, the aim was to investigate experimentally the effects of certain organizational climates on performance and on the structure of the in-basket factors (Frederiksen, Jensen, & Beaton, 1972). The subjects were 260 male executives who were employed by the state of California in a wide variety of administrative positions, ranging from forestry to prison service and from middle managers to heads of departments (appointed by the governor). In the simulation, each subject served as Chief of the "Field Service Division" of the "Department of Commerce." Data were collected during a two-day "Research Institute."

All subjects faced exactly the same in-basket problems, had the same supervisors, colleagues, and subordinates, and (except for experimental variations) worked under the same conditions. The experimental treatments were variations in the climate of the organization. There were two intersecting climate dichotomies: one dichotomy involved two contrasting "administrative" climates, one that encouraged innovation and originality and another that required one to follow rules, regulations, and SOP. The other dichotomy included two "supervisory" climates, one that encouraged a type of supervision in which subordinates were given a good deal of freedom in the way they carried out assignments ("global" supervision) and another that involved monitoring the details of the subordinate's performance ("detailed" supervision). One-half the subjects were randomly assigned to the rules climate and one-half to the innovation climate; similarly, one-half were assigned to the detailed-supervision and one-half to the global-supervision climate. The two dichotomies overlapped, as shown in Figure 1, to form four treatment combinations.

| | | Supervisory Climate | |
		Global	*Detailed*
Administrative Climate	*Innovative*	A	B
	Rules	C	D

Figure 1. Climate combinations.

Cell A, for example, contains subjects who performed under conditions where they were expected to supervise globally and administer innovatively, and Cell D contains subjects expected to use detailed supervision and to follow rules and SOP in their own work. In these cells the climate conditions are *consistent* with regard to amount of freedom allowed. In cells B and C, the climates are *inconsistent* in that freedom is encouraged in one climate and constraints on freedom are implied in the other.

An organizational climate, as we conceived it, is a set of expectations or understandings held in common by most members of an organization as to a kind of uniformity in behavior that is seen as appropriate. The climate conditions were represented in the study by materials included in the background documents given the subjects to study as part of their orientation.

One method of presenting climate conditions, for example, involved annotations and underlining that were added to a set of administrative memoranda
by Mr. Veep. For the rules climate, the annotations called attention to such
things as deadline dates, use of forms, and standard procedures; while for
the innovation climate they called attention to general goals and policies.
Other communications, both direct and subtle, called attention to the desired
kind of behavior. Additional problems (unscored) were included in in-baskets
to reinforce the perception of a climate condition. A questionnaire given at
the end of the last in-basket session indicated that most of the participants
had correctly perceived the climate conditions to which they had been
assigned.

The first principal component resulting from a factor analysis of in-basket
scores for the 260 subjects was clearly a productivity or amount-of-work
factor. Such a factor has appeared as a second-order factor in previous
analyses. In this study we decided to retain it as a primary factor and to set
it orthogonal to all the other factors, which were rotated to oblique simple
structure. This in effect partialed out the effects of productivity from all the
other factors. The names of most of the factors are by now familiar:

Productivity   Defers Judgment and Action
Acts in Compliance with   Interacts with Peers
   Suggestions   Orderly Work
Interacts with Supervisors   Informality
Thoughtful Analysis of Problems   Accepts Administrative
Plans and Discusses   Responsibility

The correlations of in-basket factor scores with measures of cognitive
abilities, personality, and biographical variables tended to be very low. The
highest correlations involved factor scores representing Productivity and
Thoughtful Analysis of Problems. Productivity was best predicted by Ideational Fluency ($r = .22$) and a test called Hidden Patterns ($r = .22$), a
measure of flexibility of closure. And for Thoughtful Analysis the highest
correlations were with Vocabulary ($r = .21$), Hidden Patterns ($r = .19$), and
two biographical variables called dead-end seniority ($r = -.18$) and staff
(as contrasted with line) officer ($r = .18$). The low correlations, as compared
with the school in-basket, may perhaps be attributable to the variability of
the subjects with regard to their background, training, and work experience
and their lack of experience and knowledge about the specific in-basket
setting.

It was found that the consistency of climate conditions significantly influenced the productivity score; productivity was higher when the climate
conditions were consistent (for those in cells A and D rather than B and C).
The effect was most pronounced for cell B; subjects in the inconsistent
innovative-detailed supervision condition accomplished substantially less
work. The row and column effects were small in comparison, but there was

evidence that, for example, those in cell A (innovation with global supervision) were less likely to interact with superiors, and that deferring judgment and action was increased in the rules row and decreased in the innovation row.

The influence of climates on the factor structure of in-basket scores was also investigated. The factor structure was found to be significantly different in each of the three comparisons: innovation vs. rules, global vs. detailed supervision, and consistent vs. inconsistent climates. The factor called Thoughtful Analysis figured most strongly in these comparisons. For example, in both the innovative and global-supervision climates (as contrasted with rules and detailed supervision), Thoughtful Analysis was negatively correlated with Interacts with Superiors and was positively correlated with Interacts with Peers. It appears that climates that provide more freedom of thought and action encourage the more thoughtful subjects to deal directly with their peers – typically heads of other divisions who are the source of many of the problems, while in the more restrictive climates the thoughtful people are more inclined to work through their superiors and the members of their own department.

The research again identifies a number of categories of performance quite unlike those elicited by conventional tests. Most of these categories appear to represent stylistic or strategic approaches to problem solving; they can be measured reliably, and they appear quite consistently for different groups of subjects and different simulated organizations. Hoban (1976) found a similar list of factors in her study of student personnel administrators.

The Department of Commerce study showed that it is feasible to use simulation techniques experimentally in studying the influence of situational variables on performance. Variations in the climate of the organization not only influenced the level of performance in certain categories, but also changed the factor structure of the scores.

Summary

The research described in the preceding sections is summarized here in terms of four topics: (1) the feasibility of using simulations of real-life problems as tests of intelligence, (2) comparisons of multiple-choice and free-response modes of responding, (3) relationships of scores based on simulations to cognitive abilities and to other personal characteristics, and (4) the influence of the situation in which tasks are embedded on levels of performance and on the structure of the performance variables.

Feasibility

It has been shown that it is possible to use simulations of real-life situations as psychological tests. The protocols resulting from such tests can be used to discover inductively the salient attributes of the behaviors elicited and to derive scores reflecting those attributes, scores that have reasonably good psychometric properties. Reliabilities vary widely, depending to a large extent on the frequency of occurrence of the relevant behaviors; but many scores were found to compare favorably in reliability with those from conventional tests. Some of the less reliable scores could no doubt be made more reliable by lengthening the test or otherwise increasing the number of opportunities to display the behavior in question.

The only available approach to validation is that of construct validity; about all that can be said is that correlational relationships with other personal characteristics appear to be generally consistent with reasonable interpretations of the meanings of the scores. When essentially the same in-basket scoring categories were used in simulations of three different organizations, the factor structures were relatively similar, suggesting that the relationships among scores are to some extent generalizable.

The use of simulations as tests makes it possible (although not necessarily efficient or economical) to gather data about intelligent behavior that would be difficult to obtain by other means and that might broaden considerably the psychometric conception of what constitutes human intelligence.

Simulations of course put some constraints on a subject's behavior, although far less than do conventional tests of intelligence. Some constraint is usually necessary in order to improve the likelihood of eliciting the desired kinds of behavior, to make the data more interpretable and the scores more reliable, and to achieve some degree of efficiency and economy in data collection. The amount of constraint imposed might vary with the purpose of the investigator: for exploratory work, a great deal of freedom might be desirable; while for work in areas where we already have a good understanding of the phenomenon under study it may be better to narrow the range of possible behaviors in order to achieve better experimental control.

Influence of test format

When simulations of problem-solving situations that called for free responses were converted to a form that allowed subjects to choose responses from lists (a type of multiple-choice format), correlations with measures of cognitive abilities were different. The major difference is that correlations with measures of ideational fluency were considerably higher for the free-response form. We interpret this finding in terms of the kind of search of the memory store that is required. Free-response problems require broad searches of memory for relevant information, while the multiple-choice version makes possible a directed search for a match to each multiple-choice option. If a match is found, the option is chosen.

Relationships of scores on simulations to other personal characteristics

The correlations of scores based on simulations with conventional tests of aptitude vary widely, depending on the nature of the simulation and the scores derived from it. Problem-solving tasks presented in FH or PMP format are quite highly structured in comparison with interviewing and in-basket problems, and their correlations involve reasoning and verbal ability, as one might expect. Ideational fluency is involved when a free-response format is used. In contrast with FH and PMP tests, the interviewing and in-basket tasks permit a good deal of freedom – about as much as would be found in a real-life job. For interviewing, the only substantial correlations with cognitive abilities were negative: warmth of the interview was inversely related to knowledge of science. For in-basket simulations, correlations varied considerably; many of the scores correlated with fluency, verbal ability, and reasoning, whereas others were quite independent of the cognitive domain. On the other hand, substantial correlations were found with measures of interest, personality, and biographical history. It would seem that there are many attributes of intelligent behavior that are not measured by conventional intelligence tests and not included in psychometric representations of the structure of intellect.

Influence of situational factors. The effects of situational variables were systematically studied in only one study, where the organizational climate was varied experimentally. It was found that climate conditions involving freedom in administration, freedom in supervising subordinates, and, especially, the interaction of these two conditions did indeed influence performance, particularly the behaviors contributing to a factor called Thoughtful Analysis of Problems. Variations in climate not only influenced the level of performance but also changed the factor structure of the performance categories.

The extent to which the area of expertise required for a set of problems matches the expertise of the subjects may perhaps be thought of as a situational variable, although the match–mismatch is a function of subject status as much as of the problem setting. An experimental study of the influence of a match–mismatch comparison was made in the medical school study, where the same students dealt with both medical and nonmedical problems in similar free-response formats. It is clear from the correlational data that quite different cognitive processes were involved. For the medical problems, knowledge was of primary importance, and there was apparently little need for making broad searches of long-term memory; while for the nonmedical problems, ideational fluency was of primary importance. The knowledge required for solving the nonmedical problems was not organized in memory for quick retrieval, and broad searches of the memory store were necessary.

Such findings as these are consistent with theories about how problem-solving skills develop (Anderson, 1982). At an early stage, problem-solving is a slow and laborious task that requires close attention and frequent review of what is known, and much search of long-term memory for relevant information and ideas. With practice, procedural units are combined to form larger units, and a pattern-recognition system begins to develop, one that links recognizable problem characteristics to the more efficient procedures. With much more experience and practice, much of the problem-solving activity may be carried out automatically, rapidly, and with a minimum of attention. Broad searches of long-term memory are less necessary because appropriate pattern-recognition skills automatically bring to mind the appropriate informational content and procedures that have been found to be successful in the past.

The differences in predictability of performance in the three in-basket situations may also be related to degree of match between expertise of subjects and expertise required by the simulation. Correlations with cognitive abilities were much higher for elementary school principals working in a simulated elementary school than for the other in-basket simulations in which there was no match.

Such findings suggest that no structure of intelligence should be considered as a fixed entity, since the interrelationships among the elements in the structure may vary with requirements of various situations and problems.

Discussion

Investigations of the kind described in this chapter suggest that our knowledge of human intelligence, at least as viewed from a psychometric point of view, is extremely limited in comparison with the manifestations of intelligent behavior that are observable in the world outside the domain of conventional psychological tests. Intelligence tests are predominantly concerned with academic abilities, including both the abilities that are taught in school and the "aptitudes" thought to be predictive of academic success. Such tests (with few exceptions) are composed of multiple-choice items, they are scored in terms of the number of correct or "best" answers chosen, and they are ordinarily administered in standardized settings where subjects are expected to follow the instructions and do their best. In real-life settings, where such restrictions generally do not apply, a much wider variety of behaviors may be displayed in response to the problems that arise.

Methods for broadening the concept of intelligence

There are at least three major ways by which the data base for the study of intelligence could be broadened. One is to use real-life problems, or simulations of real-life problems, as a method for observing and measuring aspects of intelligent behavior; another is to make use of the methods of cognitive psychologists for exploring the various processes involved in carrying out intellectual tasks; and the third is to investigate the influence of situations on performance by varying the settings in which intelligent behavior occurs.

Use of simulations. As we have seen, it is possible to create reasonably realistic simulations of real-life problem situations that are feasible for use in research on intelligence. Protocol analysis of responses to simulated problems makes it possible to discover inductively the salient dimensions of the performance elicited by the simulation, and the use of category-scoring methods makes the scoring of protocols sufficiently economical for use in research. A number of dimensions of performance have been identified by such methods that clearly belong in the domain of intelligence, but which are not found in the psychometric model of intelligence and have little correlation with psychometric factors.

Research on cognition

Cognitive psychologists have given some attention to discovering the processes that are involved in responding to the items in intelligence tests, such as verbal analogies or number-series items. Such processes may include, for example, decoding orthographic symbols, retrieving information from long-term memory, and educing relationship between elements of a problem (e.g., Jacobs & Vandeventer, 1971; Pellegrino & Glaser, 1980; Sternberg & Weil, 1980). Correlational methods are sometimes used to verify the results of such studies, by examining the relationships of the information-processing elements to the scores on the test as a whole (e.g., J. Frederiksen, 1982; Hunt, Lunneborg, & Lewis, 1975; Lunneborg, 1978; Pellegrino, Alderton, & Shute, 1984). But few cognitive psychologists limit themselves to studying items in tests; they investigate information processing as it occurs in a very wide variety of situations including, for example, reading, writing, learning a foreign language, proving propositions in geometry, playing chess, and solving puzzles (cf. Sternberg, 1985). Their research is concerned not only with the elementary processes involved in problem solving, but also the broader strategic and planning processes, sometimes called executive functions, that are presumed to control the more detailed activities. Thus the research in cognitive psychology is helping to create a hierarchical structure of human abilities (Sternberg, 1984) that is quite different from the structures that result from second- and third-order factoring of the intercorrelations of aptitude tests.

    Research aimed at integrating psychometric and information-processing conceptions of intelligence is beginning. Pellegrino (1984) describes a series of experiments showing that differences in spatial ability as revealed by psychometric measures are interpretable in terms of information-processing models and theories; introducing the psychometric (individual differences) approach into information-processing theory makes it possible to test certain basic assumptions of the method. Similar results have been found in studies of reasoning and verbal ability. Pellegrino (1984) believes that

psychometric theory and practice . . . is no longer sufficient to address the theoretical and applied issues associated with intellectual ability. Information processing theory . . . alone or in combination with developmental theory is also insufficient to address these issues. An integration of perspectives and disciplines is needed to achieve progress in tackling . . . the theoretical and programmatic issues associated with the construct of intellectual ability. (pp. 36–37)

Influence of situations on performance. There is evidence from research on creativity that a playlike atmosphere encourages the production of unusual ideas more than does a regimented testing administration, and it also reduces the correlation between creativity tests and measures of intelligence (e.g., Wallach & Kogan, 1965). But in general little is known about how changes in the environment alter the behavior of a subject engaged in test-taking activities. However, interest in studying behavior in its natural settings is growing. In a paper called "Toward an ecologically oriented cognitive science," Neisser (1986) comments that cognitive psychologists are beginning to study intelligent behavior in real life rather than in testing rooms and artificial laboratory settings. For example, such topics as how scientists solve actual scientific problems, what are the prescientific concepts of children, and how adults try to remember the names of their high-school classmates have been studied. Neisser believes that a commitment to take seriously an ecological approach to the study of cognition might have radical consequences – one can never be sure where new directions will lead. The research here reviewed suggests that studying intelligence in a variety of life-like, if not real-life, settings may indeed change our conception of human intelligence.

Defining intelligence

Intelligence has been variously defined in terms of one's ability to think abstractly, to acquire knowledge, to adapt to one's environment, to profit from experience, and to acquire new abilities – to paraphrase very briefly some of the many definitions that have been proposed. Recently Sternberg (1982) has defined intelligence as "goal-directed adaptive behavior," which he believes represents a common theme in research on intelligence. He suggests that researchers should select tasks "to assure that they do measure what constitutes intelligent behavior for a given individual or set of individuals" (p. 25). No doubt a definition would be useful to some degree in guiding the work of researchers in the field of human intelligence. However, definitions are always subject to change as more information is acquired. Eventually the best definition may be some sort of taxonomic model that describes not only the interrelationships of various cognitive skills and abilities, as do current models of the structure of intelligence, but also represents what is known about the cognitive processes that underlie and control these skills; and, in addition, the model might incorporate the relationships of all these things to those environmental influences that help to determine the nature of one's behavior.

The development of taxonomic systems is far more advanced in the biological sciences than in psychology. Hierarchical classifications of plants and animals have eight or nine levels of generality, ranging from phylum or kingdom to species or subspecies. They are useful in identifying specimens and developing retrieval systems; but their greatest value is theoretical. Since the time of Lamarck, a goal of taxonomists has been to find classifications that reflect evolutionary development. Modern taxonomic systems in biology take account not only of morphology and evolutionary relationships, but also genetic, physiological, and ecological factors. Multivariate methods are used by some biologists (Sneath & Sokal, 1973; Sokal & Sneath, 1963), but they are controversial and by no means the predominant method.

The heuristic value of a taxonomic approach to research on intelligence may be as great for psychologists as it has been for biologists. We should go beyond the use of correlational methods and attempt to build a taxonomy of cognitive abilities based not only on intercorrelations of test scores, but also on individual differences in the cognitive processes involved in thinking and on ecological considerations. Eventually, genetic, physiological, and biochemical factors might contribute to the taxonomy as well. A taxonomy based on such considerations might come to represent a general theory of cognitive behavior.

References

Anderson, J. R. (1982). Acquisition of cognitive skill. *Psychological Review, 89*, 369–406.

Barker, R. G. (1968). *Ecological psychology: Concepts and methods for studying the environment of human behavior.* Stanford, CA: Stanford University Press.

Bartlett, F. C. (1932). *Remembering: A study in experimental and social psychology.* Cambridge: Cambridge University Press.

Elstein, A. S., Shulman, L.S., & Sprafka, S. A. (1978). *Medical problem solving: An analysis of clinical reasoning.* Cambridge, MA: Harvard University Press.

Findley, W. G., Frederiksen, N., & Saunders, D. R. (1954). *An analysis of the objectives of an executive-level educational program.* Maxwell Air Force Base, Alabama: Human Resources Research Institute Technical Training Report No. 22.

Ford, M. E. (1979). The construct validity of egocentrism. *Psychological Bulletin, 86*, 1169–1188.

Frederiksen, J. R. (1982). A componential theory of reading skills and their interactions. In R. J. Sternberg (Ed.), *Advances in the psychology of human intelligence* (Vol. 1) (pp. 125–180). Hillsdale, NJ: Erlbaum.

Frederiksen, N. (1959). *Development of the test "Formulating Hypotheses": A progress report.* Princeton, NJ: Educational Testing Service.

Frederiksen, N. (1962a). Proficiency tests for training evaluation. In R. Glaser, (Ed.), *Training research and evaluation* (pp. 323–346). Pittsburgh: University of Pittsburgh Press. (Reprinted 1965, New York: Wiley.)

Frederiksen, N. (1962b). Factors in in-basket performance. *Psychological Monographs, 76,* (22, Whole No. 541).

Frederiksen, N. (1966). Validation of a simulation technique. *Organizational Behavior and Human Performance, 1,* 87–109.

Frederiksen, N. (1984). The real test bias: Influences of testing on teaching and learning. *American Psychologist, 39,* 193–202.

Frederiksen, N., Carlson, S., & Ward, W. C. (1984). The place of social intelligence in a taxonomy of cognitive abilities. *Intelligence, 8,* 315–338.

Frederiksen, N., & Evans, F. R. (1974). Effects of models of creative performance on ability to formulate hypotheses. *Journal of Educational Psychology, 66,* 67–82.

Frederiksen, N., Jensen, O., & Beaton, A. E. (1972). *Prediction of organizational behavior.* New York: Pergamon.

Frederiksen, N., Saunders, D. R., & Wand, B. (1957). The in-basket test. *Psychological Monographs, 71,* (9, Whole No. 438).

Frederiksen, N., & Ward, W. C. (1978). Measures for the study of creativity in scientific problem solving. *Applied Psychological Measurement, 2,* 1–24.

Frederiksen, N., Ward, W. C., Case, S. M., Carlson, S. B., & Samph, T. (1981). *Development of methods for selection and evaluation in undergraduate medical education* (ETS RR 81–4). Princeton, NJ: Educational Testing Service.

Ghiselli, E. (1966). *The validity of occupational aptitude tests.* New York: Wiley.

Guilford, J. P. (1967). *The nature of human intelligence.* New York: McGraw-Hill.

Hemphill, J. K., Griffiths, D. E., & Frederiksen, N. (1962). *Administrative performance and personality.* New York: Bureau of Publications, Teachers College, Columbia University.

Hoban, M. F. (1976). *Identifying student personnel administrators' decision-making style through use of in-basket simulation.* Unpublished doctoral dissertation, School of Education, Health, Nursing and Arts Professions, New York University.

Hunt, E., Lunneborg, C., & Lewis, J. (1975). What does it mean to be high verbal? *Cognitive Psychology, 7,* 194–227.

Hunter, J. E. (1980). Construct validity and validity generalization. In A. P. Maslow & R. H. McKillip (Eds.), *Construct validity in psychological measurement: Proceedings of a colloquium on theory and applications in education and measurement* (pp. 119–125). Princeton, NJ: Educational Testing Service.

Hunter, J. E., & Hunter, R. F. (1983). *The validity and utility of alternative predictors of job performance* (OPRD 83–4). Washington, DC: U.S. Office of Personnel Management.

Hunter, J. E., Schmidt, F. L., & Jackson, G. B. (1982). *Advanced meta-analysis: Quantitative methods for cumulating research findings across studies.* Beverly Hills, CA: Sage.

Jacobs, P. I., & Vandeventer, M. (1971). The learning and transfer of double-classification skills: A replication and extension. *Journal of Experimental Child Psychology, 12,* 140–157.

Keating, D. P. (1978). A search for social intelligence. *Journal of Educational Psychology, 70,* 218–223.

Klein, S. P., Frederiksen, N., & Evans, F. R. (1969). Anxiety and learning to formulate hypotheses. *Journal of Educational Psychology, 60,* 465–475.

Lave, J., Murtaugh, M., & de la Rocha, O. (1984). The dialectic of arithmetic in grocery shopping. In B. Rogoff & J. Lave (Eds.), *Everyday cognition: Its development in social context* (pp. 67–94). Cambridge, MA: Harvard University Press.

Levine, H. G., McGuire, C. H., & Nattress, L. W. (1970). The validity of multiple-choice achievement tests as measures of competence in medicine. *American Educational Research Journal, 7*, 69–82.

Lord, F. M., & Novick, M. R. (1968). *Statistical theories of mental test scores*. Reading, MA: Addison-Wesley.

Lunneborg, C. E. (1978). Some information-processing correlates of measures of intelligence. *Multivariate Behavioral Research, 13*, 153–161.

McClelland, D. C. (1973). Testing for competence rather than for "intelligence." *American Psychologist, 28*, 1–14.

McGuire, C., & Babbott, D. (1967). Simulation techniques in the measurement of problem-solving skills, *Journal of Educational Measurement, 4*, 1–10.

Neisser, U. (1986). Toward an ecologically oriented cognitive science. In T. M. Shlechter & M. P. Toglia (Eds.), *New directions in cognitive science* (pp. 17–32). Norwood, NJ: Ablex.

Pellegrino, J. W. (1984). *Information processing and intellectual ability*. Invited address presented at the American Educational Research Association annual meeting in New Orleans.

Pellegrino, J. W., Alderton, D. L., & Shute, V. J. (1984). Understanding spatial ability. *Educational Psychologist, 3*, 239–253.

Pellegrino, J. W., & Glaser, R. (1980). Components of inductive reasoning. In R. E. Snow, P. A. Federico, & W. E. Montague (Eds.), *Aptitude, learning, and instruction: Vol. 1. Cognitive process analysis of aptitude* (pp. 177–217). Hillsdale, NJ: Erlbaum.

Schmidt, F. L., & Hunter, J. E. (1977). Development of a general solution to the problem of validity generalization. *Journal of Applied Psychology, 62*, 529–540.

Scribner, S. (1984). Studying working intelligence. In B. Rogoff & J. Lave (Eds.), *Everyday cognition: Its development in social context* (pp. 9–40). Cambridge, MA: Harvard University Press.

Simon, H. A. (1973). The structure of ill-structured problems. *Artificial Intelligence, 4*, 181–201.

Simon, H. A. (1978). Information-processing theory of human problem solving. In W. K. Estes (Ed.), *Handbook of learning and cognitive processes: Vol. 5. Human information processing* (pp. 271–295). Hillsdale, NJ: Erlbaum.

Sneath, P. H. A., & Sokal, R. R. (1973). *Numerical taxonomy: The principles and practice of numerical classification*. San Francisco: Freeman.

Sokal, R. R., & Sneath, P. H. A. (1963). *Principles of numerical taxonomy*. San Francisco: Freeman.

Sternberg, R. J. (Ed.) (1982). *Handbook of human intelligence*. Cambridge: Cambridge University Press.

Sternberg, R. J. (1984). What should intelligence tests test? Implications of a triarchic theory of intelligence for intelligence testing. *Educational Researcher. 13*, 5–16.

Sternberg, R. J. (Ed.) (1985). *Human abilities: An information-processing approach*. New York: Freeman.

Sternberg, R. J., & Weil, E. M. (1980). An aptitude x strategy interaction in linear syllogistic reasoning. *Journal of Educational Psychology, 72*, 226–239.

Thorndike, R. L., & Hagan, E. (1959). *10,000 careers*. New York: Wiley.

Traub, R. E., & Fisher, C. W. (1977). On the equivalence of constructed response and multiple-choice tests. *Applied Psychological Measurement, 3*, 355–369.

Tversky, A., & Kahneman, D. (1973). Availability: A heuristic for judging frequency and probability. *Cognitive Psychology, 5*, 207–232.

Tversky, A., & Kahneman, D. (1974). Judgment under uncertainty: Heuristics and biases. *Science, 185*, 1124–1131.

Tversky, A., & Kahneman, D. (1983). Extensional vs. intuitive reasoning: The conjunction fallacy in probability judgment. *Psychological Review, 90*, 293–315.

Vernon, P. E. (1962). The determinants of reading comprehension. *Educational and Psychological Measurement, 22*, 269–286.

Wallach, M. A., & Kogan, N. (1965). *Modes of thinking in young children*. New York: Holt, Rinehart, & Winston.

Ward, W. C. (1982). A comparison of free-response and multiple-choice forms of verbal aptitude tests. *Applied Psychological Measurement, 6,* 1–12.

Ward, W. C., Carlson, S. B., Case, S. M., Frederiksen, N., & Samph, T. (1982). *Developing and validating measures of interpersonal skills for medical school applicants*. Final report to the Josiah Macy, Jr., Foundation. Princeton, NJ: Educational Testing Service.

Ward, W. C., Frederiksen, N., & Carlson, S. (1980). Construct validity of free-response and multiple-choice versions of a test. *Journal of Educational Psychology, 17,* 11–29.

Part II

Intelligence in daily life

6   Academic and nonacademic intelligence: an experimental separation

Stephen J. Ceci and Jeffrey Liker

To place our personal biases on the table, we begin by stating our beliefs on the relationship between measured IQ and "intelligence." We believe that there exists some human capability that properly can be called "intelligence" and that, despite the failure of the research community to agree on its definition, it is not distributed evenly across the population. Rather, personal experience suggests to us that some people possess more "intelligence" than others. Where we differ from many researchers, however, is in our belief that IQ and intelligence are not necessarily related. Our thesis is that there exist multiple intelligences, each an underlying capacity to acquire knowledge, detect relationships, and monitor our ongoing cognitions in a given cognitive domain, in order to adapt to the changing demands of the learning context. Whereas *intelligence* sets the limit on *how much* can be acquired in a particular cognitive domain, the environmental challenges and opportunities that one faces during their development determines *what* shall be acquired. Only when the environmental challenges, opporunities, and motivation is similar will individual differences in cognitive abilities reflect differences in underlying intelligence.

IQ is viewed as a reflection of one set of cognitive abilities formed in response to a specific set of environmental challenges and opportunities (and the motivation to benefit from both). As we shall demonstrate, many other sets of cognitive abilities are not adequately reflected by IQ, despite their high level of complexity and abstraction. An implication of this view of intelligence is that individuals possessing low IQs may exhibit high levels of cognitive abilities in nonacademic settings, whereas those with high IQs may display less cognitive ability in nonacademic matters because of varying environmental challenges leading to differential deployment of their under-

We wish to acknowledge gratefully the kind cooperation of the Brandywine Raceway staff and patrons and especially the assistance of Hap Hansen and Larry Molloy, without whose help this study could not have been conducted. Many colleagues read earlier versions of this manuscript and contributed valuable comments and suggestions, several of which have been incorporated. Special thanks goes to Professors Michael Berzonsky, Rainert Silbereisen, Urie Bronfenbrenner, and Donald Arnstine.

119

lying intelligence. (The distinction between academic and nonacademic intelligence is taken up later in this chapter.

In stating our beliefs in this way we are certainly not advancing a strong
scientific argument. We openly admit we cannot agree on the definition of
the various underlying intelligences, yet we maintain not only that they exist
but that not all members of society exhibit them to the same degree. How
can one assess the distribution of entities that can not even be defined? In
this chapter we shall try to define one type of intelligence, provide evidence
for its existence, show how it is manifested in different levels by different
individuals, and finally, examine its relationship to a traditional index of
intelligence, the IQ test. Our intent is to sidetrack the rather thorny and
often passionate arguments surrounding the traditional assessment of intelligence by providing evidence that a "hallmark" characteristic of what one
normally thinks of as one type of intelligence, that is, abstract problem solving with novel data, can be found in very high levels among persons who
perform rather unremarkably on IQ tests. We will conclude by suggesting
that the assessment of one's multiple intelligences cannot be separated from
a consideration of the important environmental challenges faced in one's
development and the relationship between the skills needed to meet these
challenges successfully, and the skills necessary for performance on standard IQ tests and their surrogates (e.g., SATs, GREs).

Several years ago, in a chapter provocatively entitled, "Do IQ tests measure intelligence?" Hans Eysenck suggested that the critical information
required to answer this question was whether the IQ test possesses external
validity. That is, is there a congruence between the measurement of IQ and
external criteria that are agreed to be relevant to intelligence (Eysenck, 1979,
p. 78)? Eysenck acknowledged the difficulty involved in measuring these
"external criteria" but proceeded to argue that "some relationship there
ought to be and we would feel disinclined to call something intelligence that
did not correlate with external criteria such as success at school and university, or in life or at work" (Eysenck, 1979, p. 78).

Eysenck's review of the literature relating IQ to both academic and nonacademic performance led him to conclude that IQ tests do indeed measure
intelligence. He argued that IQ scores not only predict academic success
but also predict aspects of one's nonacademic life such as income levels,
occupational prestige, and job performance. In expertly wading through the
hordes of potentially relevant correlations, however, Eysenck did not provide a scientifically adequate test of the relationship between IQ and nonacademic intelligence.

That low IQ individuals do not typically impress us with their mental
complexity in academic settings is well known. Economic, motivational, and
experiential reasons have been put forward to account for this finding. But
is performance in nonacademic settings tantamount to practical intelligence

in all spheres of life – that is, does IQ also predict the complexity of individuals' mental processes in their social and work worlds?

As Eysenck notes (but subsequently seems to forget), measures such as job success and the prestige of one's occupation are rather imperfect indices of real world intelligence. To say as he does that because the public perception of carpentry as a profession is lower in prestige than accounting, and furthermore that carpenters as a group have lower IQs than accountants, is not proof (or even a titillating suggestion) that IQ is measuring nonacademic intelligence. The most parsimonious conclusion one might draw from such correlations is that professions composed of individuals with high IQs (e.g., university professors) tend to be esteemed by the public. Such factors as education, social class, and personality may well be the true source of the relationship between IQ and socioeconomic status attainments such as occupational prestige and income (McClelland, 1973).

To address the issue of the relationship of IQ to mental processes, what is needed is a direct means of indexing mental complexity in nonacademic settings and demonstrating the congruence between fluctuations in such mental complexity and IQ. If one were to provide this form of evidence, it would put the issue to rest. Later, we shall present some data that show that the issue is not yet ready for bed. Before proceeding to a description and discussion of our research evidence, we shall present a brief review of what little is known about the mental complexity of individuals in social and work settings and surmise what this might tell us about the nature of the relationship between IQ and various types of intelligence. Next, we shall present the results of our own recently completed study. Third, we will present a summary of the evidence that bears on the relationship of IQ to schooling. Finally, we will conclude by sketching a contextual account of intelligence that postulates multiple specific underlying cognitive potentialities that become differentially realized as a function of experience and motivation.

What is known about practical intelligence?

A little more than a decade ago, researchers began to supply descriptions of the mental processes underlying expertise in such areas as chess (Chase & Simon, 1973), physics (Larkin, 1978), and memory (Hunter, 1976). An analysis of the information processing requirements of expertise in these domains led to an appreciation of the cognitive sophistication of experts (see Chi, Glaser, & Rees, 1982, for a good review). However, the modal subjects in these experiments were either college students, college graduates, or the children of college-educated parents, with relatively little variation in their IQ scores. Thus, it was not possible to make a meaningful examination of the relationship between subjects' level of cognitive sophistication in these domains and their IQs. More recently, researchers have brought the study of expertise to the workplace, showing that the performance of expert psychologists and businesspersons (Wagner & Sternberg, 1985), dairy factory workers (Scribner, 1984), and chief executive officers (CEOs) of large corporations (Streufert & Streufert, 1978) all appear to be guided by fairly sophisticated cognitive processes. Despite the sophistication of the planning strategies used by experts in these areas, however, there does not appear to be any relationship between them and traditional measures of competence such as school achievement and IQ.

As an example, Streufert and Streufert (1978) showed that expert business executives differ from their less successful peers in their willingness to make planning decisions that take into account their past and prospective plans. Moreover, they are less reluctant to make a decision in the absence of new information. Rather, expert business executives appear to "model run" rather than "model fit," to use decision theory terminology. That is, they mentally try out their model before data are available instead of waiting for data and then retrospectively "fitting" a model to them. Interestingly, the IQ scores of executives do not predict this sort of real-world expertise.

Scribner's (1984) fascinating study of dairy factory workers provides a second example. She demonstrates that the ability to fill milk orders in the most economical manner (in terms of physical labor) involves a rapid assessment of the various possibilities created by partially filled cases in close proximity. Her subjects reported that they often do this in a visual gestalt manner and not by actually counting how many empty slots were available in the partially filled cases. Importantly, it is not a skill that can be predicted from high school mathematics scores. In fact, if one analyzes the entire scientific literature on expertise, one is struck with the impression that what separates experts and nonexperts is less a matter of general aptitude (e.g., as reflected by IQ, speed of processing, memory) than it is of specific knowledge gained on the job (Chi et al., 1982; Wagner & Sternberg, 1985).

Recently, Dörner and colleagues reported an interesting series of experiments that come closer to an experimental separation of intelligence and IQ than any with which we are familiar (Dörner, Kreuzig, Reither, & Stäudel, 1983; Dörner & Kreuzig, 1983). Dörner and colleagues asked their subjects to solve various types of real-world problems that enable one to consider many variables for their solution. For example, subjects were asked to decide the optimal number of camels that can be supported on a stretch of fertile land in the desert – the so-called Sahara problem. Beyond a specifiable number of camels, the land will begin to erode, and consequently agricultural income will be jeopardized as well as the future likelihood of grazing. A second example involves managing a mythical city called Lohhausen and accomplishing numerous, often competing, errands in a time-efficient manner. In the Lohhausen problem there are hundreds of variables that one potentially might consider, for example, the effect that raising revenues for road construction (in order to transport services more efficiently) will have on Lohhausen's rate of unemployment.

Dörner and his colleagues classify different ways of reasoning about these problems using a hierarchy of cognitive skills, from the most simple to the most elaborate. The research question is whether subjects with relatively high IQs tend to use relatively complex cognitive skills. They have repeatedly failed to discover a relationship between their subjects' cognitive skills (as reflected in their performance on these real-world tasks) and their IQ scores.

It is tempting to conclude from these results that IQ is a poor predictor of intelligence and is unrelated to the ability to perform "intelligently" on complex real-world tasks. Later, it will be argued that IQ is related to a specific facet of mental complexity and this specific type is not required for successful performance on many real world tasks.

The studies conducted by Dörner and colleagues provide the most rigorous evidence to date that certain types of complex reasoning are not measured by standard IQ tests. Unfortunately, because of the time lag in translating their work from German to English it will be some time before their work can be critically evaluated by non-German scholars. The most serious concern that has been raised is the issue of construct validity. That is, do the assigned levels in Dörner's hierarchy really reflect their subjects' reasoning complexity on the Lohhausen and Sahara problems? Another concern is the restriction of range in Dörner's sample. In one study, subjects were college students representing a fairly restricted range of IQs (see Tent, 1984, for criticisms). This restriction, of course, reduces the likelihood of discovering a relationship between IQ and mental complexity, if one does in fact exist. If one combines several of Dörner's samples, however, this restriction of range does not appear to us to be problematic, as he has obtained similar results using the Lohhausen problem with university students ($n = 30$), senior high students ($n = 70$), and a group of volunteers ($n = 30$) to undeveloped countries (something akin to our Peace Corps but made up of young persons who have attended neither senior high nor college yet have good practical skills like carpentry).

Despite our high regard for the work of Dörner and associates, we believe that alternative tests of the same hypothesis are needed. Ideally, one would want to examine variations in performance on tasks that require complex cognitive operations for their successful completion by subjects sampled over a wide range of IQs. We turn now to our study of racetrack handicapping, which presents just such an opportunity.

Racetrack handicapping: separating IQ and intelligence

Between 1981 and 1984 we carried out a study of racetrack handicappers in which we modeled the complexity of the judgment processes involved and also measured each subject's IQ. Our subjects were quite unlike the ubiquitous college freshmen upon whom most models of intelligence have been based. Subjects in this study were middle aged and older men who were ardent horse-racing fans. On average, these men had been attending horse races at least twice per week during the sixteen years preceding the start of this study. (Some actually had attended races nearly every day of their adult lives, with occasional absences due to illness, marriage of children, and so forth.)

Selecting and classifying subjects

The first phase of this research entailed selecting groups of handicappers with relatively high levels of knowledge and skill. We restricted the sample in this way in an effort to eliminate complete novices (e.g., people who bet the numbers on their license plates or who pick horses by the color of their warm-up blankets) and to ensure that all subjects had enough experience at handicapping to have had the opportunity to develop complex algorithms. In addition, we wanted to sample experts more heavily because we suspected they represented only a small percentage of the betting public but one that was most likely to employ cognitively complex algorithms.

We gave a test of racing facts to 110 men who were attending an East Coast race track. We had reason to believe these 110 men were considerably more knowledgeable about racing facts than the average gambler because they were selected from a subset of gamblers who were observed purchasing copies of what is known as the *Early Form*, a preraceday publication that contains all of the relevant past performance statistics for the next day's racing card but does not contain official assessments of probable favorites, post-time odds, or any other evaluative information. The *Early Form* should not be used to guide actual wagers at post time, however, because it is unofficial and can contain disparities with the *Official Form*, published on the day of racing (e.g., horses listed in the *Early Form* may be "scratched" by post time, or drivers may be changed). Thus, purchasors of *Early Forms* subsequently must purchase the *Official Form*, too. Nonhandicappers typically would not purchase an *Early Form*, as they would be content to wait until the day of the races to examine the official racing card, whereas serious handicappers endeavor to study a racing card for an extended period.

The screening questions we presented to these men involved such facts as the comparative speed ratings of various race tracks around the United States (various track surfaces and sizes yield different speed ratings that must be considered when comparing two horses that raced at different tracks), horse and mare record holders in each division, track records, sires and dams of various fillies and colts, and so forth. On the basis of their answers to such questions, we selected a small group of thirty men for further study; these were the most knowledgeable of the 110 men we tested.

We devised two direct measures of handicapping skill and administered them to these thirty men. The first measure of skill required that the men predict the probable favorite in each of ten upcoming races and estimate it's probable payoff odds based only on information contained in the *Early Form.* (Because the *Early Form*, unlike the *Official Form*, contains no estimated probable odds and is published one day before the appearance of racing columns in the local newspapers, it is safe to assume that the men performed the probable odds estimation task without the benefit of sportswriters' evaluations.) A second measure of handicapping skill was based on these same ten races but this time they were asked to predict the top three horses' post-time odds in each race in their correct order of finish (i.e., making a "trifecta" selection).

Not all these highly knowledgeable men were equally proficient on these two tasks. Fourteen of them proved excellent, correctly selecting the top horse in 93% of the races and selecting the top three horses in their correct order of finish in 53% of the races. We refer to these fourteen men as *experts.* The remaining sixteen men were distinctly inferior to the experts, correctly selecting the top horse in only 55 percent of races and making the correct trifecta selection in only 8 percent of the races. We refer to these sixteen men as *nonexperts.* The probabilities associated with the two tasks attributable to chance alone are 12 percent and .00025 percent, respectively. Thus, even the nonexperts were clearly far better at handicapping than chance would predict.

Relationship of handicapping skill to IQ

What does all of this have to do with the validity of IQ tests? We gave our subjects one final task, the Wechsler Adult Intelligence Scale so we could assess the relationship between the complexity of one's handicapping process and IQ. The first question was whether handicapping skill is related to IQ and the second question is whether, in the absence of such a relationship, expert handicapping is cognitively complex.

To answer the first question, we simply examined the zero-order correlations between IQ and our measures of handicapping skill – their success in picking the favorite and top three favorites in the ten races as described above. The results can be summarized easily: There was no correlation between IQ and either of these measures of handicapping skill.

It was certainly impressive to us that persons with quite modest IQs could so consistently handicap races, picking not only the "winner" but the trifecta. However, the second question remained unanswered: Does successful handicapping really involve high-level reasoning processes, or is it merely the result of rote associative learning? Our interest in this relationship transended curiosity. Jensen and others have argued cogently that an IQ score is a reflection of the amount of cognitive effort deployed between a stimulus and a response (Nichols, 1981). The argument can be reduced to the following synopsis: Whereas the ability to process information in a rote untransformed manner is independent of IQ, high-IQ individuals are thought to have a greater capacity to go beyond a stimulus, reduce it, supplement it, even transform it.

Complexity of the task

A racing program contains a great deal of information about each horse. In the case of standardbred or harness racing (i.e., horses that pull sulky carts with drivers, as opposed to thoroughbred racing where jockeys ride atop the backs of horses), there are between twenty and thirty categories of information about each horse, depending on how one chooses to do the coding. Figure 1 is a partial reproduction of the instruction page from a typical harness racing program. Each of these categories of variables contains between three and twenty-nine levels. For example, there are twenty-nine levels of the variable called *lifetime speed*.[1] On the other hand, the variable known as track size (unlabeled but represented in Fig. 1 by the number $\frac{5}{8}$ following Brd) contains only four levels (tracks can be either $\frac{1}{2}$ mile, $\frac{5}{8}$ mile, $\frac{3}{4}$ mile, or 1 mile in circumference), but the racetrack size must be considered in combination with the horse's speed to meaningfully compare horses. (This form of reasoning is known in statistics as an "interactive effect.") All harness races are 1 mile in length, so a horse must circumvent a $\frac{1}{2}$-mile track twice versus only once for a 1-mile track. Because smaller size tracks (e.g., $\frac{1}{2}$-mile and $\frac{5}{8}$-mile tracks) have more curvature, they generally add several seconds to a horse's finish time. Thus, all other things being equal, a horse that was clocked at 1:59 and $\frac{2}{5}$ seconds on a $\frac{1}{2}$-mile track most likely ran faster than one clocked at 1:58 and $\frac{2}{5}$ seconds on either a $\frac{3}{4}$-mile or 1-mile track, even though the latter ostensibly ran one full second faster.

Although we could not be certain, on the basis of our interviews, we suspected that the process of successful handicapping was quite complex, involving between ten and twenty variables (with multiple levels of each) that are combined into some sort of multiplicative model – that is, configurations of factors were considered rather than a simpler additive model. If correct, this would provide strong evidence that handicapping is a cognitively demanding exercise, perhaps even similar to the sort of multivariate thinking that scientists often employ when they use such terms as "interactive effects," "unique variance accounted for," and "partialing." This was little more than a hunch, however, and we searched for a method of providing scientifically adequate evidence.

Our initial intention was to attempt to understand our subjects' handicapping process by means of a probing, open-ended clinical interview. It

HOW TO READ PROGRAM

The horse's head number, saddle cloth number, program number, mutuel number and post position are the same except where there is an entry in the race. The initials immediately following the horse's name represent color and sex, figures denote age. The names following are the horse's sire, dam and sire of dam in that order. Under the horse's name are his lifetime earnings and lifetime record preceded by his age when record was made up to January 1 of the current year. Following the lifetime earnings is the name of driver, his date of birth, weight and his colors. Next is the horse's best winning time on a half-mile, five-eighths, three-quarter or mile track for last year and the current racing season, followed by his starts and the number of wins, seconds, thirds in purse races and his money winnings. Beneath the horse's name are records of his eight most recent races. They read from bottom to top, therefore the top line is the horse's last race.

The date of the race is followed by the name of the track. All tracks are half-mile unless followed by the figure (1) which means that it is a mile track or (¾) which is a three-quarter mile track, etc. Then is noted the Purse, condition of the track on the day of the race, the Conditions of the race or if a Claiming Race the Claiming Price. Race distance, time of leading horse at the ¼, ½ and ¾ follow, then comes the winner's time. The figures that follow in order show the post position of the horse, his position at the ¼, ½, ¾, stretch with lengths behind except for the leading horse whose number denotes lengths ahead, and finish with beaten lengths. If he was a winner, it shows how far ahead of the second horse and the losers show how far they were behind the winning horse. The next figures shows the horse's actual time in that race. Whenever a small "°" appears after the calls, it denotes that the horse raced on the outside at least one-quarter of a mile. In some instances these figures won't appear because the track at which the horse raced did not have its races charted. Then follows the closing odds to the dollar, the horse's driver, and the order of finish, giving the names of the first three horses. On most past performance lines at extreme right the post time temperature and weather allowance can be found. Example: 64-2 means 64 degrees and the track is rated as two seconds slower than normal.

KEY TO ABBREVIATIONS

Horses' Colors
b—bay
blk—black
br—brown
ch—chestnut
gr—gray
ro—roan

Horses' Sex
c—colt
f—filly
g—gelding
h—horse
m—mare

Track Conditions
ft—fast
gd—good
sy—sloppy
sl—slow
my—muddy
hy—heavy

Finish Information
P—Placing
ns—nose
hd—head
nk—neck
dh—dead heat
dis—distanced (over 25 lengths behind winner)

Wagering Information
N.B.—No Betting
N.R.—Not Reported
*—favorite
e—entry
f—field

Racing Information
°—Raced on outside for at least ¼ mile
°°—Parked three wide
x—horse broke at this point
‡—Free-Legged Pacer
‡—Hoppled Trotter
ix—break caused by interference
i—horse interfered with at this point
Qua (dr)—Qualifying Race for Driver
Qua (h-d) Qualifying Race for both horse and driver.
†—moved up in position at finish due to the disqualification of another horse.
(P)—before driver's name indicates driver holds Provisional License issued to those with limited experience and subject to the approval of the Judges.
T.Dis.—Time for race was disallowed on this horse because of a placing due to other than a lapped on break at finish.
be—broken equipment
ax—break caused by accident
acc—accident
ex—equipment break
dnf—did not finish
BAR—Barred in wagering
R—Record
(F)—after sire denotes foreign horse
(1)—Mile Track
(⅝)—⅝ Track
z—horse claimed
★—Denotes afternoon race

Race Classes
Cd—Condition Race
3000 clm—Actual Claiming price on this horse
Clm cd—Claiming Allowance
Ec—Early closing event
FA—free for all
JFA—Junior Free for all
Hcp—Handicap Race
Inv—Invitational Race
Lc—Late Closing Event
Mdn—Maiden Race
Mat—Matinee Race
nw—Non-Winners
nw300ps—Average Earnings was less than $300 per start
Opn—Open To All
Opt Clm—Optional Claiming
Pref—Preferred
Qua—Qualifying Race
Stk—Stake Race
T—Time Trial
W—Winners

PROGRAM and HEAD NUMBER / Date of Race / Track Raced on / Purse / Track Condition / Type of Race / Condition or Claiming Price / Distance of Race / Time at ¼ / Time at ½ / Time at ¾ / Time of Winner / Post Position / Position at ¼ / Position at ½ / Position at ¾ / Stretch Position and Lengths / Finish Position and Lengths / Horse's Actual Time / Equivalent odds to 1.00 / Driver / Best Win Time of Year / Name of Winner / Name of Second Horse / Name of Third Horse

5 | **RAMBLING WILLIE** — b g, 7, by Rambling Fury—Meadow Belle by Meadow Gold — Trainer-Ro. Farrington
V. Farrington Stables, Inc. & Paul Seibert, Richwood, Ohio — Brd(⅝)$1{:}54^3$ 1977 21 9 7 3 339,125
$668,516 — 6, $1{:}55^3$ (1) — Driver-ROBERT FARRINGTON, 7-15-29 (145) RED-GREY — M(1)$1{:}55^3$ 1976 25 12 5 4 295,750
9- 4 Brd⅝ 40000 ft Inv ml 28 :57 $1{:}26^1$ $1{:}54^3$ 5 2° 1 1 1^1 1½ $1{:}54^3$ *.60 (Ro.Farrington) Rmb.Willie,Arm.Rngr.,Mdw.B.Chip

TRACK ABBREVIATIONS AND COMPARATIVE RATINGS

Track	Abbrev.	Time	Track	Abbrev.	Time	Track	Abbrev.	Time
Arlington Park, Ill. 1⅛	ArlZ	$2{:}04^1$	Frontenac Downs, Can.	FD⅝	$2{:}04^1$	Monticello Raceway, N.Y.	MR	$2{:}03^1$
Audobon Raceway, Ky.	Aud	$2{:}05^2$	Garden City, Can.	GdnC⅝	$2{:}04^3$	Northfield Park, Ohio	Nfld	2:05
Aurora, Ill.	Aur	2:07	Goshen (Historic), N.Y.	Gosh	2:05	Northville Downs, Mich.	Nor	2:05
Balmoral Park, Ill.	Bmlp⅝	2:06	Greenwood Raceway, Can.	GrR⅝	2:04	Ocean Downs, Md.	OD	$2{:}04^3$
Batavia Downs, N.Y.	Btva	$2{:}05^1$	Harrington, Del.	Har	$2{:}05^2$	Pocono Downs, Pa.	PcD⅝	$2{:}03^1$
Bay Meadows, Cal.	BM^1	2:04	Hawthorne Park, Ill.	Haw^1	$2{:}03^4$	Pompano Park, Fla.	Ppk⅝	$2{:}03^2$
Bloomsburg, Pa.	Blom	$2{:}06^1$	Hazel Park, Mich.	HP⅝	2:04	Quebec City, Can.	Que	$2{:}05^4$
Blue Bonnets, Can.	BB⅝	$2{:}03^1$	Hinsdale, N.H.	Hin	$2{:}06^1$	Raceway Park, Ohio	RP⅝	$2{:}03^3$
Brandywine, Del.	Brd⅝	$2{:}02^3$	Hollywood Park, Cal.	Hol^1	$2{:}01^4$	Richelieu Park, Can.	Rich	$2{:}04^4$
Buffalo Raceway, N.Y.	BR	$2{:}05^1$	Indianapolis, Ind.	Ind^1	$2{:}01^4$	Rideau Carlton, Can.	RidC⅝	$2{:}04^1$
Cahokia Downs, Ill.	CKA¾	$2{:}04^1$	Jackson Raceway, Mich.	Jack	2:05	Rockingham Park, N.H.	Rock	$2{:}04^4$
Carlisle, Pa.	Carl	2:05	Latonia, Ky.	Lat^1	2:03	Roosevelt Raceway, N.Y.	RR	$2{:}03^2$
Centennial, Col.	Cen^1	$2{:}05^2$	Laurel Raceway, Md.	Lau⅝	$2{:}03^1$	Rosecroft Raceway, Md.	RcR	$2{:}03^3$
Connaught Park, Can.	Conn	$2{:}06^1$	Lebanon Raceway, Ohio	Leb	$2{:}06^2$	Saratoga Raceway, N.Y.	Stga	$2{:}03^2$
Delaware, Ohio	Dela	$2{:}04^3$	Lewiston, Me.	Lew	$2{:}05^2$	Scioto Downs, Ohio	ScD⅝	$2{:}02^2$
Detroit Raceway			Lexington, Ky.	Lex^1	$2{:}01^2$	Seminole, Casselberry, Fla.	Sem¾	$2{:}03^2$
(Wolverine), Mich.	Det^1	$2{:}01^2$	Liberty Bell, Pa.	LB⅝	$2{:}02^3$	Sportsman's Park, Ill.	Spk⅝	$2{:}02^4$
Dover Downs, Del.	DD⅝	$2{:}04^2$	Los Alamitos, Cal.	LA⅝	$2{:}03^2$	Springfield, Ill.	Spr^1	2:01
DuQuoin, Ill.	DuQ^1	$2{:}01^1$	Louisville, Downs, Ky.	LouD	$2{:}05^2$	Syracuse, N.Y.	$Sycs^1$	$2{:}01^4$
East Moline Downs, Ill	QcD⅝	2:04	Maywood Park, Ill.	May	2:04	Vernon Downs, N.Y.	VD¾	$2{:}01^4$
Fairmount Park, Ill.	FP^1	$2{:}03^3$	The Meadowlands, N.J.	M^1	$2{:}01^2$	Washington Park, Ill.	Was^1	$2{:}03^1$
Foxboro Raceway, Mass.	Fox⅝	2:03	The Meadows, Pa.	Mea⅝	2:03	Windsor Raceway, Can.	WR⅝	$2{:}03^1$
Freehold Raceway, N.J.	Fhld	2:04	Mohawk Raceway, Can.	Moh⅝	$2{:}04^1$	Yonkers Raceway, N.Y.	YR	$2{:}03^3$

Figure 1 Instruction page from a typical racing program.

quickly became apparent, however, that this would not be a satisfactory approach. First, these interviews did not provide us with a basis for quantifying and validating our hunches about the complexity of handicapping. But even more importantly, our subjects found it quite difficult to introspect about the details of their handicapping models and to verbalize them. Often subjects would respond to our questions with superficial or cryptic answers. For example, subject MM, a 62-year-old crane operator with an eighth grade education, gave the following reply to the question, "Which horse do you think will win in the next race?"

A: The 4-horse should win easy; he should go off 3-to-5 or shorter or there's something wrong.

Q: What exactly is it about the 4-horse that makes him your odds-on favorite?

A: He's the fastest, plain and simple!

Q: But it looks to me like other horses in this race are even faster. For instance, both the 2-horse and the 6-horse have recorded faster times than the 4-horse haven't they?

A: Yeah, but you can't go by that. The 2-horse didn't win that outing, he just sucked-up.

Q: Sucked-up?

A: You gotta read between the lines, if you want to be good at this. The 2-horse just sat on the rail and didn't fight a lick. He just kept on the rail and sucked-up lengths when horses in front of him came off the rail to fight with front runners (i.e. attempt to pass them on the outside).

Q: Why does that make his speed any slower, I don't get it?

A: Now listen. If he came out and fought with other horses do you think for one minute he'd have run that fast? Let me explain something to you that will help you understand. See the race the 4-horse ran on June 6 (pointing to the relevant line of the racing program)?

Q: Yes.

A: Well, if the 2-horse had to do all of this fighting (pointing to indications of attempts to pass other horses) he'd run three seconds slower. It's that simple. There ain't no comparison between the 2-horse and the 4-horse. The 4 is tons better!

Q: I think I see what you're saying. But how about the 6-horse, didn't he do some fighting and still run faster than the 4-horse (pointing to indications of attempts to pass front runners)?

A: Yeah. I like the 6-horse a little, but you can't bet him against this field because he's untried. . . . He's been running in cheap company (pointing to the 6-horse's purse sizes).

Q: Why is purse size that crucial? He's still running faster than the 4-horse and fighting front runners while he's doing it. What difference does the purse make?

A: It only makes all the difference in the world, that's all. Do you think for one minute that he can pull those stunts with good horses (pointing to an indication of the 6-horse going around a "wall" of three horses)? Hell, if he tries to go three-wide in $15,000 company they'll eat 'em up.

Q: What do you mean?

A: You can't do these cheap tricks with horses of this caliber. They'll sit back and wait for him to get even with them on the outside then they'll speed-up and make him stay on the outside. You see, horses of this caliber ($15,000 claimers) can generate the speed to keep you parked outside the whole race. $10,000 claimers don't have the stamina, as a rule, to do that.

Q: And the longer you're on the outside the longer the race you have to run, right? In other words, the shortest route around the track is along the rail and the farther off it you are, the longer the perimeter you have to run.

A: Exactly. Now with $10,000 claimers, the 6-horse is a different story. He can have it all his way. But there's another horse in this race that you have to watch. Do you know who I mean?

Q: The 5-horse?

A: No! He'll still be running this time tomorrow. No, I'm talking about the 8-horse. He don't mind the outside post because he lays back early. Christ, he ran a monster of a race on June 20th. He worries me because if he repeats here, he's unbeatable.

Q: Do you like him better than the 4-horse?

A: Not for the price. He'll go off even money. He isn't that steady to be even money. If he's geared-up, there's no stopping him but you can't bet on him being geared-up. If he were 3 to 1 I'd bet him because he'll return a profit over the long run. But not at even money [i.e, 1 to 1].

Statistical modeling of reasoning complexity

As can be seen, the interviews, although "rich" with insights, are not sufficient for rigorously testing the relationship between IQ and reasoning complexity. Subsequent questions intended to elucidate the way in which experts weighted and combined such variables as fighting (i.e., attempts at passing front-running horses), purse size, and odds were unsuccessful. Many of the men did not have vocabularies that could easily support descriptions of their thoughts, especially those men with little formal education. We, therefore, decided that the best way of determining whether handicapping is a cognitively complex activity would be to ask our subjects to handicap races that we constructed by varying levels of the different variables that appeared to be important in the interviews. In this way we could assess whether experts employed implicit algorithms to handicap races. Would they, for example, systematically assign weights to a large number of variables? Can this cognitive process be accounted for by a purely additive model, or are some factors combined in a process better represented by a multiplicative model?

Because of the large number of variables and levels of each variable, a fully crossed factoral design was not feasible. (It would require hundreds of thousands of races!) Rather, we decided to employ what is known as a "factorial survey approach" to the construction of the races (Rossi & Nock, 1982). Using this approach we sampled various points along the ranges of variables and ended up with fifty races that our subjects were asked to handicap.

By designing our own racing program, made up of the fifty constructed races, we were able to determine precisely which of the thirty variables expert handicappers utilize and how each gets weighted (i.e., the relative contribution of a variable to an expert's selection algorithm) so as to sample the full range of permutations that arise by crossing every level of a variable with every level of the other variables.[2] Presented here is a summary of this study as a detailed description of our methods and analyses would take us beyond the scope of this chapter (the interested reader should see Ceci & Liker, *in press*, for these details).

At this point we had fifty races, but only one horse per race. To capture the true reasoning complexity of handicapping would require including data on eight horses per race. But it would be virtually impossible to model the reasoning process used in comparing all eight horses to each other. Moreover, we wanted to be able to compare the fifty races along a common dimension. This problem was solved by creating a description of a standard horse that was presumed to run in all fifty races. Thus, for each race, this standard horse was compared with the horse uniquely described in that race. In short, the task posed to our subjects was to compare the horse described in each of fifty races with the same standard horse and predict the winner between this two horse matchup as well as its likely odds. (After each selection, subjects were also asked to state their confidence in their selection on a seven-point scale.)

To recreate the process by which subjects handicapped races, multiple regression models were estimated predicting our subjects' probable odds estimates (as well as their professed confidence ratings of their estimates) with racing variables (e.g., speed, breeding, driver, purse size). Since we suspected that experts used a different (and more complex) reasoning process compared to nonexperts, we estimated separate regression equations for experts and nonexperts. Partial results of the statistical analysis are reproduced in Table 1.

Standard multiple regression assumes that variables are weighted and combined in a linear, additive process. Our arguments above (as well as the interview data) suggested, however, that influences of certain key variables were qualified by the levels of other variables – an interaction effect. Moreover, these are not simply two-variable interactions, but interactions involving many variables – as best we can tell, six variables are typically considered in combination by expert handicappers. Nor can they be modeled by simply multiplying the six variables and including this product term in the regression analysis. To capture this complexity, we sorted the fifty horses into seven categories using the six variables in the way we suspected experts use these variables (as we had learned in the open-ended interviewing in the first phase of the study). This is called the "interactive model variable" in Table 1, as it is the complex model we hypothesized experts used to handicap the horses.[3]

The results in Table 1 confirmed our hypothesis. For experts, the single best predictor of probable odds (log of odds ratio) was the "interactive model variable," as shown in Table 1 by the size of the standardized coefficient relative to other standardized coefficients. This variable had a large significant effect over and above the additive effects of all variables presented to the subjects in the constructed race forms. Experts appeared to assess the unique variance associated with each level of a given variable then proceeded

Table 1. *Regression of log-odds on racehorse characteristics by expertise of the rater.*[a]

Independent variable	Experts			Non-experts		
	b	SE	Standardized coefficient	*b*	SE	Standardized coefficient
Career characteristics						
Lifetime earnings (1–20)	.02	(.020)	.215	.01	(.026)	.07
Lifetime speed (1–20)	.02	(.021)	− .026	.05	(.028)	.26
Percentage races came-in money	.01	(.043)	.060	.00	(.057)	.01
Current jockey ability (1–3)	.20	(.121)	.310	.31	(.162)	.28
Prior race characteristics						
Purse size (1–10)	.11	(.070)	.003	.15	(.094)	.24
Position of finish (1–10)	.02	(.056)	− .045	.00	(.074)	.00
Payoff/dollar waged (1–11)	.01	(.027)	.050	− .030	(.037)	− .04
Overall speed (1–20)	.02	(.021)	.132	− .04	(.028)	.221
First quarter-mile speed (1–10)	.00	(.040)	.027	− .014	(.053)	− .06
Last quarter-mile speed (1–10)	− .05	(.036)	− .177	− .222[e]	(.048)	− .02
Number of moves (1–4)	.05	(.090)	.197	.10	(.120)	− .13
Race trace size (1–4)	− .07	(.073)	.027	.03	(.098)	.05
Trace surface condition (1–3)	.06	(.122)	.216	− .04	(.163)	.076
Jockey ability (1–3)	− .07	(.125)	.010	.08	(.168)	.032
Interactive model variable (1–7)[b]	.23	(.03)	.259	.10	(.03)	.10

Experts: Constant = .031, R^2 = .786, N = 700

Non-experts: Constant = − .040, R^2 = .744, N = 800

[a] A high score on "Log-odds" (log of odds ratio) means the horse being judged has a relatively good chance of coming in ahead of the standard horse. The dependent variable has been standardized for each subject to remove differences in the mean and variance of ratings across races.

[b] A statistical test of the difference in the metric coefficients for the "interactive model variable" across experts and nonexperts is significant at the .001 level (t = 2.93).

[c] $p = .05$.

[d] $p = .01$.

[e] $p = .001$.

to qualify this contribution through its interactions with other variables and groups of variables. For nonexperts, the interactive model variable did not predict probable odds to the same extent. Rather, it appears that each variable was considered independently for its unique contribution to the horse's chances of winning.

The sheer volume of raw data processed by the experts and nonexperts was quite impressive, but even more impressive is the cognitive sophistication of the algorithms experts used to weight each variable and in some cases consider them in combination with others. Our analyses indicated that experts were fairly homogeneous in this regard. They all were remarkably consistent in the variables they used and the weights they assigned to these variables. We doubt that any profession – be it scientists, lawyers, or bankers – engages in a more intellectually demanding form of decision making than these expert handicappers.

If anything was clear from our many analyses it was that expert handicappers invested great cognitive effort transforming and supplementing data in the racing programs. Our study was designed to confront experts with novel configurations of data that they could not have been expected to have ever seen in their many years of experience, let alone become familiar with. We wanted to be sure that expertise in harness handicapping entailed more than simply recognizing winning constellations of data based on one's ample past experience, otherwise one might legitimately argue that expert handicapping is little more than a form of low-level, rote associative learning whereby one forms a mental template of a "winning" horse's data and compares it with each entrant's configuration of data. Our analyses, however, demonstrated that experts do not use such a simple device to handicap races; rather, they go beyond the raw data in the racing program, assigning "weights" to each variable, systematically combining the various variables in complex, nonadditive ways, and computing a rough odds/probability equivalent for each horse. If this approach sounds cumbersome and time consuming, it is. Experts typically devote six to eight hours handicapping ten eight-horse races. Because time is limited between races (twenty to thirty minutes only), experts typically purchase an *Early Form* the day before a race in order to have sufficient time to handicap. Most experts realize that the task of handicapping is simply too complex to wait until one goes to the racetrack to purchase an *Official Form* racing program.

Having found that experts used a more complex reasoning process than do nonexperts, an obvious test of the relationship between IQ and reasoning complexity is the difference in IQ between experts and nonexperts. There was virtually no difference! A more direct test of this relationship would be to actually measure the complexity of each subject's decision process and see if this relates to his IQ. Experts' decision processes were well captured by a regression equation that contained the above-described complex six-variable interaction effect. Because the ability to reason in such a complex manner closely resembles what one normally thinks of as intelligence, we correlated this measure of reasoning complexity (i.e., the b weight measuring the extent to which each subject took into account the six-variable interaction effect) with their IQ scores. There was essentially no relationship between this assessment of mental complexity and IQ ($r = -.07$)! From these results we conclude that whatever it is that an IQ test measures, it is not the ability to think in a complex, interactive manner in the presence of novel combinations of data. And, we repeat, the manner in which the fifty races were constructed ensured that the different levels of the variables were combined in a novel way, one that could not have previously been encountered by experts, in spite of their ample experience.

Academic versus nonacademic intelligence

One might ask, "What is the conceptual basis for the distinction we have suggested in our title between academic and nonacademic intelligence?" Are there really two (or more) distinctive forms of intelligence or might there be a simpler explanation of our handicapping study? Many theorists (e.g., Neisser, 1979; Sternberg, 1985; Gardner, 1983) have suggested the existence of multiple forms of intelligence that are at least partly independent of one another; even the earliest "unitarian" factorists acknowledged the existence of specific factors in addition to *g*. Traditionally, we have been preoccupied with what is here being referred to as academic forms of intelligence. This preoccupation partly reflects historical forces (after all, Binet's commission was to develop a means of identifying children at risk for academic failure), but it also partly reflects a convenience of thinking on the part of researchers that seldom led them to challenge unitary models of intelligence.

Although the IQ test was developed with academic needs in mind, subsequent researchers clearly provided some evidence that intelligence appeared to be a unitary construct, with individuals who score high on one index of intelligence also scoring high on others. This was accomplished by demonstrating that an impressive array of academic and vocational achievements were moderately to highly correlated with each other and with IQ as well. It made little sense to maintain a differentiation between academic and nonacademic intelligence when nearly all of the tests that had been used were moderately to highly intercorrelated. However, the likelihood of accounting for a large part of the covariance among tests with the first principle component (*g*) is a funtion of the nature of the test data themselves. That is, factor analysis will yield a large first factor to the extent that the tests that are employed are similar and tightly clustered in the hyperspace, as Jensen himself clearly recognized: "as the tests change, the nature of *g* will also change, and a test which is loaded, say, .50 on *g* when factor analyzed among one set of tests may have a loading of .20% or .80%, or some other value, when factor analyzed among other sets of tests" (Jensen, 1969, P. 11).

Our view is that factor-analytic studies of intelligence presupposed the potential range of factor solutions by the limited nature of the cognitive tests employed and by the even more limited range of contexts used. To our knowledge, no one ever sought to validate certain crucial, but implicit, assumptions. For example, are such basic cognitive processes as memory, perception, inferencing, and problem solving *acontextual*? That is, can one be certain that a deficit exists in one of these operations simply on the basis of an examination of a child's performance on academic tasks that ostensibly "tap" them, usually undertaken in a classroom or a psychologist's office?

Recently it has been shown that even microlevel cognitive processes (e.g., memory strategies) are under the influence of contextual variables. The likelihood of using such a cognitively efficient strategy has been demonstrated to depend on the nature of the task (e.g., its interest level and sex-role expectations) and the setting in which the task is presented (one's own home versus an unfamiliar home versus a university laboratory). A frequent observation from such research has been that children who appear deficient in the use of microlevel cognitive strategies in one setting or on one task will deploy them spontaneously in a different setting or on a different task (Ceci & Bronfenbrenner, 1985). If such microlevel components of cognition are susceptible to contextual influences, is it not even more likely that macrolevel cognitive activities (thinking and reasoning) are similarly under the influence of contextual variables? This would seem to imply that whereas performance on academic tasks might be taken at their face value, they ought not to be taken beyond that; poor performance on a digit span test may be uncorrelated with auditory short-term memory for digits in another context, such as gambling.

Recently, Jean Lave and her students provided some fascinating evidence that the context in which a cognitive activity is undertaken determines not only the perceived nature of the problem but the shape of the solution as well. The ability to make "intelligent" choices among similar items at a supermarket, where the basis of the choices often required mental arithmetic in order to equate two items of differing size and cost, was unrelated to a subject's score on a formal arithmetic test that assessed the same arithmetic operations (Lave, Murtaugh, & de la Rocha, 1984). This led Lave and coworkers to conclude that the traditional acontextual emphasis in cognitive psychology, on problem-solving operations as forms of "disembodied mental activity," was ill-wrought because of the crucial importance of the context in creating perceptions of problems and shaping their solutions. Anthropologists have long recognized this fact, as Clifford Geertz, writing in Jordan Scher's *Theories of the Mind*, stated: "the human brain is thoroughly dependent upon cultural resources for its very operation; and those resources are, consequently, not adjuncts to but constituents of mental activity" (Geertz, 1962, p. 730).

The above argument regarding contextual influences on cognition leads us to the "bottom line" of our thesis on the relationship between IQ and intelligence. That is, the cognitive abilities that one acquires will depend on the particular environmental challenges and opportunities that one deals with (i.e., contextual variables) as well as the underlying mental capacity for such acquisition (i.e., intelligence). This thesis is analogous to Cattell's distinction between fluid and crystallized intelligence, with the additional assumption that there exist not one generic underlying intelligence but multiple underlying intellectual capabilities. Only when people have been exposed to comparable environmental challenges and opporunities will their underlying level of intelligence influence the extent to which various cognitive abilities are crystallized in one person but not in the other. Thus, intelligence will be expressed differently depending on the particular constellation of one's environmental demands and opportunities, and perhaps the personal motivation to benefit from both. This view implies that, given the relevant opportunities, demands, and motivation, our expert handicappers would show dramatic gains on IQ tests over time. In keeping with the sense of the second sentence of this chapter, we do not believe that everyone exposed to the same opportunities, demands, and motivations would benefit equally. Thus, it is our view that an IQ score is an acceptable indicant of one underlying type of intelligence, but only when discussing differential rates of acquisition of cognitive abilities that become crystallized in response to schooling experiences (e.g., vocabulary, verbal concept formation, paradigmatic classifications, chunking/recoding of linguistic stimuli,) and only between those with similar environmental challenges and opportunities (and similar levels of motivation to benefit from both).

The relationship between intelligence and schooling

If we conceptualize intelligence in terms of Cattell's crystallized and fluid distinction, then it is reasonable to suppose that the abilities that are crystallized will depend on the particular environmental challenges and opportunities (and motivation to benefit from these). In this context, schooling is seen as an environment that induces specific knowledge and modes of cognizing that are relevant for performance on tests of academic intelligence (e.g., paper-and-pencil tasks, IQ tests, achievement tests) but is not necessary for successful performance on tasks that do not depend on academic learning. That is, schooling conveys various direct and indirect benefits to academic intelligence without necessarily affecting nonacademic intelligence. That both factual and conceptual modes of cognizing are inculcated through Western types of schooling cannot be overestimated in the issue under discussion. For example, a good deal of what an IQ test tests is a rote reproduction of factual knowledge gained either directly or indirectly through the schooling process.

If one doubts this assertion, consult the INFORMATION subtest of the Wechsler Intelligence Scales for Children (WISC-R) or Adults (WAIS). Questions abound for which a knowledge of geography ("In what continent is Egypt?"), history ("Who discovered America?"), science ("What is the boiling point of water?"), and literature ("Who wrote Hamlet?") is essential.

Contrary to the traditional belief that these questions tap knowledge potentially available to all individuals, regardless of their home and school environments (Jensen, 1980), it has been clear for some time that performance
on them is directly affected by schooling. For example, it is largely overlooked that children appear to lose IQ points whenever they are not in school.
The most trivial example of this is the small but reliable decline in IQ produced by summer vacation, especially for low-income children who are less
likely to be involved in academic activities during their summers (Jencks et
al., 1972).

On a more significant level, numerous studies (that tend not to have been
widely read by psychologists) have demonstrated a large, detrimental impact
of school removal (DeGroot, 1951; Harnquist, 1968; Husen, 1951; Lorge,
1945; Ramphal, 1969). For example, Harnquist (1968) compared Swedish
men at the time of military registration (18 years of age) who previously had
been tested at the age of thirteen. After controlling for their IQs and social
class at age thirteen, boys who did not finish high school lost, on average,
nearly two IQ points for each year of missed school – between seven and
eight points for those who did not receive any secondary schooling. Thus
two boys who had equivalent IQs at age thirteen ended up with substantially
different IQs at age eighteen if only one of them had dropped out of school.
In Ramphal's study of Indian children living in South African villages whose
schooling was delayed because of teacher unavailability, the loss was nearly
five IQ points per year, as compared with Indian children in nearby villages
whose schooling was not delayed.

Another source of evidence for the direct impact of schooling on IQ can
be seen in the plight of blacks who migrated North between the World Wars
I and II. After controlling for selective migration, it was shown that the
offspring of these blacks gained between .5 and .7 IQ points for each year
they were enrolled in Philadelphia schools (Lee, 1951).

Finally, Bronfenbrenner's (1974) reanalysis of the seminal data on identical twins reared apart, which is usually taken as strong evidence for the
high heritability of IQ, showed a correlation of .87 for twins attending the
same schools versus only .66 for those attending different schools (and often
receiving different levels of schooling).

Taken together, the above studies constitute a fairly strong case for the
impact of schooling on IQ. How could we ever have thought differently?
While not denying the pervasiveness of some of these facts in many of our
daily lives (e.g., questions about the author of *Hamlet* may occasionally
appear on television game shows), surely one is most likely to have learned
about Egypt, *Hamlet*, and so forth in school (including being in the school
play). Furthermore, it would be incorrect to confine the effects of schooling
on IQ to the mere dissemination of factual knowledge. Cole & Scribner
(1974), Super (1980), and others (e.g., see several chapters in Rogoff and

Lave, 1984) have shown that entire modes of cognizing are associated with formal schooling, such as the shift from thematic/perceptual sorting to taxonomic/conceptual classifying. This shift becomes relevant when one is required to generate a relationship between two items, as in the case of the similarities subtest of the WISC-R (e.g., "In what way are an apple and an orange alike?"). Note that perceptual classifications (e.g., "they both have seeds and are round") are scored lower than taxonomic classifications ("they are both fruits").

One further way in which schooling influences IQ scores is through the style of cognizing enforced in school, for example one that values reflectiveness over impulsiveness. It is instructive to administer an IQ test to children who differ along this dimension. What one finds is that the impulsive child, while occasionally being rewarded for an exceptionally fast, correct response, is usually penalized. An actual case best illustrates this point.

An impulsive seven-year-old boy named Charlie was asked the first six questions on the SIMILARITIES subtest. He was consistently given credit for one-point answers (i.e. he generated perceptual similarities, as in the example about the apple and the orange both being round). Despite repeated encouragements to slow down, he continued to supply his answer almost as fast as the question was stated. As he progressed through the subtest, the questions become more difficult. IQ questions are normed in an age-graded manner, so that each new question is slightly harder than its predecessor. A structural assumption of such age grading is that children should never, as a rule, do better on harder questions than they do on easy ones. Yet, this is precisely what happened. When the questions became too difficult for Charlie to quickly provide an obvious perceptual commonality between two items (e.g., "How are scissors and a copper pan alike?"), he was forced to become more reflective. Consequently, he began receiving two-point scores on the more advanced questions (e.g., "they're both made of metal").

During the easy part of the subtest, it was as though Charlie had presumed a certain level of conceptual understanding on the Tester's part and proceeded to supply additional (perceptual) commonalities. For instance, he may have recoded the question, "How are an apple and orange alike?," to "How are these two fruits alike?" Thus, he would be likely to ignore supplying the obvious, that they are both fruits, and as a result be penalized, not for his lack of intelligence or knowledge but for his impulsive cognitive style. (It was revealing that Charlie was quite capable of picking out an apple and an orange in response to the question: "Can you find the fruits in the box?") When the questions became too difficult for Charlie to easily recode, however, he was suddenly forced to pause and reflect on the question and, in particular, on the shared attributes of the items in it. As a result, he began to be credited with higher scores, indicative of "conceptual thinking." Had Charlie not performed well enough on the first part of this subtest, however, he would not have even had the opportunity to demonstrate his ability to think conceptually because each section of the IQ test is discontinued after several consecutive wrong responses. Thus, were it not for his answers on the more difficult questions, we might have arrived at a rather erroneous conclusion regarding Charlie's conceptual ability.

Toward a contextual model of intelligence

The above observations have led us elsewhere (Ceci & Liker, *in press*) to suggest that a contextual account of intelligence is long overdue. According to this view, persons develop in context, and it is important to know something about their developmental contexts before we pass judgment on their intelligence. Each context carries with it a set of environmental challenges and opportunities that one strives to meet. Intelligence is best seen as the extent to which individuals have successfully met the most important environmental challenges in their lives. The degree to which the skills required to meet one's important environmental challenges overlap those required to meet academic challenges, including IQ test performance, is the degree to which an IQ score begins to reflect one's intelligence. A corollary of this statement is that many real-world challenges require the development of specific styles and modes of cognizing that may not only be unrelated to those required for successful academic performance, but actually be antithetical to it. For such persons it makes little sense to speak of their IQ score as anything more than a measure of probable academic readiness.

As stated in the Introduction to this chapter, we are of the opinion that various types of intelligence exist and are not distributed evenly in the population. We believe our expert handicappers were intelligent men, probably more so than our nonexperts, though we hesitate to press the claim terribly hard without knowing more about the nonexperts. One thing seems certain, though: An expert with an IQ of 80 exhibited far more cognitive complexity than a nonexpert with an IQ of 130, even though both men were equally matched in terms of prior experience and basic factual knowledge. (We do not believe that the underlying intelligences and/or motivation of all individuals are equal; we therefore do not expect everyone to benefit equally from the same level of experience.) Our experts developed richer, more differentiated models of racing than our nonexperts and showed their ability to apply these models consistently, even in the face of new constellations of data. When you put all of these things together, you emerge with a picture of men who approached their environmental challenges in a planful manner, developing complex algorithms that were capable of correctly predicting racing odds from novel sets of data. In short, when faced with a task that was important and exciting to them, these men even exhibited one of the hallmarks of academic intelligence: abstract reasoning. This leaves us with a rather obvious conclusion with regard to their failure to display similar complexity on an IQ test. The attainment of vocabulary skills and the acquisition of large amounts of general information, though important for successful performance on IQ tests, apparently was not of ample interest to these expert handicappers during their development to encourage their acquisition.

An implication of the above argument is that each of us possesses some underlying level of innate intelligence that can be funnelled into various cognitive activities, the outcomes of which are a function of one's opportunities and motivation to achieve. We have no quarrel with such a view – as far as it goes. We prefer to think of "multiple underlying intelligences" as opposed to a single underlying intellectual force, however. According to such a view, each of us possesses innate potentialities for achievement in abstract reasoning, verbal analysis, creative expression, quantification, visual-spatial organization, and so on (see Gardner, 1983, for a description of various independent types of intelligence). Additionally, each of us are exposed to multiple contexts for expressing these potentialities. In the types of environments that are typically seen as "enriched," there are opportunities to develop most or even all of one's potentialities. For most, however, the opportunities that are relevant for the actualization of even a single potentiality may not have been available during critical periods of development. Such a view of multiple underlying intelligences and varying opportunities and motivations for developing each, goes a long way toward accounting for the seemingly contextual nature of cognitive complexity. Most of us perform on a complex level in one or two areas in which the requisite ingredients are simply a good underlying potential in this area, ample opportunities to exercise this potential, and the motivation to take advantage of these opportunities. We do not function in a complex manner in all areas of intelligence or even on all tasks that appear to "tap" the same area of intelligence, as some of these will have flourished and others wilted because of environmental and motivational differences. Thus, similar forms of analytic reasoning might underpin philosophical inquiry and certain fantasy games (no slur intended against the former) but cognitive complexity on one does not guarantee complexity on the other.

This last observation leads us to our concluding argument. It has been argued by some researchers that intelligence is not contextually dependent, as we have tried to represent it, but rather acontextual. According to these researchers anyone might become competent (even cognitively sophisticated) in a specific domain. What separates the truly intelligent from those with only pockets of isolated achievements is that the former are able to generalize their complexity to all domains. Intelligence, according to the view of these researchers, is general, not specific. There are solid reasons for rejecting this belief in the generality of intelligence, however. Perhaps the most interesting reason is the failure of most individuals, including researchers themselves, to exhibit the same complexity in their personal lives (e.g., finances) that they exhibit so magnificently in their professional lives (see Nisbett & Ross, 1980, for examples). The generality of intelligence is probably more illusory than any of us would like to admit.[4]

Notes

1 In Figure 1, Rambling Willie's life-time speed record was 1:55 and $\frac{3}{5}$ seconds, recorded on a 1-mile track: Between the range of the fastest horse's lifetime speed mark of 1:55 and $\frac{3}{5}$ seconds and the slowest horse's lifetime mark of 2:01 and $\frac{1}{5}$ seconds are twenty-nine one-fifth second increments.

2 Although the factorial survey approach calls for random sampling of levels of variables, we chose instead to select data from actual race forms that represented a range of combinations of levels. (We searched through approximately 2,200 races and selected fifty.) We reasoned that randomly generating races would present subjects with implausible combinations of levels that would make the handicapping task artificial and undermine the value of the complex algorithms employed by expert handicappers. However, we sacrificed the orthogonality that the factorial survey method provides, and in some cases there were substantial correlations between variables. A complex series of tests were run to evaluate the effects of collinearity and the results of these tests indicated that our conclusions appear to be valid (Ceci and Liker, *in press*).

3 That the "interactive model variable" represents the results of a complex reasoning process is best demonstrated by example. In order to predict a horse's closing speed, experts considered how fast each horse had run during the earlier part of the race, because this sets the limit on how much energy the horse still has available to sprint the final quarter-mile. It is important, however, to take into consideration not only how fast the horse ran, but its behavior while running. For example, if a horse in the program appeared to have run fast while trying to pass front runners, it is likely that it ran even faster than was indicated in the program because it would be necessary for it to move away from the rail while passing these other horses. (The length of the race is 1 mile for a horse that stays on the rail but it can actually expand in excess of 1 and $\frac{1}{16}$th mile in the case of a horse that spent much of the race on the outside.) Experts are adept at adjusting a horse's earlier speed to take into consideration its behavior, the track size, and the turf conditions.

4 A nice example of this can be found in some of our unpublished work with children who were asked to predict the distance that was likely to be traversed by a microdot on a computer monitor. The solution requires that one simultaneously take into consideration the size of the dot, its color, and its speed, because each variable can potentially influence the value of the others. Not surprisingly, perhaps, young children found this prediction task very difficult. They consistently failed to estimate the correct distance the dot would travel. Yet, when they were given what was essentially the same task except that the prediction was embedded in a video gamelike format, they performed substantially better. In the latter task children were told to "fire a missile" at the likely location on the computer screen that a spaceship of a specified color, shape, and size would appear. The two tasks ostensibly tapped a similar ability to think in terms of a three-way interaction, but the context of the task determined whether a child would exhibit this ability. Thus, complexity on one task did not guarantee complexity on the other, even though both tasks presumably tapped similar higher-order reasoning skills.

References

Bronfenbrenner, U. (1974). Nature with nurture: A reinterpretation of the evidence. In Montague, A. (Ed.), *Race and IQ*. New York: Oxford University Press.
Ceci, S. J., & Bronfenbrenner, U. (1985). Don't forget to take the cupcakes out of the oven: Strategic time-monitoring, prospective memory and context. *Child Development, 56*, 175–190.
Ceci, S. J., & Liker, J. (in press). A day at the races: A study of IQ, expertise, and cognitive complexity. *Journal of Experimental Psychology: General.*
Chase, W., & Simon, H. A. (1973). Perception in chess. *Cognitive Psychology 1*, 55–81.
Chi, M. T. H., Glaser, R., & Rees, E. (1982). Expertise in problem solving. In R. J. Sternberg (Ed.), *Advances in the psychology of human intelligence* (Vol. 1, pp. 7–75). Hillsdale, NJ: Earlbaum.
Cole, M., & Scribner, S. (1974). *Culture and thought.* New York: Wiley.
DeGroot, A. D. (1951). War and the intelligence of youth. *Journal of Abnormal Social Psychology, 46*, 596–597.
Dörner, D., & Kreuzig, H. (1983). Problemlösefähigkeit und intelligenz. *Psychologische Rundschaus, 34*, 185–192.
Dörner, D., Kreuzig, H., Reither, F., & Stäudel, T. (1983). *Lohhausen: Vom Umgang mit Unbestimmtheit und Komplexität.* Bern: Huber.
Eysenck, H. (1979). *A model for intelligence.* New York: Springer-Verlag.
Gardner, H. (1983). *Frames of mind: The theory of multiple intelligences.* New York: Basic.
Geertz, C. (1962). The growth of culture and the evolution of mind. In Scher, J. M. (Ed.), *Theories of the mind.* New York: Free Press.
Harnquist, K. (1968). Relative changes in IQ from 13 to 18. *Scandinavian Journal of Psychology, 9*, 50–64.
Hunter, I. M. L. (1977). An exceptional memory. *British Journal of Psychology, 68*, 155–164.
Husen, T. (1951). The influence of schooling upon IQ. *Theoria, 17*, 61–88.
Jencks, C., Smith, M., Acland, H., Bane, M. J., Cohen, D., Gintis, H., Heyns, B., & Michelson, S. (1972). *Inequality: A reassessment of the effect of family and schooling in America.* New York: Basic.
Jensen, A. R. (1980). *Bias in mental testing.* New York: Free Press.
Jensen, A. R. (1969). How much can we boost IQ and scholastic achievement? *Harvard Educational Review, 39*, 1–123.
Larkin, J., McDermott, J., Simon, D. P., & Simon, H. A. (1980). Expert and novice performance in solving physics problems. *Science, 208*, 1335–1342.
Lave, J., Murtaugh, M., & de la Roche, O. (1984). The dialectic of arithmetic in grocery shopping. In B. Rogoff & J. Lave (Eds.), *Everyday cognition: Its development in social context.* Cambridge, MA: Harvard University Press.
Lee, E. S. (1951). Migration: A Philadelphia test of the Klineberg hypothesis. *Sociological Review, 16*, 227–232.
Lorge, I. (1945). Schooling makes a difference. *Teacher's College Record, 46*, 483–492.
McClelland, D. C. (1973). Testing for competence rather for "intelligence." *American Psychologist, 28*, 1–14.
Neisser, U. (1979). The concept of intelligence. *Intelligence, 3*, 217–227.
Nichols, R. C. (1981). Origins, nature, and determinants of intellectual development. In M. Begab & C. Haywood (Eds.), *Psychosocial influences in retarded performance* (Vol. 2, pp. 127–154). Baltimore: University Park Press.
Nisbett, R. & Ross, L. (1980). *Human inferential ability.* NY: Appleton-Century-Crofts.
Rogoff, B. & Lave, J. (1984). *Everyday cognition: Its development in social context.* Cambridge, MA: Harvard University Press.
Rossi, P. H., & Nock, S. L. (1982). *Measuring social judgments: A factorial survey approach.* Beverly Hills, CA: Sage.

Scribner, S. (1984). Studying working intelligence. In B. Rogoff & J. Lave, (Eds.), *Everyday cognition: Its development in social context* (pp. 166–189). Cambridge, MA: Harvard University Press.

Sternberg, R. J. (1985). *Beyond IQ: a triarchic theory of human intelligence.* NY: Cambridge University Press.

Streufert, S. & Streufert, S. C. (1978). *Behavior in the complex environment.* Washington, DC: Winston.

Super, C. (1980). Cognitive development: Looking across at growing up. In C. Super, & S. Harkness, (Eds), *New Directions for Child Development: Anthropological Perspectives on Child Development, 8,* 59–69.

Tent, L. (1984). Intelligenz und problemlösefähigkeit. *Psychologische Rundschaus, 35,* 152–155.

Vernon, P. (1979). *Intelligence: heredity and environment.* San Francisco: Freeman.

Wagner, R. K. & Sternberger, R. J. (1985). Practical intelligence in real-world pursuits: The role of tacit knowledge. *Journal of Personality and Social Psychology. 49,* 436–458.

7 Some lifelong everyday forms of intelligent behavior: organizing and reorganizing

Jacqueline J. Goodnow

One of the odd features to traditional measures of intelligence is the extent to which they concentrate on tasks or questions that are novel, that is, are seldom encountered in everyday life or likely to be so. The occasions are rare, for instance, when one is asked to recall numbers backwards, say what is similar between an ant and a bush or, as an adult, put together the pieces of a wooden puzzle. It is true that some tests or subtests tap more directly into past knowledge: asking one to name the days of the week, for example, or to state the best thing to do when you find a stamped, addressed envelope on the street. Most of the time, however, the standard tests and measures are designed to avoid tapping in any direct fashion into accumulated knowledge. Most of the time, also, they avoid tapping into the use of that knowledge for problems that people actually face. I have no interest, for instance, in knowing how many miles there are between New York and Paris (a question on the Wechsler–Bellevue) and have always found the question "silly," a pretentious way of playing Trivial Pursuit. By contrast, I have a lively interest in how many hours of flying time are involved – that is what I feel one "needs to know" – but that is not the question asked.

Are there alternatives to such approaches to intelligence? One alternative takes the form of arguing that we should pay more attention to practical intelligence or "everyday intelligence": – that is, to situations where people can use, and have some interest in using, their past knowledge to solve a real-life problem.

That alternative may raise two spectres. One is the possibility of having to abandon the hope of comparable measurement situations (comparable in their content or in the kinds of demand that they make), developing instead a long list varying with age group and social group and perhaps having to be individualized. That kind of alarm might be generated, for example, by noting that people interested in the development of everyday intelligence

I am especially indebted to Jeannette Lawrence of Murdoch University for several stimulating discussions on this topic. The chapter was completed while the author was at the Center for Advanced Study in the Behavioral Sciences, Stanford, California and the support of the Spencer Foundation is gratefully acknowledged.

have begun to analyze the specific skills and demands of being a carpenter, a tailor, a packer of milk cartons, or a skier (examples from Rogoff & Lave, 1984). At first sight there appears to be a danger of accumulating signs of intelligence in occupational groups as we once did with national groups.

The other ghost is the possibility of having to abandon all formal or laboratory analysis of intelligent behaviors, leaving no effective points of contact between studies based on tasks encountered in everyday life and studies based on tasks designed to highlight particular aspects of practical intelligence. At first sight again, it seems easy to identify interest in everyday intelligence with the exclusive use of ethnographic or qualitative methods, an identification that both Rogoff (1982) and Scribner (1984) see as unnecessary.

The main burden of this chapter is that both spectres can be avoided. It is possible to locate situations that call for practical intelligence and that recur in the lives of many. It is also possible to bring together formal and more naturalistic approaches and – an issue in practical intelligence for every researcher or scholar – to use the combination as a way of emerging with fresh perspectives and new questions.

This chapter concentrates on two intelligent behaviors observed in the daily life of children and adults. They are the behaviors of organizing and reorganizing, called for on many occasions; for example, when a number of errands have to be packed into a short time, an extra task has to be fitted into a tight schedule, a car breaks down, a child falls ill on a busy day, or one sleeps beyond an appointed time. I shall consider both organizing and reorganizing but shall stress the latter and its particular demands for repair, recovery, and a rearrangement of activities or people.

The material is presented in several sections. The first asks, Why these behaviors? This question calls for a short review of gaps and directions in earlier studies of intelligence. The second, third, and fourth sections look at some everyday situations in which children face a demand for reorganization. These sections primarily serve the purpose of asking, What are the components of these intelligent behaviors? How do they emerge? What kinds of learning are called for in their development and display?

Each section reviews briefly some formal studies, mostly emerging under the label of planning, and asks about links between what has been observed in these studies and what is suggested by the dissection of the everyday situations. The underlying argument is that the study of intelligence and intelligent behavior benefits from combining studies, regardless of whether these focus on behavior displayed in psychometric testing, in laboratory studies of cognition, or during the course of everyday problem solving. Such combining is facilitated however when we study behaviors called for in several such situations, a criterion met by organizing and reorganizing behaviors.

The background of interest

The section is in two parts, representing two lines of questioning: (1) Why change from traditional approaches to the study of intelligence?, and (2) Why focus on organizing and reorganizing?

A shift from tradition

I shall summarize several changes, noting for each the way that a shift in perspective brings about a shift in research questions. The first shift is a move away from the concept of intelligence as an absolute (readily recognized by all) to the notion of intelligence as socially defined. In the latter case, one person's view of what represents intelligent behavior may well not be the same as another's. The socially-defined notion has its origin in cross-cultural studies (cf. Goodnow, 1976). Perhaps because of that origin, it first gave rise to research on the extent to which people in several cultures vary in their definitions of intelligence or in the values they place on particular intellectual skills (e.g., Chen, Braithwaite, Huang, 1982; Gill & Keats, 1980; Serpell, 1974), and then to questions about consensus within a culture (e.g., Sternberg, Conway, Ketron, & Bernstein, 1981).

A second shift may be phrased as a question: Who makes judgments about degrees of intelligence? In other terms, who makes assessments? The older view stressed psychologists. The more novel view is that psychologists have no monopoly and that assessments are not limited to formal testing situations. During the course of daily life, both children and adults happily make judgments about others or themselves, labeling some actions or people as "dumb," "slow," "stupid," or "facile" and others as "smart," "quick," "clever," or "deep." This shift in perspective encourages questions about the comparability of formal and informal assessments (e.g., Nerlove, Roberts, Klein, Yarbrough, & Habicht, 1974; Serpell, 1974) and about the opinions one group has of the assessment procedures of another (a topic so far neglected although touched on in the work of Chen, Braithwaite, & Huang, 1982). The shift encourages also the questions: Which people are most likely to carry out assessments? At what ages and for what purposes? The U.S. parents observed by Fischer and Fischer (1963), for instance, made early assessments as part of their duty to "divine the potential" in each individual child and to arrange the environment so as to "maximize the potential." By contrast, the Baoule mothers interviewed by Dasen (1985) initially declined a request for early assessment, on the grounds that intelligence is a quality one ends up owning rather than a quality one starts with.

A third shift moves away from the idea of intelligence as a quality residing within the individual and toward the notion of intelligence as a judgment or an attribution, made in formal or informal situations. We make the judgment "intelligent", the argument runs, just as we make judgments about a remark being witty or a person well-informed. From this perspective, the interesting questions are then not about the amount of intelligence someone has but about the nature of the judgment. The questions may be about the people making the judgment: the distinctions drawn (e.g., between being "smart," "wise," or "clever"), the cues used, the signs of bias or error. They may also be about the person being judged: the strategies used to present oneself as intelligent or to protect oneself from unflattering judgments (cf. Covington & Omelich, 1979; Goodnow, 1976, 1984).

The final shift to be noted has to do with the measures or procedures used to study intelligent behaviors. Psychologists have traditionally been attracted to stripped-down tasks, forcing the individual to work completely "in the head" (Goodnow, 1976) and alone. The result is that we know little about the intelligent use of physical and social resources. A striking contrast can be seen in observations of the competent divisions of labor that some people establish in a group situation (e.g., Cole & Traupmann, 1980; McDermott, Cole, & Hood, 1978) and in the theoretical argument that social interaction is not only a mark of intelligence but also its primary basis (e.g., Doise, 1978; Doise & Mugny, 1981; Doise & Palmonari, 1984).

Psychologists have also preferred tests or questions that are "new" – that cannot be solved by repeating something learned from past experience. A contrasting and more recent approach is to analyze performance on repeated, familiar tasks, drawn from outside the laboratory.

Some of these studies stem from the recognition that skills are often context bound (tied to specific materials or situations), so that assessment in an unfamiliar context provides no reasonable way of assessing any general skill or process. Members of the Laboratory of Comparative Human Development have made this argument with special force (Scribner, Gay, Glick, & Sharp, 1971; Cole & Scribner, 1974; Laboratory of Comparative Human Development, 1982). Other studies of familiar tasks have emerged in analyses of the development of "expertise," acquired in the course of repeated experience with physics problems (e.g., Chi, Feltovich, & Glaser, 1981), judicial decisions (Lawrence, 1986), filling milk orders (Scribner, 1984), playing cards (Davidson, 1979) or cutting cloth (Lave, 1977). The focus of interest in all such cases is the acquisition of "tricks of the trade" (Goodnow, 1972). This shift in measures or in the situations one studies is of particular importance for this chapter and will be given somewhat closer attention than the previous three shifts have been given.

The first point to be noted is the background to the "novel task" tradition. It was seen as giving all people a relatively equal chance of success (no one individual was more likely than another to have met the task before) and as building on a distinction between "intelligence" and "learning." It also fitted well with the values and perceived needs of the societies to which most test makers belong. In these, a high value is placed on being innovative, on rising to the challenge of new problems in a world in which change is seen as inevitable and as desirable. Out of that orientation toward definition and measurement have come most of the formal measures psychologists use: intelligence tests, problem-solving tasks, Piagetian measures of cognition development.

Many of these novel measures work extremely well as predictors of performance in settings that also specialize in presenting questions that can seldom be answered by drawing directly on past everyday experience: school settings, for instance. At the same time, there has emerged the realization that all is not well with this approach, especially if used as the only approach to the study of intelligent behavior.

For one thing, the measures seem still to give an advantage to some people rather than to others. The link to past experience may have been attenuated but it has been far from eliminated. For another, the approach leads us away from any understanding of everyday life and the way people make sense of it – topics Armistead (1974) has described as "the very stuff" of what psychology should be about. More subtly, the approach leaves us with little understanding of the effects of experience. Once we begin to think about it, it is clear that we do improve or change in our performance when we meet the same kind of problem several times. It is difficult to study such effects, however, if we regularly use tasks or problems in which the links to past experience have become more and more indirect.

Finally, an exclusive reliance on novel tasks makes it difficult to study the effects of socialization. Once pointed out, it is easy to recognize that most of us learn to present an "intelligent self," to vary Goffman's (1959) phrase. Most of us learn to be "bright," "smart," or "talented" in ways that our society expects of us: developing our musical, mathmetical, spatial, verbal, and nonverbal skills in some accord with what is thought to be appropriate or important for our age, gender, or station. Most of us also learn when to display various kinds of "smart" behaviors: when to be flippant or serious, when to stress ideas or data, when to stay task oriented at some risk to social relationships, when to accept that social relationships are the real heart of a meeting's agenda, and when – as Covington and Omelich (1979) note – to avoid effort so that some room is left for an attribution to ability if one would only try. The nature of all this socialization is relatively neglected as a research topic. It is probably closest to the surface in studies of how people come to regard skill in mathematics as not "natural" to women and as requiring more effort from females than from males (cf. Parsons, Adler, & Kaczala, 1980). There are undoubtedly many other cultural messages about appropriate intelligent behaviors, all inviting research on the way such messages are delivered and absorbed at various ages.

Should we then abandon traditional approaches to the study of intelligence, or study only behaviors as they occur in naturalistic situations? That would seem unwise. The old tradition is a source of both data and concepts. Moreover, the new tradition of work on repeated tasks also has its limitations. The work deals so far with only a limited set of cognitive skills (e.g., arithmetic and memory skills). Social aspects and social cognitive skills have yet to be considered. The work is also, at this stage, restricted to the skills of adults.

A more moderate alternative is to find ways of combining work on intelligence tests, on problem solving with laboratory tasks, and on everyday behaviors. How to achieve such mergers is not an obvious next step. One way forward, however, lies in selecting for study behaviors with qualities that allow one to build on past work and at the same time to explore the neglected topics of daily life, socialization, display rules, and the effects of experience. What would such behaviors need to be like? To begin with, they should be observable in everyday life. They should be potentially observable in several everyday situations, so that there is some chance to ask about conditions that make them more or less likely to be displayed in one context as against another. They should evoke individual differences, and they should be observable at several ages or at several levels of skill, so that one has some chance to see how the skills emerge, what the components are, and how it is that a social context shapes or socializes us into the display of various kinds of skill. They should involve some aspect of "social intelligence" – a phrase acknowledging that we develop an understanding of people as well as of objects. Finally, the behaviors should be amenable to some forms of formal study, so that one might bring together the results of naturalistic and experimental approaches. I hope to show that the behaviors of organizing and reorganizing meet these several criteria.

The choice of organizing and reorganizing

One of the rewards of thinking about everyday life is the recognition that for some incidents in daily life we have little available psychological theory. The incidents may often seem small, but the sense remains of a phenomenon that is important but poorly understood.

For me, some organizing and reorganizing incidents have had that quality. The first feature to catch my eye was the presence of large individual differences. Some people appear to be better organizers and reorganizers than others are. Reorganizing is especially intriguing. In the face of a demand for change, some people panic. Some become stubbornly resistant to change. Some cannot see beyond the "ruin" of their plan or the pain of a change in their habits. Some nibble at the edges of the problem, making little changes here and there with no substantive success. A few are able to see quickly that the problem can be met by what I have come to call "locating the moveable bits and squeezable pieces'' (Goodnow & Burns, 1985) – changing the order of various segments, cutting down the time for one and expanding the time for another, shifting a task from one person to another, re-ordering priorities, deferring or abandoning all but the "essentials."

The second observation to catch my eye came from a novel, from the ending to John O'Hara's *From the Terrace*. A man once prominent and powerful, but now retired, is asked at short notice if he can pick up someone at the airport. The person to be picked up is a closer friend of the person who makes the request than of the person being asked. In effect, the request is to change one's own plans in order to solve the problems in someone else's schedule. The request is immediately understood as a telling sign that status and power have been lost. In the old days, no one would have assumed that this person was "available," "had time on his hands," or "had nothing better to do." I knew of little in the psychological literature that dealt with these social aspects of problem solving, but I again had the sense that the incident signaled something worth understanding if one were to try studying social intelligence or linking formal psychology with everyday life.

These observations – of individual differences and of delegation as a sometimes acceptable form of problem solving – suggested that organizing and reorganizing behaviors met some of the criteria I had in mind for "intelligent behaviors worth studying." None of these observations, however, had much to do with children, and my ideal was a set of behaviors that could be traced through a life-span. The gap has been filled by some material on children that allows analysis of what organizing and reorganizing involve in their lives. One source is a study of children's tasks about the house that has raised some interesting questions about acceptable delegation to others (Goodnow, et al., 1986). The other is a large-scale survey of primary school children in Australia, conducted by the Australian Department of Social Security and containing several questions about the course of the day and about areas of change: What would you change if you could change one thing in the morning? At school? In the world for other children? Details of the children's answers to these and other questions are contained in Goodnow and Burns (1985). For the present paper, I shall use only comments that provide examples of early reorganization tasks and that help clarify the nature of the demand and of the skill.

A first component: learning some physical constraints

Consider the task of getting ready for school. It is an everyday version of many planning tasks in the sense that a number of activities have to be fitted into a reasonable sequence within a limited time period. In the words of a fourth-grader:

You have to have a shower, get dressed, have breakfast, clean your teeth, make your bed, feed the cat, catch the bus. And you must not be late. By the time you get to school, you're already tired.

In short, organization is called for. So also is reorganization, if one sleeps late or takes more than the time usually allocated for a particular task.

What do the children's comments tell us about the nature of organizing and reorganizing? The comments highlight the recognition of options: of solutions by way of combining, dropping, moving, or compressing various activities. They also highlight the recognition that some activities, by virtue of their perceived qualities or features, are more open than are others to different options. I shall trace out some of these perceived qualities.

Units as combinable or incompatible

The children often use the word "instead." "I wish instead of school I could go fishing, play at home, stay in bed, watch television" are frequent wishes. The term "instead" implies a recognition that two activities are incompatible. They cannot be combined. The one means that the other has to go. The same understanding is implied by the use of "but" as in the comment: "I wish I could have more time in the morning to have a swim, but I don't want to get out of bed any earlier." By contrast, there are few comments on what might be combined. Those that occur are mainly in the form of combining television with some other activity. I wish, some children say, that "I could eat breakfast in front of the TV" or that "I could stay in my snuggly bed and watch television." The real extent of combining segments may be larger than the comments suggest. The combinations that do receive spontaneous comment seem to do so largely because they have been vetoed but remain as attractive ways of what Wilensky (1981) has called the "piggybacking" of goals.

Units as more or less malleable

Other than by combining segments, how could one solve problems caused by not waking up on time or by misjudging the time that some morning task might take?

The children's comments suggest that part of the first inspection consists of tagging some pieces as unchangeable. Out of the 2,000-odd suggestions for change in one's morning, only two are for getting up earlier, and one of those is quickly ruled out ("but then I would be even more tired"). The largest set of suggestions is that the piece at the far end of the sequence should change. All would be well, the children argue, if school would start a little later. To take one example:

I wish school didn't start until about a quarter to eleven so that we can make our beds, tidy our room, have a shower, clean our teeth and have a good breakfast. Then you might have time to watch a little television and you don't have to rush.

It is unlikely, however, that school will start later or "come to me" as one child suggested. In effect, the units at each end of the sequence turn out to be unalterable. Some middle unit will have to give way.

One candidate is the route to school. "I wish I was the fasts [sic] runner in the world so I would not be late," says one child. "I wish my mother could drive me to school," says another. "I wish I could make the bus go faster," says a third. "I wish I could fly to school at a trillion miles per second and never get tired or exhausted. I should make sure where to land," says a fourth. A fifth hopes more simply the "mum would sometimes do seventy miles per hour."

The most frequently mentioned candidate for change is breakfast. Time and again, it is mentioned as the squeezed or sacrificed activity. To choose a few comments:

I wish I had enough time in the morning to have a full breakfast.
I wish I could sleep in and have a big breakfast and still get to school on time.
I wish I could sleep in and get up when I want. And I wish when I did that, I would not have to rush and would still have a big breakfast.

These nominations for squeezing particularly prompt one to ask, What features of a unit mark it as a candidate for particular kinds of change? Take the dropping or the compressing of breakfast as an example. One possibility is that breakfast catches attention because it is a segment that can be reduced. Among children, at least, it is usually easier to eat half a breakfast than it is to go out the door half-dressed. Another possibility is that breakfast stands out because it takes up such a large part of the available time that change in this segment would have considerable freeing up effect on others. "I wish a machine could be invented so it would dress me and give me breakfast in tablets so I could get up late," to use the words of a fifth-grader. To these information-processing possibilities, one should add another that is less cognitive. Breakfast may stand out because it is the piece where the necessary squeezing is most regretted. Few children would lament having less time to tidy one's room in terms such as the following:

I wish that I could sleep in longer than I do. I wouldn't have to do the dishes and make my bed. And I would have more time for breakfast and not have it taking [sic] away when I am halfway.

At this point, we have an example of an everyday demand for reorganization appearing early in life. Some environments may make this demand less strongly than do others. It seems feasible, however, that even in the most traditional and routinized settings one could locate examples of this type of demand.

We also have an indication that when this type of demand is made some units or some activities are seen as better candidates for combining, moving, and squeezing than are others. And we have the suggestion that underlying this choice is the early recognition that activities have qualities that give rise to physical and time constraints on what is possible or that allow particular kinds of change. How does this information fit in with more formal analyses of planning?

Links to the formal literature on planning

Some of the formal literature deals with theoretical analyses of planning as a process. The concern is sometimes directed toward the possible description of planning behaviors (e.g., Miller, Galanter, & Pribram, 1960; Wilensky, 1981) and sometimes toward the analysis of the kinds of knowledge that planning generally requires. This required knowledge may be about the planning process itself – knowledge usually considered under the heading of "metacognition" or "cognitive monitoring" (e.g., Brown, Bransford, Ferrara, & Campione, 1983; Brown & De Loache, 1978) or "metaplanning" (Wilensky, 1981). It may also be in the form of "world knowledge": the knowledge, for instance, that "asking for something is a way of getting something from someone" (Wilensky, 1981, p. 200).

Available also are some empirical analyses of plans offered by people for various activities. I shall concentrate on studies using tasks that parallel most closely the start of the morning. In these studies, subjects are given a map showing the location of several places and a list of errands that might be fitted into a given time (Hayes-Roth & Hayes-Roth, 1979; Lawrence, Dodds, & Volet, 1984; Oerter, 1981). Between 11 a.m. and 5 p.m., for instance, how could one meet a friend for lunch, see a film, go to the bank, buy a book, choose a birthday gift, and be in time to pick up the car at a given garage? Such tasks have brought out developmental changes in attention to time constraints (Oerter, 1981), the benefits of experience (housewives in the study by Lawrence et al. plan more effectively and fit in more errands than do adolescents), and the presence of two forms of planning: a hierarchical top-down style, and a more "opportunistic" mode in which some top-down planning is combined with side steps and on-the-spot revisions to take advantage of being in a particular spot (Hayes-Roth & Hayes-Roth, 1979).

To this material, the children's comments add the need for research on two aspects. One is the acquisition of the "world knowledge" that allows particular plans or opportunistic variations to be considered. One does need to learn, for example, how much time it takes to carry out any morning activity, and that parents do not usually approve of watching television while eating breakfast.

The other aspect is the perception of segments as having particular features or qualities that suggest or restrict various kinds of options and changes. These perceptions stand out very clearly in the children's comments. They are, however, given little or no place in current studies of planning, even though they must have a strong influence on the points at which one makes opportunistic revisions (Hayes-Roth & Hayes-Roth, 1979) or attempts to overlap and piggyback goals (Wilensky, 1981). To take account of these perceptions, one needs in fact to reach back to an older literature: to the argument by Polya (1957) and by Duncker (1945) that the essence of problem solving is the way people perceive tasks or segments of tasks as having particular qualities, and to empirical work on the way some segments come to be regarded as "fixed" and unavailable for a change in function (Duncker, 1945) or come to be "cognitively embedded" and seen as unavailable for separation into detachable and moveable segments (Scheerer & Huling, 1960).

In short, we are led to a new concern with the developmental aspects of these feature perceptions or feature analyses, and to the recognition that an older literature on such feature perception among problem-solving adults may be profitably combined with a more recent literature on planning. There remains, however, a major aspect of planning or problem solving in daily life that is poorly represented in any set of formal studies. This is the social aspect. The children's comments on the start of the day highlight the way that organizing and reorganizing are often social in nature. They involve other people. In fact, the solution to problems may consist of turning to other people as resources. The nature of this social aspect is the topic of the next sections.

A second component: social aspects

It must be rare in everyday life that organizing and reorganizing take place without other people being involved. What is the nature of that involvement? And what needs to be learned to cope with it or work with it?

The children's comments on starting the day and on household tasks suggest four aspects.

First, other people may provide you with nicely varied experiences. These may differ in such a way that you can identify some pieces as always occurring and others as sometimes happening, a patterning of experience that allows the identification of "fixed" and "changeable" slots within the scripts of everyday life (Nelson, 1973).

Second, other people may point out to you what can be changed. Their inspection of the sequence rather than your own active inspection and thought may give rise to your knowledge of what can be moved or squeezed.

In such cases, the skills needed are mainly those called for in implementing someone else's suggestions or in knowing who to turn to for suggestions.

Third, other people may need to give approval to your choice of pieces to be moved or squeezed. To take the start of the day again as an example, not all parents agree that breakfast should be the prime candidate. In the words of one child, "I wish that every morning instead of my mother pushing me to have breakfast I could fly and be free." In fact, many mornings seem to involve a great deal of negotiation as to what can be dropped, deferred, or given "a lick and a promise." In such cases, the skills most needed appear to be negotiating skills. One needs to learn the arguments and justifications that will persuade whoever holds the seal of approval.

Fourth, the most appealing solution may be to alter someone else's pattern of work: to change their schedule or to have them take over tasks. The latter behavior (shifting tasks from one person to another) is the form of change I wish to stress. It is a form of problem-solving that appears under many everyday labels (off-loading, delegating, subcontracting, doing favors, helping out) but is seldom formally studied.

The example from O'Hara's novel points to one direction of potential shifting: from others to you. The appropriate learning in such positions must consist either of defensive action (heading off the request or learning to say "no" effectively) or in making clear the conditions of acceptance. I wish to place more stress on the other direction of shifting: from oneself to others. What does it involve?

To shift tasks effectively, I propose, one needs to learn what can be most easily moved. The children's comments point to the acquisition of several rules about what can and cannot be delegated. In their everyday life, the first rule seems to be that you should not ask other people to clean up after you. A special reason has to be produced if you wish to ask someone else to make your bed, put away your toys, pick up your dirty clothes, tidy up a mess you have made. Such requests, the children and their mothers imply, run the risk of placing the other individual in the category of servant. They violate a rule that people in Australian society are expected to learn and follow unless there are good reasons not to, such as "You used it, you put it away" or "you made this mess, you clean it up." There are as well hints of a second rule: "You started it, you finish it," but that seems to be applied more gently and to be qualified by how far it is reasonable to expect an anticipation of future problems, especially if they are children or novices.

In order to shift tasks effectively, one also needs to learn who may legitimately and reliably be asked to do what. If the children's comments are a guide, you might in current Australian society ask your mother or a sibling to make your bed on a rushed morning, but you would seldom, if ever, ask your father. You might ask your father to give you a lift to school, but even that seems more likely to be asked of mothers. Mothers, in fact, seem to play a special role in everyday reorganization, serving as the area of "give" or "slack" in the system. That may be because mothers react more kindly to requests (rejecting fewer as illegitimate) or because mothers are more available and can more often vary their schedules. In fact, the only lament heard for a "working mother" was from a fourth-grader who said he "used to be lucky; when my mum didn't work, she used to pick me up after school on rainy days."

Finally, to shift tasks effectively, what needs to be learned is the expected exchange, the expected pattern of reciprocity. At this homely level, children are already acquiring the knowledge that "favors" need to be paid for or "returned." The exchange may vary. It may consist only of being properly appreciative or grateful, or it may take the form of being willing, if asked, to take on the same or an equivalent task. The mothers in our study of household tasks seemed to place particular stress on this aspect of learning, perhaps because the exchange is subtle (not always an exact quid pro quo) or because there is often some time delay between the first favor and its return – conditions that make the learning of rules or conditions more difficult than if the return is an identical favor or if consequences are immediate.

In short, one can begin to see at this everyday level in the lives of children the outlines of learning about the limits and the niceties of an always tempting way of solving problems, namely, passing some pieces to someone else.

Some links to the formal literature

If we are to understand the social aspects of organizing and reorganizing in everyday life, we shall need to know more about negotiating skills and about delegation: prime skills in the use of social resources or in coping with social constraints. I shall focus on delegation, a form of problem-solving that has received some mention in the planning literature although much remains to be discovered.

Delegation as a possible move in an errand-running task is mentioned by Oerter (1981) in connection with data from unpublished work by Dreher and Dreher (1978, cited by Oerter, 1981). Subjects ranged from age 10 years to adulthood. With age, they showed an increase in consideration for time limits and in the use of a bicycle that was available. They also showed a slight increase in "delegation" (sending someone else to the bank), although the solution was used infrequently even by adults.

Oerter (1981) raises some interesting questions. One is the issue of what determines the selection of people to whom one delegates. The material cited from Dreher and Dreher suggests a development from family members to friends, acquaintances, and people for whom the primary qualities are their "qualification and eligibility" (Oerter, 1981, p. 75). The interaction of that progression with the specific qualities of various tasks would be interesting to pursue. A further issue is the possibly late appearance of delegation. Oerter (1981, p. 75) concludes that "the delegation principle appears relatively late in the cognitive development of planning strategies." Our "at-home" data suggest that the notion of delegation may appear quite early in everyday life. That impression would fit also with the mention of some young subjects solving the problem of remembering things for school by asking their mothers to remember for them (Kreutzer, Leonard, & Flavell, 1982). Rather than seeing delegation as a late achievement, it seems more reasonable to consider that the degree of use varies with the perception of its being, for a particular task, feasible and proper.

The most explicit attention to delegation I have so far found is within an article by Fikes (1982) on the way in which "informal cooperative work proceeds." The specific concern of Fikes and his colleagues was with the extent to which office procedures might be regarded as "analogous to a collection of computers executing a program" (Fikes, 1982, p. 332) and hence amenable to fairly straightforward automation. Their conclusion was an even stronger turning away from a simple computer model than was the Hayes-Roths' (1981) turning away from a top-down model for an account of errand-planning. "Simple-program execution" was eventually discarded as "an inadequate basis for automating" and as "misleading as a metaphor for understanding the skills and knowledge needed by computers or people to do the work" (Fikes, 1982, p. 333). What gave rise to such a conclusion was the fluidity of work arrangements and the significance of "social process" in determining the "negotiated agreement between the client and contractor" (p. 333) or between contractor and subcontractor. The delegation of authority, the possibilities of subcontracting and of "one-time agreements," and the presence of complex agreements among three parties were particularly difficult to account for in usual automation terms and strongly influenced the conclusion that "standard computer program description techniques (e.g., flowcharts) are hopelessly inadequate" (Fikes, 1982, p. 339).

What kind of approach might be a viable alternative? Fikes (1982) suggests that the analysis of informal cooperative work requires the analysis of "commitments" that give the agents involved considerable freedom "to decide how and whether a given commitment has been fulfilled" (p. 343). The approach is described in theoretical terms only, but it offers so far the best fit to tasks such as getting oneself ready for school in the morning (with the general commitment to "being ready") and to mothers' reports of children's work around the house (the general commitment is to "taking a share"; the negotiations about that share and the possibilities of exchange and subcontracting can be intricate). In effect, if we were to study delegation or other social aspects of organizing and reorganizing, the concepts proposed by Fikes (1982) would provide a good starting point.

A third component: facilitating conditions

So far I have suggested that one part of learning to be competent or intelligent in organizing and reorganizing consists of coming to understand the physical, time, and social constraints on what may be dropped, combined, substituted, moved, squeezed, or given to someone else. It is easy to imagine that age and experience affect such learning. It is also easy to imagine that some situations allow easier organizing and reorganizing than others do.

Some forms of difference among situations are the topic of this section. They are of interest not only because they alter the likelihood of intelligent behavior being displayed at a particular time, but also because they provide a way of breaking down those mysterious variables: "experience" or "social context." One person's experience may differ from another's largely in the extent to which situations of a particular type have been encountered.

Some possibilities are highlighted by the contrasting quality of children's answers to two questions: "If you could change one thing at school, what would you change?" "If you could change one thing in the world for other children, what would you change?" Suggestions for changes in school were fluent, assured, and packed with creative ideas for moving pieces around (Goodnow & Burns, 1985). Suggestions for changes in the world were either unimaginative or vague and uncertain. The children suddenly seemed less intelligent. Why should this be so?

Suggested changes at school

From an early age, children are able to generate suggestions for changes in a school timetable. They make such proposals as these (second- third-, and fourth-graders):

Easy things right after lunch. (grade 2)
Spelling on Sunday, because then I would not be there. (grade 3)
School for an hour and fifteen minutes, and that would be big lunch and little lunch (recess). (grade 3)
Math's first thing when you're fresh. (grade 4)

In addition, children often put their proposals in the form "less this, more that," pointing to a recognition that change in one part of the system needs to be offset by change in another.

How is it that this type of reorganizational thinking can be so free and so specific? The setting seems to have three features: (1) a clear value to moving pieces; (2) relatively few social constraints, for instance, few questions about the legitimacy of moving a school subject from one time slot to another, at least from the child's point of view (teachers may struggle to keep "prime time''); and (3) the availability of many models. A few teachers may treat timetables as sacred, but most school settings provide many examples of moving activities around to accommodate assemblies, examinations, visiting dignitaries, absent teachers, or rainy days. In effect, the climate is relatively conducive to thinking freely about reorganization possibilities even if one is seldom asked in most schools to propose changes.

Suggested changes in the world

By contrast, thinking about world changes places one at a great disadvantage. Understanding the nature of the disadvantage helps bring out sources of difficulty likely to apply to many reorganization problems. To bring out the difficulties, I shall propose first that the question about change in the world is an everyday version of some classical formal problems – problems known as "cannibals and missionaries," "foxes and geese," or "Tower of Hanoi." The pieces in these puzzles must be moved around from one place to the other (one side of the river to another or one tower to another). Some constraints must be observed (cannibals must not outnumber missionaries on any one side, large pieces must not sit above smaller pieces in the tower). Despite its surface difference, the question about social change has much the same form as those laboratory problems. The question is readily understood (after grade 2) as implying two groups ("haves" and "have nots") and the need to rearrange pieces so that the "have nots" improve their position, usually by some shift of goods from the "haves."

Why do the children appear less competent with this kind of problem than with the school problem? The first thing to note is that there is little confusion about the people who would benefit from changes. The children have readily available to mind a set of categories, a set of named groups: "the poor," "the blind," "the starving children," "the Kampucheans," "the retarded."

There is less clarity and confidence about what should be moved toward these groups, how the moves should occur, and what the constraints are on effective moves. Some children see these problems as coped with by a third party. The "haves" give to the "have nots" by contributing to charitable organizations that arrange the collection and the distribution. This delegation occasionally gives rise to some odd perceptions of what is moved where: for example, one second-grader suggested, "we should give food to the blind." For the most part, however, these conventional solutions are relatively straightforward. The only constraints are presumably that the "haves" should not be asked to give so much that it would be painful or would convert them into "have nots."

Once the suggestions move away from these conventional and relatively "unthinking" solutions, the children are in difficulty. The moveable pieces are mostly things (food, clothes, money, schools, hospitals) and occasionally people (mainly in the form of moving refugees from one country to the other). The children express reservations about both forms of movement. They are not sure about value, as reflected by such statements as "My dad says money and stuff don't always get there," "It won't do any good if people don't learn to care for one another," and "We could bring them here, but we don't have many jobs." They are not sure about cost: "They might like it better in their own place," "We have a lot of unemployed and they would take our jobs." They are not sure about feasibility: "The rich should give money, but they are pretty stubborn," "All the governments should change so there are no wars – but they won't."

Such uncertainties make it difficult to appear intelligent in the face of the request to think about this social problem. There are also some further negative factors. One is that the surrounding society is often of little help. Even if "the poor" or "the needy" were part of a child's direct experience of the world, rather than simply being read about or heard about, the information provided is not conducive to clear thinking about novel moves. The information often comes in packaged form ("food for the starving children") that invites no inventiveness, no novel solutions, and no questioning. Where questions are raised, they may not be about other ways to proceed but about the very legitimacy of all the moves children have heard about – "the poor should help themselves," "the money goes into someone's pockets" – comments likely to stop thought rather than provoke it.

The second feature has to do with the nature of the question and with the way in which a successful answer is defined. In a sense, the question about "change in the world" is actually two questions. The adult is asking, Can you come up with a sensible suggestion? The adult is also asking, Can you at the same time display your compassion, your awareness that there are people less fortunate than you, your lack of smugness? In all life, I suggest, solutions or answers that have to succeed on double sets of criteria are difficult. They range from "what are you going to be when you grow up?" (your anser should be sensible; it should also display a proper mixture of modesty, ambition, and an awareness that you should seek a job) to "what do you think of my chances for this job?" (be thoughtful, show interest, and be careful of my feelings). By contrast with such double-standard questions, proposing changes in the school timetable is far less taxing and allows far more opportunities, with fewer risks, for appearing both intelligent and interesting.

Some links to the formal literature

One of the recent moves in developmental psychology concerns the nature of the environment or social context in which knowledge is received or constructed. The classical view, represented especially in Piagetian theory, treats the environment as if it benignly offered all the information one might seek. The major limitation to learning then lay in the individual's capacity to absorb what was offered. A more recent position within psychology is to argue that environments are often not so benign. They may in fact restrict access to knowledge, labeling some knowledge as restricted, confidential, or not proper for a particular individual to acquire.

This difference in positions has been commented upon in an earlier paper (Goodnow, Knight, & Cashmore, 1986). I now wish to add a suggestion from the sociologist Peter Berger (1977). Berger regards all societies as designating some domains as not open for innovation and some as allowing individual variation (the latter usually labeled "private" as in "the private sector" or "the privacy of one's home"). Modern society, Berger argues, more and more rules out innovation in one's job but encourages in compensation the free reign of imagination in organizing and decorating one's house or home. A certain degree of individuality in these domains becomes almost mandatory within some social groups. Part of socialization, in Berger's analysis, consists of learning the domains that encourage, permit, or forbid innovation. Specifying the nature of such social learning – the acquisiton of ideas about domains where "doing one's own thing" will meet with varying reactions – would be an interesting step towards uncovering more about the everyday, real life aspects of organizing and reorganizing.

Some open questions

I began this chapter with the hope that tracing a particular behavior across both formal studies of cognition and some everyday situations would provide a way of linking at least two current approaches to the study of intelligent behaviors – one stressing the everyday social contexts of intelligent behaviors and the other stressing behaviors observed in laboratory settings. In both approaches, one might proceed by way of either naturalistic observation or focused questions and experimental arrangements. The choice of method has not been my concern so much as the questions one might be prompted to ask. These are questions so far not well covered by formal research on intelligence or on cognitive development: questions, for instance, about the early recognition of several planning solutions and the feature perceptions that give rise to regarding some activities as more open than others to particular forms of change, about the social aspects of organizing and reorganizing (negotiation and delegating skills especially), and about the conditions that give rise to a readier display of intelligent reorganizing on some problems than on others. All these questions are amenable to research. Their emergence is one sign of the feasibility and the benefits of seeking to combine approaches to the study of specific intelligent behaviors, whether these appear in the laboratory, the testing room, or the course of everyday life.

References

Armistead, N. (Ed.) (1974). *Reconstructing social psychology*. Harmondsworth: Penguin.

Berger, P. (1977). *Facing up to modernity*. Harmondsworth: Penguin.

Brown, A. L., Bransford, J. D., Ferrara, R. A., & Campione, J. C. (1983). Learning, remembering and understanding. In J. H. Flavell & E. M. Markman (Eds.), *Handbook of child psychology* (4th ed.) (Vol. 3, pp. 77–166). New York: Wiley.

Brown, A., & De Loache, J. (1978). Skills, plans and self-regulation. In R. S. Siegler (Ed.), *Children's thinking: What develops?* (pp. 3–36). Hillsdale, NJ: Erlbaum.

Chen, M. J., Braihwaite, V., & Huang, S. I. (1982). Attributes of intelligent behaviour: Perceived relevance and difficulty by Australian and Chinese students. *Journal of Cross Cultural Psychology, 13*, 139–156.

Chi, M. T. H., Feltovich, P., & Glaser, R. (1982). Categorization and representation of physics problems by experts and novices. *Cognitive Science, 5*, 121–152.

Cole, M., Gay, J., Glick, J., & Sharp, D. W. (1971). *The cultural context of learning and thinking*. New York: Basic.

Cole, M., & Scribner, S. (1974). *Culture and thought*. New York: Wiley.

Cole, M., & Traupmann, K. (1980). Comparative cognitive research: learning from a learning disabled child. *Minnesota Symposium on Child Development* (Vol. 12). Minneapolis, MN: University of Minnesota Press.

Covington, M. V., & Omelich, C. L. (1979). Effort: The double-edged sword in school achievement. *Journal of Educational Psychology, 71*, 169–182.

Dasen, P. (1984). The cross-cultural study of intelligence: Piaget and the Baoule. *International Journal of Psychology, 19*, 407–434.

Davidson, G. (1979). An ethnographic psychology of aboriginal cognition. *Oceania, 49*, 270–294.

Doise, W. (1978). *Groups and individuals*. Cambridge: Cambridge University Press.

Doise, W., & Mugny, G. (1981). *La construction sociale de l'intelligence*. Paris: Intereditions.

Doise, W., & Palmonari, A. (1984). *Social interaction in individual development*. Cambridge: Cambridge University Press.

Duncker, K. (1945). On problem-solving. *Psychological Monographs, 58*, No. 270.

Fikes, R. E. (1982). A commitment-based framework for describing informal cooperative work. *Cognitive Science, 6*, 331–348.

Fischer, J. L., & Fischer, A. (1963). The New Englanders of Orchardtown. In B. B. Whiting (Ed.), *Six cultures: Studies of child rearing*. New York: Wiley.

Gill, R., & Keats, D. M. (1980). Elements of intellectual competence: Judgements by Malay University students. *Journal of Cross Cultural Psychology, 11*, 233–243.

Goffman, E. (1959). *The presentation of self in everyday life*. Garden City, NY: Doubleday.

Goodnow, J. J. (1972). Rules and repertoires, rituals and tricks of the trade: Social and informational aspects to cognitive and representational development. In S. Farnham-Diggory (Ed.), *Information processing in children* (pp. 83–102). New York: Academic Press.

Goodnow, J. J. (1976). The nature of intelligent behaviour: Questions raised by cross-cultural studies. In L. B. Resnick (Ed.), *The nature of intelligence* (pp. 169–188). New York: Erlbaum.

Goodnow, J. J. (1984). On being judged intelligent. *International Journal of Psychology, 19*, 391–406.

Goodnow, J. J., & Burns, A. (1985). *Home and school: Child's eye view*. Sydney, Australia: Allen & Unwin.

Goodnow, J. J., Knight, R., & Cashmore, J. (1986). Adult social cognition: Implications of parents' ideas for approaches to development. In M. Perlmutter (Ed.), *Minnesota Symposia on Child Development* (Vol. 18, pp. 287–324). Hillsdale, NJ: Erlbaum.

Hayes-Roth, B., & Hayes-Roth, F. (1979). A cognitive model of planning. *Cognitive Science, 3*, 275–310.

Kreutzer, M. A., Leonard, S. K., & Flavell, J. H. (1982). Prospective remembering in children. In U. Neisser (Ed.), *Memory observed: Remembering in natural contexts* (pp. 343–348). San Francisco: Freeman.

Laboratory of Comparative Human Development. (1983). Culture and cognitive development. In W. Kessen (Ed.), *Handbook of child development* (4th ed.) (Vol. 1, pp. 346–356). New York: Wiley.

Lave, J. (1977). Cognitive consequences of traditional apprenticeship training in West Africa. *Anthropology and Educational Quarterly, 7*, 177–180.

Lawrence, J. A. (1986). Expertise on the bench: Modelling magistrates' judicial decision-making. In M. T. H. Chi, R. Glaser, & M. Farr (Eds.), *The nature of expertise*. Hillsdale, NJ: Erlbaum.

Lawrence, J. A., Dodds, A., & Volet, S. (1983). An afternoon off: A comparative study of adults' and adolescents' planning activities. *Proceedings of the Australian Association for Research in Education*. Canberra, Australia: A.A.R.E.

McDermott, R. P., Cole, M., & Hood, L. (1978). "Let's try to make it a good day" – Not so simple ways. *Discourse Processes, 3*, 155–168.

Miller, G. A., Galanter, E. H., & Pribram, C. H. (1960). *Plans and the structure of behaviour*. New York: Holt.

Nelson, K. (1973). Social cognition in a script framework. In J. Flavell & L. Ross (Eds.), *Social cognitive development* (pp. 97–118). Cambridge: Cambridge University Press.

Nerlove, S. B., Roberts, J. M., & Klein, R. E., Yarbrough, C., & Habicht, J. B. (1974). Natural indications of cognitive development: An observational study of rural Guatemalan children. *Ethos, 2*, 265–295.

Oerter, R. (1981). Cognitive socialization during adolescence. *International Journal of Behavioral Development, 4*, 61–76.

Parsons, J. E., Adler, T. F., & Kaczala, C. M. (1982). Socialization of achievement attitudes and beliefs. *Child Development, 53*, 310–321.

Polya, G. (1957). *How to solve it: A new aspect of mathematical method*. Garden City, NY: Doubleday.

Rogoff, B. (1982). Integrating context and cognitive development. In M. Lamb & A. Brown (Eds.), *Advances in development psychology* (Vol. 2, pp. 125–167). Hillsdale, NJ: Erlbaum.

Rogoff, B., & Lave, J. (Eds.). (1984) *Everyday cognition: Its developmental and social context*. Cambridge, MA: Cambridge University Press.

Scheerer, M., & Huling, M. D. (1960). Cognitive embeddedness in problem solving: A theoretical and experimental analysis. In B. Kaplan and S. Wapner (Eds.), *Perspectives in psychological theory: Essays in honor of Heinz Werner* (pp. 256–302). New York: Interecnational Universities Press.

Scribner, S. (1984). Studying working intelligence. In B. Rogoff & J. Lave (Eds.), *Everyday cognition: Its development in social context* (pp. 9–40). Cambridge, MA: Harvard University Press.

Serpell, R. (1974). Estimates of intelligence in a rural community of Eastern Zambia. *Human Development Research Unit Reports*, No. 25.

Sternberg, R. J., Conway, J. L., Ketron, J. L. & Bernstein, M. (1981). People's conception of intelligence. *Journal of Personality and Social Psychology, 41*, 37–55.

Wilensky, R. (1981). Meta-planning: Representing and using knowledge about planning in problem solving and natural language understanding. *Cognitive Science, 5*, 197–283.

8   The theory of multiple intelligences: some issues and answers

Joseph M. Walters and Howard Gardner

A fable

Two Martians were sent on an expedition to Earth to investigate what Earthlings were calling "issues of the mind." The first Martian landed quite by chance on the campus of a major university. He stopped people who were passing by and asked them about "the mind." Even though he spent most of the morning in this fashion, the answers were so confusing that he was nearly forced to give up. Then he came upon the Educational Psychologist.

The Educational Psychologist was eager to help. The key to the "mind" is Intelligence, she explained. An individual who is intelligent will do well in school and will be successful throughout his life. To measure this intelligence, she continued, psychologists have recently invented special tests, in which subjects are asked questions that require short answers: "Who wrote the Iliad?" or "Repeat the following digits: 2 5 6 7 9 3 4 2." And so on. Those subjects who answer many questions correctly on these tests are the very ones who will succeed at almost anything they try. The Martian asked why that might be. The psychologist explained that intelligence was a general talent that could be turned in the direction of most any task including the task of answering short-answer questions. Measuring this talent with such tests, she concluded, was quite reliable. The Martian was just about to ask about how the short-answer questions informed a theory of "mind," when the Educational Psychologist hurried off to teach her next class.

Meanwhile, the second Martian was pursuing a different kind of investigation. The "mind," he reasoned, should be related to tasks that humans performed. Moreover, different individuals may have different minds, which in turn could account for why they perform various tasks differently. The Martian concluded that the most straightforward investigative technique

Acknowledgments. The research reported in this chapter was supported by grants from the Bernard van Leer Foundation of The Hague, the Spencer Foundation of Chicago, and the Carnegie Corporation of New York. We would like to thank Robert Sternberg and Richard Wagner for their careful reading of an earlier draft of this manuscript.

163

would be a simple observation of humans performing tasks, in which he would pay special attention to those things that some humans did exceptionally well.

The second Martian landed first in the South Seas. During a brief tour of the Islands, he came upon a sailor who had developed extraordinary skills at navigation without the use of sophisticated equipment. The next stop found him in Africa, where he observed an elaborate hunting society. Later he landed in a Japanese city, where he watched an expert computer programmer at work, on to India to visit a prominent religious leader, and then to Europe to watch two great tennis players compete. He listened to a musician, observed a biologist, met a businessman, a seer, and a poet. And then it was time to return to Mars.

The Martian stopped at the university campus, where he picked up his colleague, who was playing frisbee with the Educational Psychologist. The second Martian described the people he had seen and the marvelous things they had created. He pointed out that in many cases, these exceptional individuals had taken intelligence tests and had done quite poorly – this was especially true of the South Seas sailor and the musician. He asked the Educational Psychologist about these other "intelligences."

The Educational Psychologist was amused at this innocence and patient in her response. She explained that she and others used the term in a different sense. Tasks involving music, sports, navigation, politics, and so on required "talent" or "skill," but not necessarily intelligence. Moreover, although perhaps some talented individuals do poorly on the special tests of intelligence, most people who are successful, regardless of their occupation, do relatively well. Intelligence, in addition to whatever special skill is required, is necessary in any problem-solving setting.

Then she paused. The special tests are only one indicator, she added. For example, when we choose graduate students in educational psychology we consider many other things as well. We want good "problem finders" as well as good "problem solvers." And before the Martians could ask her to explain this, she rushed off to a faculty meeting.

The Martians climbed into their ship and took off. They had quite a bit to think about on the way home. They had learned a great deal about the "mind" of earthlings. And they had learned that this "mind," whatever it was, did not as yet understand itself.

This fable is a caricature. We have used it to question the standard view of intelligence, as it has come to be accepted almost unreflectively by the society as a whole and by most professionals as well. We will present our critique as an alternative theory, developed over the past several years: we call this alternative approach the theory of Multiple Intelligences (MI theory).

We elected the approach taken by the second Martian. We wanted a way of looking at the matter that was not biased by either a prior commitment to a certain mode of testing or our Western point of view. This chapter will summarize the results of that investigation.

Like the second Martian, we prefer to examine performances and products that are prized by various cultures. We analyze how individuals of exceptional talents fashion these products and we look for signs of similar, if more modest, skills in the rest of the population. We have also examined the neurological literature, evidence from special populations, information about child development, clues from evolutionary history, as well as data from psychometrics and from psychological testing. We think that the abilities to fashion a poem, sonata, or geometric proof, to build a computer or a bridge, to organize a political campaign or direct a corporation, all require some form of intelligence, and that they may not all require the same form. If there is a plurality of abilities, as the framework of multiple intelligences would suggest, then it becomes of crucial importance to help people find suitable vocational and avocational niches. Such a brokering can provide for a more efficient and more harmonious society and can engender a population that exhibits feelings of efficacy.

As the term multiple intelligences indicates, we believe that human cognitive competence is better described in terms of a set of abilities, talents, or mental skills, which we call "intelligences." All normal people possess each of these skills to some extent; but by virtue of innate endowment and the particular history of training, individuals differ in the profile of skills and in their combination. We believe that this theory of intelligence may be more veridical and more humane than alternative views of intelligence and that it more adequately reflects the data of human "intelligent" behavior. In this chapter, we will briefly summarize the various "intelligences." We will then examine some of the questions raised by a theory that jettisons the standardized-test approach to the mind.

Multiple intelligences theory

What constitutes an intelligence?

The optimal definition of "intelligence" looms large in our inquiry. Indeed, it is in the formulation of a definition that the theory of multiple intelligences (MI) diverges from more traditional points of view. In our view, an Intelligence is an ability or set of abilities that permits an individual to solve problems or fashion products that are of consequence in a particular cultural setting. The problem-solving skill permits one to approach a situation, in which a goal is to be obtained, and to locate and pursue appropriate routes to that goal. The problems to be solved range from creating an ending to a story, to anticipating a mating move in chess, to repairing a quilt. The creation of a cultural product is the preferred route to capturing knowledge, transmitting knowledge, formulating new knowledge, and expressing views or feelings. These products range from scientific theories to musical compositions to political campaigns, and they are of consequence to the degree that the society attempts to foster their growth and development through the devotion of resources such as education, monetary reward, or high status.

MI theory is framed in light of the biological origins of each mental faculty. Only those skills that are universal to the human species are considered. Even so, the biological proclivity to participate in a particular form of mental activity must be coupled with the cultural manipulation or embodiment of that activity. For example, language, a universal skill, faculty, or "intelligence," may manifest itself particularly as writing in one culture, as oratory in another culture, and as a secret anagrammatic code in a third. Similarly, spatial ability, another universal human capacity, may be manifest as navigation in one society, hunting in a second, geometrical reasoning in a third, creation of a sculpture in a fourth.

Given the aim of identifying intelligences that are rooted in biology, and valued in one or more cultural settings, how does one actually discover an "intelligence"? In coming up with our list of intelligences, we consulted evidence from several different sources: knowledge about normal development and development in gifted individuals; information about the breakdown of cognitive skills under conditions of brain damage; studies of exceptional populations, including prodigies, idiots savants, and autistic children; data about the evolution of cognition over the millenia; cross-cultural accounts of cognition; psychometric studies, including examinations of correlations among tests; and psychological training studies, particularly measures of transfer and generalization across tasks.

Only those candidate intelligences that satisfied all or most of these criteria were selected as bona fide intelligences, and many candidates were rejected because they met only a few criteria or because one criterion refuted another. A more complete discussion of each of these "criteria for an Intelligence" as well as an account of the seven Intelligences which have been proposed so far, is found in Gardner's recent book, *Frames of Mind* (1983). In the concluding chapters of his book, Gardner considers how the theory might be disproved and compares it to alternative theories of intelligence and cognition.

In addition to satisfying the aforementioned criteria, each intelligence must have an identifiable core operation or set of operations. As a neurally based computational system, each intelligence is activated or "triggered" by certain kinds of internally or externally presented information. For example, one core of musical intelligence is the sensitivity to pitch relations, whereas one core of linguistic intelligence is the sensitivity to phonological features.

Both cases are supported by impressive evidence that all normal infants can respond to these cardinal features of an auditory signal (Eimas, Siqueland, Jusczyk, & Vigorito, 1971; Trehub, Bull, & Thorpe, 1984).

An intelligence must also be susceptible to encoding in a symbol system, that is, a culturally contrived system of meanings that captures and conveys important forms of information. A symbol system in this use of the term is an entity that either exemplifies or refers to any other entity. An intelligence is not itself symbolic but, through operation of the intelligence, symbols can be created and combined and eventually yield full-fledged symbolic products. Natural language, picturing, and mathematics – each closely identified with a particular intelligence – are but three nearly worldwide symbol systems that are necessary for human productivity. Sonnets, stories, plays, prayers, and reviews exemplify a range of symbolic products generated by the linguistic system.

The relationship of a candidate intelligence to a human symbol system is no accident. In fact, the existence of a core computational capacity anticipates the existence of a symbol system that exploits that capacity. Although it may be possible for an intelligence to proceed without an accompanying symbol system, a primary characteristic of human intelligence may well be its gravitation toward such an embodiment.

The seven intelligences

Having sketched the basic characteristics and identifying-criteria of an intelligence, we turn now to a brief consideration of each of the seven intelligences. We begin each sketch with a thumbnail biography of a person who demonstrates an unusual facility with that intelligence. These biographies illustrate the abilities central to the fluent operation of a given intelligence. Because we are using talented individuals as examples, it is important to stress that the intelligences exist in every normal person as well; we employ the "star" biographies only because they communicate the nature of an intellectual skill with particular clarity. Moreover, although each biography illustrates a particular intelligence, we do not wish to imply that in adulthood intelligences operate in isolation. Indeed, except in the case of abnormal persons, intelligences always work in concert, and any sophisticated adult role will involve a melding of several of them. After each capsule biography, we survey a few lines of evidence that support each candidate as an "intelligence."

Musical intelligence

When he was three years old, Yehudi Menuhin was smuggled into the San Francisco Orchestra concerts by his parents. The sound of Louis Persinger's violin so entranced the youngster that he insisted on a violin for his birthday and Louis Persinger as his teacher. He got both. By the time he was ten years old, Menuhin was an international performer. (Adapted from Menuhin, 1977)

Violinist Yehudi Menuhin's musical intelligence manifested itself even before he had touched a violin or received any musical training. His powerful reaction to that particular sound and his rapid progress on the instrument suggest that he was unlike other children his age and that perhaps he was biologically prepared in some way for that endeavor. In this way the unusual developmental patterns found in child prodigies support our claim that there is a biological underpinning and proclivity for a particular intelligence. Other special populations, such as autistic children who can play a musical instrument beautifully but who cannot speak, underscore the independence of musical intelligence from the others.

A brief consideration of the evidence suggests that musical skill passes the other principal tests for an intelligence. For example, certain parts of the brain play important roles in perception and production of music. These areas are characteristically located in the right hemisphere, although musical skill is not as clearly localized, or located in specifiable areas, as language. Although the particular susceptibility of musical ability to brain damage depends on the degree of training and other individual differences, there is clear evidence for "amusia," an isolated loss of musical ability.

Music apparently played an important unifying role in Stone Age societies. Birdsong provides a link to other species. Evidence from various cultures supports the notion that music is a universal faculty. Studies of infant development suggest a "raw" computational ability in early childhood. Finally, musical notation provides an accessible and lucid symbol system.

In short, evidence to support the interpretation of musical ability as an "intelligence" comes from many different sources. Even though musical skill is not typically considered an intellectual skill like mathematics, it qualifies under our criterion of yielding significant cultural products. By definition, it deserves consideration and, in view of the data, its inclusion is empirically justified.

Similar analysis support each of the other six intelligences as well. We can describe them only briefly here. Detailed accounts can be found in *Frames of Mind*.

Bodily-kinesthetic intelligence

Fifteen-year-old Babe Ruth played third base. During one game his team's pitcher was doing very poorly and Babe loudly criticized him from third base. Brother Mathias, the coach, called out, "Ruth, if you know so much about it, *you* pitch!" Babe was surprised and embarrassed because he had never pitched before, but Brother Mathias insisted. Ruth said later that at the very moment he took the pitcher's mound, he KNEW he was supposed to be a pitcher and that it was "the most natural thing in the world" for him to strike people out. Indeed, he went on to become a great major league pitcher (and, of course, achieved legendary status as a hitter). (Adapted from Conner, 1982)

Like Menuhin, Babe Ruth was a child prodigy who recognized his "instrument" immediately upon his first exposure to it. This recognition occurred in advance of formal training.

We use the term bodily-kinesthetic intelligence to refer to the abilities to use the whole body, or various portions of it (e.g., the hands or mouth) in the solution of problems or in the construction of products or displays. Dancers, athletes, actors, instrumentalists, surgeons all display significant bodily-kinesthetic intelligence. Control of bodily movements is of course localized in the motor cortex, with each hemisphere dominant or controlling bodily movements on the contralateral side. In right handers, the dominance for such movement is ordinarily found in the left hemisphere. The ability to perform movements when directed to do so can be impaired even in persons who can perform the same movements reflexively or on a nonvoluntary basis. The existence of specific apraxia, the loss of specific voluntary movements in the absence of general paralysis or loss of muscular strength and sensitivity, constitutes an intriguing line of evidence for a bodily-kinesthetic Intelligence.

Logical-mathematical intelligence. In 1983 Barbara McClintock won the Nobel Prize in medicine for her work in microbiology. Her intellectual powers of deduction and observation illustrate one form of logical-mathematical intelligence that is often labeled "scientific thinking." One incident is particularly illuminating. While a researcher at Cornell in the 1920s, McClintock was faced one day with a problem – while theory predicted 50 percent pollen sterility in corn, her research assistant (in the "field") was finding plants that were only 25 to 30 percent sterile. Disturbed by this discrepancy, McClintock left the cornfield and returned to her office where she sat for half an hour, thinking:

Suddenly I jumped and ran back to the (corn) field. At the top of the field (the others were still at the bottom) I shouted "Eureka, I have it! I know what the 30% sterility is!" . . . They asked me to prove it. I sat down with a paper bag and a pencil and I started from scratch, which I had not done at all in my laboratory. It had all been done so fast; the answer came and I ran. Now I worked it out step by step – it was an intricate series of steps – and I came out with [the same result]. [They] looked at the material and it was exactly as I'd said it was; it worked out exactly as I had diagrammed it. Now, why did I know, without having done it on paper? Why was I so sure? (Keller, 1982, p. 104)

This anecdotes illustrates two key facts of the logical-mathematical intelligence. First, in the gifted individual, the process of problem solving is often remarkably rapid – the successful scientist copes with many variables at once and creates numerous hypotheses that are each evaluated and then accepted or rejected in turn.

The anecdote also underscores the nonlinguistic nature of this particular Intelligence. A solution to a problem can be constructed before it is articulated. In fact, the solution process may be totally invisible, even to the problem solver as in this case. This need not imply, however, that discoveries of this sort – the familiar "aha" phenomenon – are mysterious, intuitive, or unpredictable. The fact that it happens more frequently to some people (perhaps the Nobel Prize winners) suggests the opposite. We interpret this cognitive breakthrough as the work of the logical-mathematical Intelligence. It is worth noting that most standardized instruments and most traditional definitions of intelligences feature the logical-mathematical faculty.

Linguistic intelligence

At the age of ten, T. S. Eliot created a magazine called "Fireside" to which he was the sole contributor. In a three day period during his winter vacation, he created eight complete issues. Each one included poems, adventures stories, a gossip column, and humor. Some of this material survives and it displays the talent of the poet. (Adapted from Soldo, 1982)

Calling linguistic skill an "intelligence" is consistent with the stance of traditional psychology. This candidate also passes our empirical tests as well. For instance, a specific area of the brain, called Broca's area, is responsible for the production of grammatical utterances. A person with damage to this area can understand words and sentences quite well but has difficulty putting them together in anything other than the simplest of utterances. At the same time, other thought processes may be entirely unaffected. Conversely, some persons who are otherwise retarded do speak normally and may even decode written texts at a very early age.

The gift of language is universal and its development in children is strikingly parallel across cultures. Even in deaf populations where a manual sign language is not explicitly taught, children will often "invent" their own manual language and use it surreptitiously. We thus see how an intelligence may operate independently of a specific input modality or output channel.

Spatial intelligence

Navigation around the Caroline Islands in the South Seas is accomplished without instruments. The position of the stars, as viewed from various islands, the weather patterns, and water color are the only sign posts. Each journey is broken into a series of segments; and the navigator learns the position of the stars within each of these segments. During the actual trip the navigator must envision mentally a reference island as it passes under a particular star and from that he computes the number of segments completed, the proportion of the trip remaining, and any corrections in heading that are required. The navigator cannot see the islands as he sails along; instead he maps their locations in his mental "picture" of the journey. (Gardner, 1983)

Spatial problem-solving ability is required for navigation as well as for the use of maps. Other spatial problem-solving capacities are brought to bear in visualizing an object seen from a different angle or in playing chess. The visual arts also require intelligence with respect to the use of space.

Evidence from brain research is clear and persuasive. Just as the left hemisphere has, over the course of evolution, been selected as the site of linguistic processing, the right hemisphere proves to be the site most crucial for spatial processing. Damage to the right posterior regions leads to impairment of the ability to find one's way around a site, to recognize faces or scenes, or to notice fine details.

Patients with damage specific to regions of the right hemisphere will attempt to compensate for their spatial deficits with linguistic strategies. They will try to reason aloud, to challenge the task, or even make up answers. But such nonspatial strategies are rarely successful.

Blind populations provide an illustration of the distinction between the spatial intelligence and visual perception. A blind person can recognize shapes by an indirect method, running a hand along the object translates into length of time of movement, which in turn is translated into size of object. For the blind person, the perceptual system of tactile modality plays the role assumed by visual modality in the seeing person. Analogies between the spatial reasoning of the blind and the linguistic reasoning of the deaf are noteworthy.

There are few child prodigies among visual artists, but there are idiots savants such as Nadia (Selfe, 1977). Despite a condition of severe autism, this preschool child made drawings of the most remarkable representational accuracy and expressive finesse.

Interpersonal intelligence With little formal training in special education and nearly blind herself, Anne Sullivan began the intimidating task of instructing a blind, deaf 7-year-old. Communication efforts were complicated by an emotional struggle as the child tried to cope with the world around her. At their first meal together, this scene occurred:

Annie did not allow Helen to put her hand into Annie's plate and take what she wanted, as she had been accustomed to do with her family. It became a test of wills – hand thrust into plate, hand firmly put aside. The family, much upset, left the dining room. Annie locked the door and proceeded to eat her breakfast while Helen lay on the floor kicking and screaming, pushing and pulling at Annie's chair. (After half an hour) Helen went around the table looking for her family. She discovered no one else was there and that bewildered her. Finally, she sat down and began to eat her breakfast, but with her hands. Annie gave her a spoon. Down on the floor it clattered, and the contest of wills began anew. (Lash, 1980, p. 52)

Anne Sullivan sensitively responded to the child's behaviors. She wrote home: "The greatest problem I shall have to solve is how to discipline and control her without breaking her spirit. I shall go rather slowly at first and try to win her love."

In fact, the first "miracle" occurred two weeks later, well before the famous pumphouse scene. Annie had taken Helen to a small cottage near the family's house where they could live alone. After seven days alone together, Helen's personality suddenly underwent a profound change – the therapy had worked:

My heart is singing with joy this morning. A miracle has happened! The wild little creature of two weeks ago has been transformed into a gentle child. (p. 54)

It was just a few weeks after this event that the first breakthrough in Helen's grasp of language occurred, and from that point on she progressed with "miraculous" speed. A significant key to that miracle was Anne Sullivan's insight into the "person" of Helen Keller.

Interpersonal intelligence builds on a core capacity to notice distinctions among others, in particular contrasts in their moods, temperaments, motivations, and intentions. In more elaborated forms, this intelligence permits a skilled adult to read the intentions and desires of others, even when these have been hidden. This skill appears in an highly sophisticated form in religious or political leaders, teachers, therapists, and parents. The Helen Keller–Anne Sullivan story suggests that this interpersonal intelligence does not depend on language.

Intrapersonal intelligence. In her essay "A sketch of the past," written almost as a diary entry, Virginia Woolf discusses the "cotton wool of existence," or the mundane events of life. She contrasts this "cotton wool" with three specific and poignant memories from childhood: a fight with her brother, seeing a particular flower in the garden, and hearing of the suicide of a past visitor. These remarks follow:

These are three instances of exceptional moments. I often tell them over, or rather they come to the surface unexpectedly. But now for the first time I have written them down, I realize something that I have never realized before. Two of these moments ended in a state of despair. The other ended, on the contrary, in a state of satisfaction.

The sense of horror (in hearing of the suicide) held me powerless. But in the case of the flower, I found a reason; and was thus able to deal with the sensation. I was not powerless.

Though I still have the peculiarity that I receive these sudden shocks, they are now always welcome; after the first surprise, I always feel instantly that they are particularly valuable. And so I go on to suppose that the shock-receiving capacity is what makes me a writer. I hazard the explanation that shock is at once in my case followed by the desire to explain it. I feel that I have had a blow; but it is not, as I thought as a child, simply a blow from an enemy hidden behind the cotton wool of daily life; it is or will become a revelation of some order; it is a token of some real thing behind appearances; and I make it real by putting it into words. (Woolf, 1976, pp. 69–70)

This quotation from Virginia Woolf vividly illustrates the intrapersonal intelligence – knowledge of the internal aspects of a person; the access to one's own feeling life, one's range of emotions, the capacity to effect discriminations among these emotions, and eventually to label them and to draw upon them as a means of understanding and guiding one's own behavior. The insights into personality illustrate the operation of the intrapersonal intelligence. Since this intelligence is the most private, it can be detected by an outside observer only through language, music, or some other expressive form of intelligence. In the above quote, for example, linguistic intelligence is drawn upon to convey intrapersonal knowledge. We note here the interaction of intelligences, a common phenomenon to which we will return later.

Both inter- and intrapersonal faculties pass the tests of an intelligence. They both feature problem-solving endeavors with significance for the individual and the species. Both can be manifested in symbol systems: the interpersonal intelligence finds expression in public rituals, whereas the intrapersonal intelligence is symbolized in the internal world of dreams. The susceptibility of intelligences to embodiment in symbol systems permits investigators to examine them, although in principle these intelligences might be detected through nonsymbolic and perhaps even physiological means.

In the individual's sense of self, one encounters a melding of inter- and intrapersonal components. Indeed, the sense of self emerges as one of the most marvelous of human inventions – a symbol that represents all kinds of information about a person and that is at the same time an invention that every individual constructs for himself or herself.

Summary: the unique contributions of the theory

As human beings, we all have a repertoire of skills for solving different kinds of problems. Our investigation has begun, therefore, with a consideration of such problems, the contexts in which they are encountered, and the culturally significant solutions or products that may be the outcome. We have not approached "intelligence" as a reified human faculty that is necessarily brought to bear in any problem setting; rather, we have begun with the problems that humans solve and worked back to the "intelligences" that must undergird the solutions.

Evidence from brain research, developmental and evolutionary investigations, and cross-cultural comparisons were all brought to bear in our search for the relevant human intelligences: a candidate was included only if reasonable evidence to support its membership was found across these diverse fields. Again, this tack differs from the traditional one: since no candidate faculty is necessarily an intelligence, we could effect our choices on a motivated basis. By contrast, the traditional approach to "intelligence" permits no equivalent opportunity for drawing on such diverse lines of evidence.

We have reason to believe that these multiple human faculties, the intelligences, are to a significant extent independent of one another. For example, research with brain damaged adults repeatedly demonstrates that particular faculties can be lost, while others are spared. This independence of intelligences implies that a particularly high level of ability in one Intelligence, say mathematics, does not require a similarly high level in another Intelligence, like language or music. This independence of intelligences contrasts sharply with traditional measures of IQ, which find high correlations among test scores. We speculate that the usual correlations among subtests of IQ tests come about because all these tasks in fact measure the ability to answer quickly on paper-and-pencil items of a logical-mathematical or linguistic sort. We believe that these correlations would be substantially reduced (if not eliminated) if one were to have the opportunity to survey in a contextually appropriate way the full range of human problem-solving skills. Such efforts are in fact now under way with a preschool population.

Nearly all traditional psychological theorizing about cognition assumes that human abilities are organized in a horizontal fashion. That is, processes of perception, learning, memory, and so on are said to obtain in a parallel fashion across the board. One radical implication of MI theory is that such capacities are better thought of in a vertical manner. Instead of a general faculty called memory, there are specific memories for music, spatial events, language, and so on. Furthermore, there need be no correlation among these various memories. Similar arguments would be made in the areas of learning, perception, attention span, and other horizontal faculties. Brain damage evidence supports this analysis quite strongly. While far more evidence must be accumulated before the vertical view can replace the horizontal view (Fodor, 1983), MI theory suggests that this possibility should at least be taken seriously.

Until now, we have supported the fiction that adult roles depend largely on the flowering of a single intelligence. In fact, however, nearly every cultural role of any degree of sophistication requires a combination of Intelligences. Thus, even an apparently straightforward role like playing the violin transcends a reliance on simple musical intelligence. To become a successful violinist requires bodily-kinesthetic dexterity as well as the interpersonal skills of relating to an audience and, in a different way, of choosing a manager; quite possibly it involves an intrapersonal intelligence as well. Successful dance requires skills in bodily-kinesthetic, musical, interpersonal, and spatial intelligences in varying degrees. Success in politics requires an interpersonal skill, a linguistic facility and perhaps some logical aptitude. Inasmuch as nearly every cultural role requires several intelligences, it becomes important to consider individuals as a collection of aptitudes rather than as having a singular problem-solving faculty that can be measured directly through short answer tests. Even given a relatively small number of such intelligences, the diversity of human ability is readily captured through the differences in these profiles. In fact, it may well be that the "total is greater than the sum of the parts." An individual may not be particularly gifted in any intelligence; yet, because of his particular combination or blend of skills, he may be able to fill some niche uniquely well. It is thus of paramount importance to assess the particular combination of skills that may earmark an individual for a certain vocational or avocational niche.

Critique of the theory of multiple intelligences

The theory of multiple intelligences challenges many of the central points of traditional theories of intelligence. We would like to consider some of the common critiques of the theory, with the aim of placing the theory in the broader context of contemporary psychology. This discussion also treats other questions that are commonly asked of the theory. For a more detailed treatment of many of these critiques and questions, see *Frames of Mind* (Gardner, 1983) and other publications (e.g., H. Weinreich-Haste, 1985).

Your "intelligences" – musical, bodily-kinesthetic, and so on – are what others call talents or gifts. Why confuse the issue by using the word "intelligence" to describe them?

There is nothing magical about the word "intelligence." We have purposely chosen it to join issue with those psychologists who consider logical reasoning or linguistic competence to be on a different plane than musical problem-solving or bodily-kinesthetic aptitude. Placing logic and language on a pedestal reflects the values of our Western culture and the great premium placed on the familiar tests of intelligence. A more Olympian view sees all seven as equally valid. To call some "talent" and some "intelligence" displays this bias. Call them all "talents" if you wish; or call them all "intelligences."

Is multiple intelligences really a "theory?" It carefully selects certain data in support of its hypotheses while ignoring others. Furthermore, it is not confirmed by experiment. Therefore, the theory cannot be disproved as it stands, nor can it be contrasted with competing theories. And since the possibility of contradiction is a prerequisite for any nontrivial theory, MI fails the test.

MI theory does not consider all data since such consideration is at best impractical. Instead it surveys a wide variety of independent research traditions: neurology, special populations, development, psychometrics, anthropology, evolution, and so on. The theory is a product of the synthesis of this survey. That the various research traditions point to and support a single theory does not confirm the theory but does support the contention that this theory is on the right track.

To be sure, the theory at best only explains existing research findings; it can be confirmed only through experiments and those experiments remain to be performed. Still, the contention that MI is not a theory until the experiments are performed is unwarranted.

Controlled experiments could either confirm or disconfirm MI. Several come to mind: a test of the independence of intelligences, for example; a test of the universality of intelligences across cultures; or a test of the developmental stability of an intelligence. There is another way that the theory can be disconfirmed, however, even before such experiments are performed. Gardner's original program, presented in *Frames of Mind*, might be described as a "subjective factor analysis," which aimed to discover a reasonably small set of human faculties that formed "natural kinds" and that had biological validity and educational utility. If other researchers, looking at the same empirical data or at new empirical data, were to come up with a list of faculties that were better supported, the current version of MI theory would be called into question. If there turned out to be a significant correlation among these faculties, as measured by appropriate assessments, the independence of the faculties would be invalidated.

Moreover, the theory could be partially discomfirmed on any number of finer points. Perhaps one or more of the candidate intelligences we have accepted will be found to be inadequately justified by further review. Perhaps there are several candidates that we have not considered. Or perhaps the intelligences are not nearly as independent as claimed. Each of these alternatives can be empirically verified and can provide means for disconfirming or reformulating the theory, although in the case of certain revisions, there might still be some utility to the theory itself.

These tests all rely on tasks developed from a careful and complete articulation of the mechanisms underlying each Intelligence. How can these tasks be constructed when MI has yet to provide an explanation of "how" each particular Intelligence works?

It is true that the focus of MI theory thus far has been on identification and description of the faculties rather than on the fine structuring and functioning of the intelligences. In principle, there is certainly no reason why information-processing accounts could not be given for each of these intelligences and their manner of interaction; indeed, this would be a worthwhile project. Certainly careful articulation of each intelligence is required in the diagnostic process. We believe that operational definitions of each intelligence along with diagnostic procedures can be constructed, and we are engaged in a four-year investigative effort that has just that objective. We realize that it may be difficult to come up with precise definitions and assessment procedures for the personal intelligences: that considerable ingenuity will be required in creating formulations that are faithful to the scope of these intelligences and yet lend themselves to some kind of objective assessment. But the difficulty of this undertaking certainly does not excuse our ignoring these forms of knowing, a practice that has been the rule in mainstream psychology in the last several decades.

There is a great deal of evidence in the psychometric literature that suggests that humans differ from one another in general intelligence. This trait, labeled g, *can be measured quite reliably through statistical analysis of test scores. There is no place for* g *in MI theory, so how can this large body of data be explained?*

We do not deny that *g* exists; instead, we question its explanatory importance outside the relatively narrow environment of formal schooling. For example, evidence for *g* is provided almost entirely by tests of linguistic or logical intelligence. Since these tests measure skills that are valuable in the performance of school-related tasks, they provide reliable prediction of success or failure in school. The tests are not nearly as reliable in predicting success outside of school tasks.

Second, these tests almost always rely on short answers. Again, a particular test taking skill, relevant to school success but not much else, contributes to the measured individual differences and the correlations that result. If reliable tests could be constructed for different intelligences, and these tests did not rely solely on short answers, often through pencil-and-paper presentations, but instead used the materials of the domain being measured, we believe that the correlations responsible for *g* would greatly diminish. Tests of musical intelligence would examine the individual's ability to analyze a work of music or to create one, not simply to compare two single tones on the basis of relative pitch. We need tests of spatial ability that involve finding one's way around, not merely giving multiple choice responses to depictions of a geometric form as depicted from different visual angles.

For example, tasks that require the memorization of letters versus digits often return correlated results, even though these tasks appear to require different Intelligences. We are dubious of the ecological significance of these measures. But putting that aside, according to our analysis, the memorization of both numbers and letters involves linguistic memory and thus both tasks tap the same underlying facility. As an alternative, one might ask subjects to memorize a poem on the one hand and a mathematical proof on the other. We predict that results from tasks of this type would show relatively low correlations. Finally, it is worth noting that students trained to memorize long strings of digits (up to 80 to 100) show no transfer when they are asked to memorize other putatively meaningless strings of information (Ericsson, 1984).

Even if g is a valid concept for describing the capacities of certain individuals, it seems to pass by many others who have striking individual talents. Consequently, from a societal point of view, a focus on g is biased and often unproductive.

In rebutting the phenomenon of g you suggest that scores from standardized tests are correlated because they assess a test-taking skill rather than a general faculty of intelligence. However, not all these test scores are equally correlated. How do you explain this variation?

Perhaps some of the differences among correlations are due to the different ways that these tests measure the various intelligences. For example, the standardized tests may capture more of the variance for logical-mathematical intelligence than for spatial or musical intelligence.

Our critique of standardized testing has two parts. First, we believe that all significant human capacities should be assessed, not just those that are valued in formal schooling. Second, we believe that the ultimate challenge to psychometrics is the construction of "intelligence-fair" tests – tests that use the materials of different domains as integral parts of their presentation.

Perhaps the strongest justification for IQ is the fact that the tests of IQ are reliable and practical (as well as profitable). Furthermore, much of the MI thesis depends on adequate diagnosis or assessment of the various intelligences in individuals. What will this diagnostic procedure look like, and how will it be made available to the measurement community at large?

Together with David Feldman of Tufts University, we are beginning to investigate the viability of a new form of assessment. Our research program will attempt to identify intellectual propensities in preschool children. As research materials, we will rely heavily on resources which are quite close to the elements used in solving problems and fashioning products in everyday life, rather than the more familiar short answer test items. Following an intensive monitoring of a child's intellectual propensities, we will produce a report that will not only summarize the child's particular strengths and weaknesses but that will also make concrete suggestions about activities that might profitably be pursued at home, at school, and in the community at large (Gardner and Feldman, 1985).

According to the theory of MI, each intelligence undergoes a complex developmental history that must be discovered through empirical investigation. The course of logical-mathematical thought, as it develops spontaneously and as it can be refined and trained, may bear little resemblance to the developmental course of musical or interpersonal intelligence. For this reason, it is necessary to assess each intelligence (as well as combinations of intelligences) in ways appropriate both to the developmental course of that intelligence and to the age or stage of the subject. It would be antithetical to the theory to attempt to ordain in advance the optimal means of testing intelligences in adolescents or adults. If our attempt to assess intellectual propensities in preschool children meets with some success, we will be emboldened to continue the investigation for other age groups as well.

What prevents the ambitious theoretician from constructing a new "intelligence" for every skill found in human behavior? In that case, instead of seven intelligences, there might be 700!

A list of 700 intelligences would be forbidding to the theoretician and useless to the practitioner. Therefore MI theory attempts to articulate only a manageable number of intelligences that appear to form natural kinds. There is every reason to expect that each natural kind will have several (or more) subcomponents. However, it is also likely that, in most normal human behaviors, the several subcomponents of an intelligence should cluster together, while they should show little inclination to correlate with subcomponents of other intelligences. This claim could and should be tested empirically.

As indicated in *Frames of Mind*, the decision to search for a small number of intelligences or faculties is a deliberate one. Without question, one might want to have a larger set of intelligences if one were pursuing other theoretical or practical ends. In this sense, the decision is a metatheoretical one.

The theory of Multiple Intelligences outlines several independent faculties but fails to provide any discussion of how these are orchestrated into the symphony of human behavior. How can diverse and independent intelligences function effectively without a leader, an executive?

A theory that does not posit an executive function has certain advantages over one that does. For one thing, such a theory is simpler; it also avoids many of the temptations of infinite regression involved in the explanation of such a function. Moreover, an executive is not a necessary attribute of such a theory. Committees, for example, can be effective without a leader. Rogers and Hammerstein were able to collaborate brilliantly with neither serving as the executive.

At the same time, however, it does appear on the basis of daily experience that many people can evaluate their intelligences and plan to use them together in certain putatively effective ways. Perhaps this is a component of the sense of self that we view as an outgrowth of the intrapersonal intelligence, leavened by the other intelligences like language and logic. In our "particle" society, individuals themselves do the planning and negotiating. But that role can be played by someone else; for example, the mother often plays the role with the prodigy, and the rest of society plays the role in many other so-called "field" societies. The phenomenal experience of an executive sense of self may make sense in our society, but it does not appear to be an imperative of successful human functioning.

Effective problem solving requires both an appreciation of the problem at hand as well as some understanding of the resources and strategies that are available. While the problem may be rooted in the "materials" of the domain (in MI parlance), the personal resources and strategies are not. These are often called "metacomponents" of intelligence, because they operate beyond the realm of the actual problem.

In fact, it may be that the "metacomponents" provide the mechanism for explaining the g discussed earlier. At any rate, how can they be incorporated into MI, if at all?

Our preference for independent intelligences leads us to believe that metacomponents may function independently in different domains. In this sense, they do not explain g except to the extent that g maps onto logical and linguistic abilities. To our knowledge, there is no research literature relevant to the discussion of metacomponents in, say, tasks of bodily kinesthetic knowledge or musical knowledge.

Certainly, this is an area in which more empirical work is needed and in which the theory can be profitably expanded or linked with other theoretical efforts (cf. Sternberg, 1984).

Why is moral or spiritual intelligence not considered?

Moral or spiritual intelligence serves as a reasonable candidate, although there is good reason to consider it as an amalgam of interpersonal intelligence and intrapersonal intelligence with a value component added. What is moral or spiritual depends greatly on cultural values; in describing intelligences we are dealing with abilities which can be mobilized by the values of a culture rather than the behaviors which are themselves valued in one way or another.

Need the intelligences be entirely independent?

The theory is simpler, both conceptually and biologically, if the various intelligences are totally independent. However, there is no theoretical reason why two or more intelligences could not overlap or correlate with one another more highly than with the others.

The independence of intelligences makes a good working hypothesis. It can only be tested by using appropriate measures in different cultures. Otherwise, one might prematurely jump to the conclusion that two candidate intelligences are correlated, only to find that the results are artifactual or culture bound.

Are the intelligences modifiable?

Possibly genetic factors set some kind of upper bound on the extent to which an intelligence may be realized or modified in the course of a human life. As a practical matter, however, it is likely to be the case that this biological limit is rarely if ever approached. Given enough exposure to the materials of an intelligence, nearly anyone who is not brain damaged can achieve quite significant results in that intellectual realm (This is the lesson of the Suzuki musical method and other "hot house" techniques.) By the same token, no one – whatever his or her biological potential – is likely to develop an intelligence without at least some opportunities for exploration of the materials that elicit a particular intellectual strength (Walters and Gardner, 1986). In sum, the surrounding culture plays a prepotent role in determining the extent to which an individual's intellectual potential is realized.

Is a rapprochement between MI and competing theories of intelligence possible?

Certainly. For example, there are many intriguing points of contact between MI and the triarchic theory articulated by Sternberg (Sternberg, 1984). Sternberg's theory distinguishes three different forms of cognition that might be mapped into different intelligences: problem solving (onto logical-mathematical), verbal (onto linguistic), and practical social competence (onto interpersonal intelligence). Expansion of these connections might provide some grounds for rapprochement (see Gardner, 1984).

Whatever the future holds, it is desirable, when a new theory is introduced, to accentuate its unique properties so that it can be more readily contrasted with its competitors. Consequently, we resist the attempt to combine MI with other theories at this point. Better a forceful and monistic theory than an all-encompassing but innocuous first attempt (see Sternberg, 1983).

Concluding remarks

The theory of MI faces two directions: toward the world of educational psychology and toward the world of everyday experience. To educational psychology, it presents a theoretical analysis of various sources of data with the aim of explaining the variety of human accomplishments. To the world of everyday experience, it provides a framework whereby practitioners, teachers, and parents may better cope with the mélange of individual differences. Throughout this chapter we have made no distinction between the "practical" intelligence and a more "general" intelligence. Indeed, according to the theory of Multiple Intelligences, all intelligent acts are (potentially) practical, and all practical activities, those involving solving problems or creating products, require at least one intelligence.

Consider again the two Martians and their fresh points of view on "the human mind." With no investment in the methods of traditional intelligence testing and unencumbered by the prejudices of any given cultural (or professional) group, they are free to study, and marvel at, human nature in all its complexity and creativity. Through this fable, we are suggesting that earth-bound psychologists might break fresh scientific ground should they become similarly unbound.

References

Connor, A. (1982). *Voices from Cooperstown,* New York: Collier. (Based on a quotation taken from *The Babe Ruth Story,* Babe Ruth & Bob Considine. New York: Dutton, 1948.)

Eimas, P., Siqueland, E., Jusczyk, P., & Vigorito, J. (1971). Speech perception in infants. *Science, 171,* 303–306.

Ericsson, K. (1984, December). Presented at the Workshop on Expertise, sponsored by the Social Science Research Council, New York City.

Fodor, J. (1983). *Modularity of mind.* Cambridge, MA: MIT Bradford Press.

Gallwey, T. (1976). *Inner tennis.* New York: Random House.

Gardner, H. (1983). *Frames of mind.* New York: Basic Books.

Gardner, H. (1984, June). Assessing intelligences: A comment on "Testing intelligence without I.Q. tests." *Phi Delta Kappan,* 699–700.

Gardner, H., & Feldman, H. (1985). *First Annual Report on Project Spectrum.*

Keller, E. (1983). *A feeling for the organism.* San Francisco: Freeman.

Lash, J. (1980). *Helen and teacher: The story of Helen Keller and Anne Sullivan Macy.* New York: Delacorte.

Menuhin, Y. (1977). *Unfinished journey.* New York: Knopf.

Selfe, L. (1977). *Nadia: A case of extraordinary drawing ability in an autistic child.* New York: Academic.

Soldo, J. (1982). Jovial juvenilia: T. S. Eliot's first magazine. *Biography, 5,* 25–37.

Sternberg, R. (1984). Toward a triarchic theory of human intelligence. *Behavioral and Brain Sciences, 7,* 269–315.

Sternberg, R. (1983). "How much Gall is too much gall? A review of *Frames of mind: The theory of multiple intelligences. Contemporary Education Review, 2,* 215–224.

Trehub, S., Bull, D., & Thorpe, L. (1984). Infants' perception of melodies: The role of melodic contour. *Child Development, 55,* 821–830.

Walters, J., & Gardner, H. (1986). Crystallizing experiences: Discovering an intellectual gift. In R. Sternberg & J. Davidson (Eds.), *Conceptions of giftedness.* Cambridge: Cambridge University Press.

Weinreich-Haste, H. (1985). The varieties of intelligences: An interview with Howard Gardner. *New Ideas in Psychology, 3,* 47–65.

Woolf, V. (1976). *Moments of being.* Sussex: The University Press.

For all practical purposes: criteria for defining and evaluating practical intelligence

Martin E. Ford

Basic definitional issues

Practical intelligence is a subset of the larger domain of intelligence. In order to identify criteria for defining and evaluating practical intelligence, it is first necessary to define, at least in a general way, what intelligence means. M. Ford (1982, 1986) provided a definition that fits in well with the approach to be developed in the present chapter. He defines intelligence as the attainment of relevant goals in specified environments, using appropriate means and resulting in positive developmental outcomes. This definition is of course incomplete since it does not specify the content of either the short-term or long-term objectives that people must accomplish in order to be considered intelligent (i.e., the relevant goals and the positive developmental outcomes) or the boundary conditions that apply to these accomplishments (i.e., the specified environments and appropriate means for goal attainment). However, because the meaning of intelligence depends on individual, contextual, and developmental factors (M. Ford, 1986; Sternberg, 1985), these content specifications can be supplied only after the precise purposes and contexts of a given assessment of intelligence are determined. Thus, the definition offered by M. Ford (1982, 1986) is a useful "generic" definition that supplies all of the parameters that must be considered in a specific operationalization of intelligence.

This definition is also useful because it enables researchers to map out subdomains of intelligence by delimiting the content specifications in certain ways. In fact, intelligence itself is often defined in this manner (i.e., the field traditionally does not include all kinds of goal attainment under the rubric of intelligence). In the case of practical intelligence, there are essentially two unique defining features.

First, the goals to be accomplished must be transactional; that is, they must refer to an effect outside of the person (e.g., fixing a flat tire; controlling someone else's behavior) rather than to an effect inside the person (e.g., understanding a concept, experiencing a sunset). This requirement is congruent with dictionary definitions of the word "practical"; for example,

183

Webster's Seventh New Collegiate Dictionary emphasizes the idea of being "actively engaged in some course of action" or of being "disposed to action as opposed to speculation or abstraction" (p. 666).

The second defining feature of practical intelligence is that the goals to be accomplished must be important either to the individual being assessed or to the cultural groups of which that individual is a part (or both). Personal or social importance is often a key criterion for defining relevance; however, people sometimes pursue goals in which they (or the culture) have little investment because they are uncertain about what goals are important or because they are in a situation that provides no opportunity to pursue important goals. Also, goals that merely facilitate the pursuit of other goals may be both relevant and quite unimportant in and of themselves.

Practical intelligence is often contrasted with academic intelligence and is sometimes even regarded as its opposite (e.g., Neisser, 1976; Wagner & Sternberg, 1985). This distinction is useful and revealing, but one must be careful in drawing the boundaries of each type of intelligence. At least some aspects of academic intelligence may be able to serve practical purposes. Specifically, academic capabilities that directly promote or that themselves represent important transactional achievements would be viewed as falling within the rubric of practical intelligence according to the perspective offered here. Whether there are many such achievements is an interesting and important question; nevertheless, one must recognize that although the prototypical features of academic and practical intelligence may be quite distinct, the two categories represent overlapping rather than mutually exclusive aspects of intelligence.

One should also resist the temptation to describe all achievements that are not practical as being "impractical." This would be appropriate if the achievement was both confined to the self and considered relatively unimportant, but when only one of these criteria is met the label can be quite misleading. For example, desired internal states such as self-esteem, peace of mind, and efficient digestive functioning may only indirectly affect a person's ability to behave in practically intelligent ways, but these accomplishments can hardly be considered impractical. Similarly, people often pursue transactional goals of little intrinsic importance because these goals are "necessary evils" that must be accomplished in order to attain other desired outcomes. These kinds of accomplishments (e.g., routine household chores, boring classroom assignments, menial work tasks) are not impractical (indeed, they usually serve practical purposes), but they are also not often mentioned as appropriate criteria for defining and evaluating practical intelligence.

Identifying transactional goals: the boundaries of practical intelligence

Conceptualizing practical intelligence as the attainment of important short-term and long-term transactional goals (within specified behavioral and environmental boundary conditions) is a critical first step in specifying criteria for defining and evaluating practical intelligence. However, this conceptualization is not sufficiently concrete for most assessment purposes. Precisely which kinds of goals involve transactional accomplishments and which kinds do not? In order to address this question in a systematic manner, it is necessary to begin by considering the full range of possible human goals. Although this is obviously impossible to do at a molecular or situational level of analysis, Ford and Nichols (in press) have developed a comprehensive taxonomy of goals in which they attempt to represent different types of human achievements at a level that is fairly abstract but still useful in further explicating the meaning of practical intelligence. This taxonomy is described in Table 1.

Before considering the details of this taxonomy, it is important to consider several points. First, there is no implication in this taxonomy that some goals are more important or more fundamental than others (cf. Maslow, 1943). Although people may vary widely in their priorities and achievements with regard to these objectives, there is no assumption that people in general will tend to pursue one type of goal over another, nor is there an assumption that some goals will serve as prerequisites for other goals. The taxonomy simply describes a number of different ways of being intelligent (or competent, if one prefers a broader term). A second point is that none of these goals is considered mutually exclusive at a general level of definition and assessment. There will be many situations in which the pursuit of one goal will foreclose the opportunity to attain another type of goal. Nevertheless, given a normal range of life contexts, it is generally possible for individuals to seek and attain almost any combination of the objectives listed in Table 1. This raises a third related point, namely, that goal-directed behavior tends to be quite complexly organized. People generally do not seek one goal at a time in a simple and straightforward manner. Rather, behavior typically serves multiple purposes simultaneously and is organized hierarchically in episodes and subepisodes of goal seeking which are woven together in a complex and variable stream of activity (D. Ford, in press). As a result, it is sometimes difficult to tell whether a person's behavior is serving a practical purpose or not.

Seven major categories of goals are described in Table 1. Achievements in three of these categories – arousal, experiential, and physiological goals – are clearly not within the rubric of practical intelligence because they focus on internal states and processes rather than transactional outcomes. In ad-

Table 1. *A taxonomy of human goals.*

Arousal goals	
Entertainment	Having fun, avoiding boredom, seeking heightened arousal
Tranquility	Peace of mind, serenity, avoiding stress
Happiness	Feelings of joy, satisfaction, or well-being
Evaluation goals	
Positive or confirmatory self-evaluations	Self-efficacy, self-esteem, self-acceptance, self-worth, self-validation
Positive or confirmatory social evaluations	Social approval, respect from others, esteem from others, social validation
Experiential goals	
Bodily sensation	Experiencing physical movement or a bodily state, feeling relaxed
Transcendence	Rising above ordinary experience, pursuing an idealized state, spirituality
Unity	Seeking coherence, harmony, or oneness
Physiological goals	Seeking feelings of physiological well-being
Safety goals	Avoiding threatening or depriving circumstances
Sex and reproduction goals	Engaging in sexual activity, seeking sexual satisfaction
Social relationship goals	
Self-assertion	Maintaining or promoting the self
Individuality	Uniqueness, separateness, individual identity
Self-determination	Personal control, freedom, autonomy
Superiority	Social status or importance, dominance, winning, comparing favorably with others
Resource acquisition	Obtaining support, assistance, advice, and other resources for oneself
Integration	Maintaining or promoting other people or social groups
Belongingness	Attachments, intimacy, friendship, community, social identity
Social responsibility	Fulfilling social roles, keeping interpersonal commitments, accepting legitimate social control
Equity	Fairness, justice, reciprocation, comparing equally with others
Resource provision	Providing support, assistance, advice, and other resources for others
Task goals	
Exploration	Curiosity, intellectual stimulation, learning
Understanding	Ordering, categorizing, explaining, making sense
Mastery	Achievement, competence, excellence
Creativity	Investing new ideas or products, expanding one's limits
Management	Handling routine tasks, organizing people or things, being productive

dition, several goals that refer to cognitive accomplishments rather than behavioral outcomes would not be considered appropriate criteria for defining or assessing practical intelligence. These include self-evaluation goals and three types of task goals: (1) exploration, where the goal is to perceive or acquire new information; (2) understanding, where the goal is to enrich or improve the accuracy, value, or meaningfulness of existing cognitive representations; and (3) intellectual creativity, where the goal is to develop new ideas or new ways of thinking about some phenomenon.

Creativity may also refer to transactional accomplishments (e.g., painting a picture, writing a book, inventing a new tool) and must therefore be considered potentially relevant to an assessment of practical intelligence (i.e., depending on how it fares on the importance criterion). Other task goals that meet the transactional criterion are mastery, where the purpose is to develop a behavioral skill or product that meets a specified standard of performance, and management, where the objective is to promote the smooth functioning of the people or things in a given context. Because most people spend considerable time pursuing mastery and management objectives, both categories of goals are strong candidates for inclusion in a comprehensive assessment of practical intelligence.

The ability to accomplish safety goals is another plausible criterion for defining and evaluating practical intelligence since it would objectively seem to be a very important part of successful everyday life. Although safety goals have a highly personal focus, they are not internal goals. They are transactional goals which refer to a desired relationship between the self and the environment. That is, safety represents a state of person–environment organization in which harmful environmental effects are unlikely to occur to the self. This can be distinguished from the internal goal of perceived safety, which in the Ford and Nichols (in press) taxonomy would be classified under the rubric of tranquility goals (a type of arousal goal).

The remaining categories of goals listed in Table 1 – sex and reproduction goals, social evaluation goals, and social relationship goals – all refer to desired outcomes of interpersonal functioning. Because social goals are important to virtually everyone, social intelligence can be regarded as an essential criterion for defining and evaluating practical intelligence. In fact, given the diversity of social goals that people can pursue and the ubiquity of social transactions in people's everyday lives (especially in modern information-based societies), it is possible that for many persons practical intelligence will be virtually synonymous with social intelligence. (Note that interpersonal effects may also be of central concern in each of the other categories of goals associated with practical intelligence.)

Sex and reproduction goals are important goals for most people during much of their lives, although they are often complicated by the desire to maintain other desired consequences (e.g., safety and belongingness). The need to accomplish all these goals simultaneously in order to be considered practically intelligent in contexts involving intimate relationships clearly illustrates the complex multidimensional nature of real-world intelligence. It is quite possible for a person to interact with other people with just one purpose in mind, but in most instances behavior is guided by several important practical considerations that must be coordinated in order to create an intelligent stream of activity (D. Ford, in press).

Social evaluation goals often seem to rank high in people's goal hierarchies, as evidenced by the attention that is given in most cultures to concerns involving physical appearance, impression management, and social propriety. On the other hand, there is evidence to suggest that at least some such matters may be viewed as being rather trivial in and of themselves (e.g., Turiel, 1983). Thus, it is not clear to what extent these kinds of achievements should be included in an assessment of practical intelligence. This may depend on the degree to which such achievements are truly necessary for the attainment of other important transactional goals.

Finally, social relationship goals are likely to be central to any comprehensive assessment of practical intelligence. There are essentially two major purposes to be accomplished here: the maintenance and promotion of the self in relationships with other people (i.e., self-assertion) and the maintenance and promotion of other people and the social groups of which one is a part (i.e., integration). These two aspects of social intelligence involve four interrelated issues central to effective human functioning (M. Ford, 1985, 1986):

1. Defining one's identity as a separate person (individuality) and as a member of various social groups (belongingness)
2. Control, both with regard to establishing personal control over life circumstances (self-determination) and accepting legitimate and necessary forms of social control (social responsibility)
3. Social comparison, both in terms of doing better than others (superiority) and in terms of promoting equality and fairness (equity)
4. Resource distribution, which refers to both the giving (resource provision) and receiving (resource acquistion) of assistance, advice, and other material, informational, or emotional supports

In sum, the Ford and Nichols (in press) taxonomy of human goals suggests that criteria for defining and evaluating practical intelligence should be selected from the following categories of transactional goals: sex and reproduction goals; safety goals; mastery, creativity, and management goals; social evaluation goals; and social relationship goals. Each criterion selected must also pass the importance test, and since importance will vary as a function of personal and cultural values (M. Ford, 1986; Sternberg, 1983), somewhat different criteria may be needed for different assessment contexts. On the other hand, there are indications that there may be more agreement about these criteria, at least at a general level of analysis, than one might expect given the extensive individual, developmental, and contextual differences that characterize human behavioral activity (e.g., Ford & Miura, 1983; Krumboltz, Ford, Nichols, & Wentzel). Thus, despite tremendous variability in the content and contexts of goal-directed behavior, and despite differences in the weights given to different types of transactional goals, there may be a considerable amount of consistency and stability in the broad categories of behavioral outcomes that people seek throughout their lives.

Identifying important transactional goals: the core of practical intelligence

Essentially two basic strategies can be used to identify the transactional goals that a person or culture values the most. One strategy is to ask people directly what goals are important to them (e.g., by having them rate or rank a set of potentially important outcomes). The other is to infer these goals by examining the content of implicit theories or "prototypes" of practically intelligent people. Researchers also often try to infer goals from people's behavior in relevant situations; however, because a given behavior usually serves multiple purposes and because the same behavior can often be used to attain different goals (D. Ford, in press), this is a very difficult task except in very simple situations (which is not the nature of most real-world contexts). Also, people sometimes do not pursue the goals they value the most due to external constraints, self-regulatory deficits, and habitual patterns of seeking other goals (M. Ford, 1986; Winell, in press).

We shall now look at two illustrative sets of research results. The first set of results comes from a pair of studies which explored people's conceptions of "everyday intelligence" (Sternberg, Conway, Ketron, & Bernstein, 1981) and "social competence" (Ford & Miura, 1983). Both studies used the prototype strategy in an attempt to identify the defining features of constructs related to practical intelligence. The second set of results comes from a recently completed large-scale survey in which a group of high school students, parents, and teachers were asked to rate and rank 170 academic and nonacademic (i.e., "personal responsibility") goals both in terms of their general importance and in terms of the schools' role in promoting each outcome (Krumboltz et al., in preparation). This research exemplifies the direct approach to identifying the criteria that should be considered in defining and evaluating practical intelligence.

The prototype studies

Sternberg et al. (1981) asked 186 people, including commuters, housewives, and students, to list attributes they considered characteristic of intelligence, unintelligence, academic intelligence, and everyday intelligence. They then enlisted a second group of twenty-eight laypersons to rate how characteristic they considered each of the 250 items mentioned by the first group for each of the three types of intelligence. A factor analysis of the ratings for everyday intelligence (on the basis of 98 particularly relevant items) yielded four factors that Sternberg and co-workers labeled practical problem-solving ability, social competence, character, and interest in learning and culture. A similar analysis of the ratings made by sixty-five experts in the field of intelligence (based on a slightly different pool of items) yielded a somewhat different result involving three factors: practical problem-solving ability, practical adaptive behavior, and social competence. However, the correlation between experts' and laypersons' characteristicness ratings of everyday intelligence over the entire set of 250 items was very high (.81).

Although the lack of a table of factor loadings for the everyday intelligence factors obtained by Sternberg et al. (1981) makes it somewhat difficult to precisely match these factors with the goals in Ford and Nichols (in press) taxonomy, it seems clear that subjects primarily emphasized characteristics pertaining to task goals and social relationship goals in their conceptions of everyday intelligence. Some of this emphasis was on internal rather than external characteristics, however. Specifically, many of the items focused on the cognitive goals of exploration and understanding (e.g., items referring to interest, insight, and openness to new information). From the present perspective, these characteristics would not be considered appropriate criteria for defining and evaluating practical intelligence per se, even though they may sometimes facilitate the attainment of certain kinds of transactional goals.

Of those items that were more behaviorally relevant, many tended to focus on morality-related aspects of practical intelligence – that is, the integrative goals of social responsibility, equity, and resource provision (Ford, Burt, & Bergin, 1984). Surprisingly, little emphasis appeared to be placed on self-assertive achievements, even though these outcomes generally require more "skill" than integrative accomplishments (M. Ford, 1986). On the other hand, a number of items referring to transactionally oriented cognitive skills may be of particular relevance to self-assertive goals (e.g., makes good decisions, determines how to achieve goals). Nevertheless, these kinds of characteristics are also likely to contribute in significant ways to the attainment of other transactional goals (e.g., mastery and management goals).

In their research on people's conceptions of social competence, Ford and Miura (1983) began by collecting descriptions of "the most socially competent person I know" from ninety-nine university students. Each respondent was asked to give a detailed description of their nominee and to include as many reasons as they could for nominating that particular (real) individual. The actual phrases used by the respondents in their nominations were transferred onto cards and then copied onto a large chart where they could more readily be combined for similarity of content. This procedure yielded a final list of twenty descriptors representing the prototypically social competent adult.

In the next phase of the study, forty-four students working in a variety of disciplines (e.g., education, psychology, english, business) and representing a fairly wide range of age and ethnic groups were asked to combine the twenty descriptors into categories they thought would provide the best representation of the interrelationships among the elements of the social competence prototype. A cluster analysis of the grouping results indicated that there were four major components in these subjects' conceptions of social competence: prosocial skills (e.g., responds to the needs of others), social-instrumental skills (e.g., knows how to get things done), social ease (e.g., enjoys social activities and involvement), and self-efficacy (e.g., has a good self-concept). These results are described in Table 2.

In a second study designed to explore the possibility that people's conceptions of social competence would vary as a function of the age of the target individual, Ford and Miura (1983) asked each child in a suburban grammar school sample of thirty-five third- and and fifth-graders to describe the most socially competent child they knew between the ages of 6 and 10. Nominations of social competence exemplars in the six to ten age range were also obtained from sixteen teachers and four room mothers assigned to first- through fifth-grade classrooms in two suburban grammar schools. The prototypes that emerged from these two sets of nominations were surprisingly similar to those obtained in the initial study, with virtually nothing being subtracted and only a few new items being added (e.g., is good in sports, has a good physical appearance).

These results are similar to those obtained by Sternberg et al. (1981) in several significant ways. First, subjects in both studies seemd to regard integrative characteristics, especially those relating to moral and prosocial behavior, as being of central importance to effective real-life functioning. By contrast, neither group placed much emphasis (at least explicitly) on self-assertive attributes. This finding suggests that social importance may be a more salient or more fundamental criterion than personal importance in people's conceptions of practical intelligence. Goals involving self-interest, although not necessarily impractical, may be regarded as having limited practical value unless they are pursued in such a way that they are linked or subordinated to broader social and cultural concerns.

Subjects in the two prototype studies also seemed to place considerable emphasis on the action-oriented processes of goal setting, decision making, planning, and problem solving. Although these instrumental skills cannot be regarded as appropriate criteria for defining practical intelligence (since they do not themselves represent transactional accomplishments), they may be useful criteria for evaluating practical intelligence, as they seem to represent an "all-purpose" set of cognitive tools that can be used to attain a wide range of transactional goals. This is congruent with the emphasis placed on these skills in theories of intelligence which focus more on transactional accomplishments than cognitive achievements. For example, "action" theory (Eckensberger & Meacham, 1984), contemporary social learning theory

Table 2. *The prototype of the socially competent adult.*

Prototypical features	Frequency of mentions (%)
I. Prosocial skills	
1. Is sensitive to the feelings of others (understanding, considerate, empathic)	66
2. Respects others and their viewpoints (open-minded, tolerant, nonjudgmental)	39
3. Is socially responsible (is willing to conform or adapt to accepted moral and social rules)	35
4. Responds to the needs of others (helpful, nurturant, prosocial)	31
5. Is genuinely interested in others (sincerely cares about people)	29
6. Is emotionally supportive (warm, tender, loving)	27
7. Can be counted on (trustworthy, dependable, honest)	24
II. Social-instrumental skills	
8. Knows how to get things done (capable, resourceful, intelligent)	57
9. Has good communications skills (listens and expresses ideas well)	40
10. Likes to set goals (self-directed, purposeful, ambitious)	31
11. Can handle stressful situations (keeps cool, can accept criticism, admit mistakes, and handle disappointments)	29
12. Has leadership abilities (can take charge of a situation, assertive, strong)	22
III. Social ease	
13. Is easy to be around (friendly, pleasant, relaxed)	56
14. Is socially adaptable (appears to be at ease with all types of people, can adjust easily to almost any situation)	55
15. Enjoys social activities and involvement (likes people and likes doing things with them)	25
16. Opens up to people (willing to share feelings with others, personal, intimate)	24
IV. Self-efficacy	
17. Has own identity and own values (independent, autonomous, self-reliant)	48
18. Has a good self-concept (likes and respects oneself, has feelings of self-worth, self-confident)	37
19. Is open to new experiences (likes challenges, continues to strive for self-improvement and personal growth)	25
20. Has a good outlook on life (optimistic, positive, enthusiastic)	25

(Bandura, 1982; Mischel, 1973), and the Fords' living systems framework (D. Ford, in press; M. Ford, 1986) all view effective activity as being produced largely by cognitive processes which function to direct, regulate, and control behavior.

Finally, the results of both prototype studies suggest that there are a number of transactional achievements that people do not commonly associate with either social competence or everyday intelligence. Evidently, accomplishments in the areas of safety, sex and reproduction, and social evaluation are not part of most people's core meaning of practical intelligence. This result is not particularly surprising for social evaluation goals, as it is congruent with the idea alluded to earlier that positive social evaluations may often be desired not so much for their own value but because they allow one to attain other desired goals such as belongingness or resource acquisition. However, the failure of subjects to mention safety or sex and reproduction goals seems rather surprising given the intrinsic desirability of these outcomes. It would seem that, as is the case for self-assertive behavior, the nature of both sexual and safety-related activity is such that these goals are more a matter of personal than social importance (except in extreme or unusual cases). They may also not be very "practical" criteria to use for evaluating practical intelligence because of the ethical and psychometric problems likely to accompany their application.

The study of the goals of education

In May 1983 a randomly selected sample of several hundred students representing five high schools in the San Francisco Bay Area participated in a study known as the Project on Schooling and Personal Responsibility (Krumboltz, Ford, Nichols, & Wentzel, in preparation). This research, which was a part of a larger collaborative project called the Study of Stanford and the Schools, was conducted to assess people's perceptions of the importance of goals in five nonacademic or "personal responsibility" domains: attitudes, interpersonal competence, moral development, health, and career development. Five academic domains (verbal, math, science, social studies, and fine arts) were also included in the study so that direct contrasts could be made between the personal responsibility goals and desired outcomes traditionally associated with schooling. The parents of the selected students and a number of teachers at each school were also invited to participate in the study.

Subjects were asked to respond to lists of statements representing goals to be achieved by the age of eighteen. These goal statements were developed by examining school district curriculum guides from around the country, by consulting with local teachers and other experts in each domain, and by applying criteria of simplicity, logic, and internal consistency to each statement. Each domain contained seventeen hierarchically organized goal state-

ments: one "global-level" goal statement (e.g., develop competence in dealing with people), four "broad-level" goal statements (e.g., get along well
with people different from themselves), and twelve "specific-level" goal
statements (e.g., get along comfortably and cooperatively with members of
different racial, cultural, and ethnic groups). Thus, there were a total of 170
different goal statements. Because pilot work indicated that subjects began
to lose interest before they had responded to the entire array of goal statements, four different survey instruments were constructed which were non-
overlapping except for the global-level goal statements, which appeared on
all four forms.

Two questions were asked about each goal statement: (1) How important
is it that people achieve this outcome by age eighteen?; and (2) How large
a role should the school play in contributing to this outcome? Subjects responded to each question by making a rating on a five-point scale. A ranking
response format was also used for the school role question; however, since
the importance results are of primary interest for the purposes of the present
chapter, neither the rating nor ranking data for school responsibility will be
reported here (see Krumboltz et al., in preparation, for a complete description
of these results).

The scale used to rate the importance of each goal statement was coded
as follows: 1 = critical, 2 = very important, 3 = somewhat important, 4
= not very important, and 5 = not important at all. The lower the score,
the higher the importance. Because a concerted and systematic effort was
made to word all goal statements in as attractive a manner as possible,
subjects rarely selected the "not important at all" response option and only
infrequently said that a goal was "not very important." However, substantial
variability was found in subjects' use of the other three response categories,
especially for the specific-level goal statements, so that meaningful differences in responses to different goal statements did seem to emerge in a fairly
clear and consistent fashion.

Except for the attitudes domain, which referred exclusively to internal
outcomes (e.g., pride, self-confidence, interest in schoolwork), all the personal responsibility domains were focused primarily on transactional goals.
Interpersonal competence was the most heterogeneous domain, as it included goal statements referring to belongingness (e.g., have good, satisfying
relationships with family and friends), resource provision (e.g., give to other
people without always expecting them to do something in return), equity
(e.g., treat people with fairness and respect even if they hold different values
or beliefs), and the acquisition of social-instrumental skills (e.g., have good
communication skills). Only one item directly involved self-assertive behavior (i.e., be able to stand up for themselves and what they believe), an
imbalance which resulted from the emphasis of school curriculum guides
and educational experts on the importance of integrative achievements (a

fact that itself may be quite revealing). The entire moral development domain also focused on integrative goals, especially those involving social responsibility concerns (e.g., avoid actions that hurt others or violate others' rights, keep promises and commitments, obey the law and respect those responsible for enforcing it).

Some of the goal statements in the health domain were primarily relevant to physiological goals (e.g., understand and avoid the harmful effects of smoking, such as heart disease and cancer), whereas others emphasized safety concerns (e.g., know and avoid the harmful effects of constant stress). However, several of these latter items were as concerned with the promotion of others' safety (an integrative goal) as with the maintenance of personal safety (e.g., know how to avoid sexually transmitted diseases and unwanted pregnancy; know how to prevent and respond to accidents, for instance, wear seat belts and know how to use emergency first aid). The career development domain included a few understanding goals (e.g., know the duties, requirements, benefits, and costs for different career possibilities), but focused primarily on the management and mastery of specific job- and career-related skills (e.g., obtain job-seeking skills; know how to obtain information and help for career problems from counselors, employment agencies, books, tests, and other available sources).

In contrast to the personal responsibility goal statements, the five academic domains tended to emphasize cognitive objectives, especially understanding goals (e.g., understand the meaning of commonly used words, understand basic principles of geometry, acquire knowledge of chemistry, understand the significance of current events, and understand how works of art are created). Thus, the importance ratings for most of the academic goal statements are not of direct relevance to the problem of defining and evaluating practical intelligence. They do allow, however, for an interesting comparison between two sets of goals (i.e., the personal responsibility and academic objectives) that can be construed as approximating the general domains of practical and academic intelligence. Also, there were a few transactionally oriented items among the academic goal statements, especially in the verbal and math domains (e.g., be able to write clear sentences and paragraphs, be able to use mathematical skills to manage personal finances).

The results for the importance ratings given by students, parents, and teachers to the 120 specific-level goal statements, aggregated to the domain level, are presented in Table 3. The most notable aspect of these data is that for each set of raters all five personal responsibility domains were regarded as more important than any of the academic domains. Although the results for the broad- and global-level goal statements were slightly less dramatic (i.e., the verbal and math domains occasionally made it into the top five), this set of findings is nevertheless rather striking, with important implications for both education professionals and intelligence researchers. Simply put,

Table 3. *Specific-level importance ratings by students, parents, and teachers for each domain in five schools.*

	Students				Parents				Teachers			
Rank	Domain	Mean rating	SD	n	Domain	Mean rating	SD	n	Domain	Mean rating	SD	n
1	Attitudes	1.61	.81	303	Moral	1.41	.68	215	Moral	1.49	.69	89
2	Interpersonal competence	1.65	.82	306	Attitudes	1.47	.68	215	Attitude	1.61	.81	89
3	Moral	1.74	.96	306	Interpersonal competence	1.55	.74	216	Interpersonal competence	1.65	.64	89
4	Career	1.78	.84	305	Health	1.65	.80	216	Career	1.84	.75	89
5	Health	1.88	.91	305	Career	1.76	.82	216	Health	1.87	.84	89
6	Math	2.06	.93	304	Verbal	1.92	.81	215	Math	1.97	.86	89
7	Verbal	2.15	.96	303	Math	1.93	.75	215	Verbal	1.98	.80	89
8	Social studies	2.19	.98	305	Social studies	2.20	.91	215	Social studies	2.13	.96	89
9	Fine arts	2.80	1.04	305	Fine arts	2.69	.85	216	Fine arts	2.67	.74	88
10	Science	2.95	.94	305	Science	2.72	.83	216	Science	2.93	.86	89

Note: Mean ratings for each domain were constructed by averaging the twelve specific-level statements for that domain. Ratings range from 1 to 5, with 1 being the highest rating.

we may not be teaching or testing the most important outcomes for competent functioning in the everyday world.

Although virtually all the personal responsibility goal statements were considered very or even critically important, the moral development and interpersonal competence objectives were generally regarded as being the most important transactional goals to be attained by age 18. This is remarkably consistent with the prototype studies' emphasis on moral and prosocial behavior. Taken together, these two sets of results provide compelling evidence for the argument that integrative achievements should be included as a part of the core definition of practical intelligence.

Within the health domain, the specific-level goal statements rated highest in importance were those having relevance to both physiological and safety concerns (e.g., know when to see a doctor and when to take care of a health problem themselves; understand and avoid the harmful effects of alcohol, including drunk driving accidents and physical diseases). This result implies that the importance of a skill or characteristic may be largely a function of the number of goals served. It also suggests that skills and achievements related to matters of personal safety are appropriate criteria for defining and evaluating practical intelligence, although the centrality of these characteristics may depend on the certainty or severity of the negative consequences likely to result from unintelligent safety-related behavior.

The outcomes considered to be the most important within the career domain were those involving mastery goals (e.g., know how to obtain training for different career possibilities; know how to improve career possibilities by obtaining job skills and experience) and management goals (e.g., practice good work habits, displaying accuracy, promptness, and so forth; know how to obtain information and help for career problems from counselors, employment agencies, books, tests, and so on). One potentially revealing aspect of these findings is that students seemed to be much more concerned about the mastery objectives than parents and teachers, while the adult raters appeared to be relatively more interested in the personal and interpersonal management skills needed to continue in a job or career after entering the world of work. This observation suggests that in order to obtain a meaningful assessment of practical intelligence somewhat different criteria may need to be used for different individuals or social groups (i.e., depending on the particular goals and contexts relevant to the persons being assessed).

Although relatively few of the academic goal statements referred directly to transactional achievements, it is interesting to note that the academic objectives rated highest in importance were those that had a more practical orientation. Specifically, there were six general "themes" that received the strongest endorsement from students, parents, and teachers: clear, grammatically correct writing; the comprehension and appreciation of written material; fluency in applying mathematics to everyday situations; the development of logical reasoning and problem-solving skills; an understanding of U.S. economics, politics, and law; and an understanding of current social problems. In contrast, the academic achievements which received the least enthusiastic endorsement of students, parents, and teachers included the following general themes: the development of complex, high-level mathematical skills; knowledge of scientific disciplines not involving people as a primary focus of study (e.g., physics, astronomy); and artistic and literary skills. Although these outcomes were not considered unimportant, that is, they were typically rated as being somewhat important, their relatively low standing in the hierarchy of academic and personal responsibility goals suggests that there may be a close association between the perceived importance of a particular skill or achievement and its practical value.

Summary and conclusions

This chapter has attempted to accomplish two purposes: the intellectual goal of explicating the nature of practical intelligence, and the practical goal of specifying criteria for defining and evaluating practical intelligence. The strategy used to try to achieve these objectives has involved three interrelated components: (1) a set of assumptions regarding the general conceptualization of practical intelligence, (2) a theoretical taxonomy of human goals, and (3) a body of evidence pertinent to the conceptual components of the chapter.

With regard to the first component, it was assumed that practical intelligence should be viewed as a subset of the larger domain of intelligence. M. Ford's (1982, 1986) definition of intelligence, which focuses on goal attainment rather than on procedures for attaining goals, was used as a starting point for defining practical intelligence. It was further assumed that practical intelligence can be uniquely identified by its emphasis on transactional goals considered important by a particular person or social group.

Ford and Nichols' (in press) taxonomy of human goals was then introduced as a heuristic tool for outlining the possible boundaries of the domain of practical intelligence. One set of goals (i.e., arousal goals, experiential goals, physiological goals, and a subset of task goals) was described as falling outside the boundaries of the domain because of its emphasis on internal states and processes. Another set of goals (i.e., safety goals, sex and reproduction goals, social evaluation goals, social relationship goals, and a subset of task goals) was characterized as being potentially relevant to the domain of practical intelligence because of its focus on transactional accomplishments.

In order to apply the importance test to this latter category of goals, the results of three relevant research studies were described. Two of these studies explored people's prototypical conceptions of intelligence or competence in the everyday world. The third study asked people to rate the importance of a large set of goals involving educationally relevant aspects of practical and academic intelligence.

Overall, the results of these three studies seemed to converge in a surprisingly consistent fashion. Three general themes emerged from these data. First, there was a strong emphasis on integrative achievements such as having good family and friendship relations, showing concern and respect for the rights of others, treating other people fairly and equitably, and being a responsible citizen. Mastery and management objectives also appeared to be regarded as core criteria for defining and evaluating practical intelligence, with the focus placed on both a set of instrumental skills closely associated with these outcomes (i.e., goal-setting, decision-making, planning, and problem-solving skills) and the outcomes themselves. Finally, there appeared to be little emphasis on any of the other transactional goals. The possible exception was safety goals, which seemed to receive some attention when the potentially harmful consequences were sufficiently serious. In sum, practical intelligence can be conceptualized as involving a social relationship component and a task component, each of which rests on a foundation of personal well being.

References

Bandura, A. (1982). Self-efficacy mechanism in human agency. *American Psychologist, 37,* 122–147.

Eckensberger, L. H., & Meacham, J. A. (1984). The essentials of action theory: A framework for discussion. *Human Development, 27,* 166–172.

Ford, D. H. (in press). *Humans as self-constructing living systems.* Hillsdale, NJ: Erlbaum.

Ford, M. E. (1982). Social cognition and social competence in adolescence. *Developmental Psychology, 18,* 323–340.

Ford, M. E. (1985). The concept of competence: Themes and variations. In H. A. Marlowe & R. B. Weinberg (Eds.), *Competence development* (pp. 3–49). Springfield, IL: Thomas.

Ford, M. E. (1986). A living systems conceptualization of social intelligence: Outcomes, processes, and developmental change. In R. J. Sternberg (Ed.), *Advances in the psychology of human intelligence,* (Vol. 3, pp. 119–171). Hillsdale, NJ: Erlbaum.

Ford, M. E., Burt, R. E., & Bergin, C. C. (1984). *The role of goal setting and goal importance in adolescent social competence.* Paper presented at the annual meeting of the American Educational Research Association, New Orleans.

Ford, M. E., & Miura, I. (1983). *Children's and adults' conceptions of social competence.* Paper presented at the annual meeting of the American Psychological Association, Anaheim, CA.

Ford, M. E., & Nichols, C. W. (in press). A taxonomy of human goals and some possible applications. In M. E. Ford & D. H. Ford (Eds.), *Humans as self-constructing living systems: Putting the framework to work.* Hillsdale, NJ: Erlbaum.

Krumboltz, J. D., Ford, M. E., Nichols, C. W., & Wentzel, K. R. (in preparation). The goals of education. Stanford University School of Education, Stanford, CA 94305.

Maslow, A. (1943). A theory of human motivation. *Psychological Review, 50,* 370–396.

Mischel, W. (1973). Toward a cognitive social learning reconceptualization of personality. *Psychological Review, 70,* 252–282.

Neisser, U. (1976). General, academic, and artifical intelligence. In L. B. Resnick (Ed.), *The nature of intelligence* (pp. 135–144). Hillsdale, NJ: Erlbaum.

Sternberg, R. J. (1983). *A contextualist view of the nature of intelligence.* Unpublished manuscript, Yale University.

Sternberg, R. J. (1985). *Beyond IQ: A triarchic theory of human intelligence.* New York: Cambridge University Press.

Sternberg, R. J., Conway, B. E., Ketron, J. L., & Bernstein, M. (1981). People's conceptions of intelligence. *Journal of Personality and Social Psychology, 41,* 37–55.

Turiel, E. (1983). *The development of social knowledge: Morality and convention.* Cambridge: Cambridge University Press.

Wagner, R. K., & Sternberg, R. J. (1985). Practical intelligence in real-world pursuits: The role of tacit knowledge. *Journal of Personality and Social Psychology, 49,* 436–458.

Winell, M. (in press). Personal goals: Key to self-direction in adulthood. In M. E. Ford & D. H. Ford (Eds.), *Humans as self-constructing living systems: Putting the framework to work.* Hillsdale, NJ: Erlbaum.

Part III

The development of practical intelligence

10 Toward life-span research on the functions and pragmatics of intelligence

Roger A. Dixon and Paul B. Baltes

Considered together, several recent reviews of adult intellectual development testify to the vast, variegated, but promising nature of theory and research in the area (Baltes, Dittmann-Kohli, & Dixon, 1984; Baltes & Labouvie, 1973; Botwinick, 1977; Denney, 1982; Dixon, Kramer, & Baltes, 1985; Horn, 1982; Schaie, 1983; Willis, 1985). This multifarious situation has begotten and nurtured several controversial issues and discordant interpretations. At the same time, however, it has generated a number of potentially fruitful new research approaches and agendas.

One major reason for the variation in the interpretation of the course of adult intellectual development is the apparent absence of biological and cultural stabilization associated with the phenomena of old age. In contrast to the overall regularity surrounding the earlier portion of the life-span (Bayley, 1970; Flavell, 1970; McCall, 1979), the biocultural dynamics associated with (or shaping) adulthood and old age are sufficiently recent and indeterminate as to permit more instability and irregularity in the developmental functions involved (Dixon et al., 1985). Our suspicion, in brief, is that many of the discordant interpretations may be accurate; they may represent legitimately an unresolved, undetermined phenomenon, one that continues to fascinate specialists and laypersons alike.

A central issue in current conceptions of intellectual development throughout adulthood is the relative emphasis to be placed on the joint processes of – or, perhaps, the dynamic between – growth and decline (Baltes, in press). There are two interrelated aspects to this issue. First, there is a preponderance of evidence for decline in psychometric test performance, and concomitant suggestive evidence regarding personal perceptions and stereotypes of decline, especially in the later years of adulthood. Second, several authorities have suggested that there are aspects of intelligence that exhibit stabilization or even progression, or that in principle could exhibit stabilization or progression, given a variety of "appropriate" testing meth-

Acknowledgment: The authors appreciate the helpful comments of Freya Dittmann-Kohli, Daniel Keating, Reinhold Kliegl, Jutta Heckhausen, and Jacqui Smith on an earlier version of this chapter.

ods or supportive performance conditions (Baltes et al., 1984; Denney, 1982; Labouvie-Vief, 1982, 1985). These aspects of intelligence are usually associated with (1) the practical, cognitively demanding situations of daily and professional life; (2) the natural course of experience and accumulation of cultural knowledge; (3) select domains of specialization or expertise; or (4) such hypostatized domains of age-related mental functioning as wisdom. Increasingly, it has been suggested that because the less pragmatic dimensions are overrepresented in, for example, standard psychometric tests, the typical finding of age-related performance decline may not be a valid indicator of the overall intellectual readiness, adaptiveness, or everyday performance of older adults (Baltes & Willis, 1979; Berg & Sternberg, 1983; Labouvie-Vief, 1982, 1984). In particular, it may underrepresent that functional mental activity that occurs in daily life and the reserve capacity of older adults that, under proper conditions, can be tapped as a source of further advancement or as a resource for compensation for other declining functions (Baltes & Kliegl, 1986; Dixon et al., 1985). However, it is also apparent that many efforts to develop measures of "practical intelligence" or of "practical problem solving" have not resulted in the expected positive age differences (Denney, 1982; Salthouse, 1982).

From this perspective, three interrelated principles of intellectual development thoughout adulthood may be derived:

1. An age-related decline in the mechanics of mental functioning occurs, especially in the later adult years, but there may be some stabilization, and perhaps even advancement, in some well-practiced, skilled, and pragmatic aspects.
2. Despite an unambiguous age-related decline in the various underlying mechanisms of intelligence, under normal conditions there is also sufficient reserve capacity so as to nurture an (at least temporary) increase in performance, especially if appreciable interest, effort, training, practice, motivation, or social support are present.
3. A concomitant adaptive – sometimes selective and sometimes automatic – compensatory feature of mental functioning allows for the inevitable decline to be less debilitating, less generalized (i.e., more localized), and less transferred to other features than might otherwise be expected.

In the present chapter we argue that these principles of intellectual development throughout adulthood are united by a handful of assumptions pertaining to human mental activity in the context of changing social conditions, the physical ecology, and the life course. We shall focus on (1) these assumptions and principles, especially as they complement and contrast with prior considerations and auger the future of research activity, and (2) selected pragmatic dimensions of intellectual functioning that may hold special promise as domains of future scholarly consideration. Our first topic, however, is the conceptual framework that appears to sponsor, in part, some of this work. Although there may appear to be of more than one such framework

– for example, contextualism (Hultsch & Pentz, 1980; Jenkins, 1974; Sternberg, 1983), functionalism (Beilin, 1984; Dixon & Hertzog, in press), and neofunctionalism (Dittmann-Kohli & Baltes, in press) – for present purposes, they are sufficiently similar to be addressed in combination. Thus, our intent is not to examine the details of the convergence of these frameworks, but rather to propose that, because they are derived from the same logical motivation, they form a certain natural convergence and that their specific points of mutuality and conflict may be left, for now, unexamined.

A functional approach to intellectual development

Since the early 1970s, the study of psychological development has been marked by considerable parlance in metatheoretical and conceptual realms (Lerner, Hultsch, & Dixon, 1983; Manicas & Secord, 1983; Reese & Overton, 1970). Within the generous context of this forum, similar deliberations have occurred in various subdisciplines of developmental psychology, such as personality and temperament (Lerner & Lerner, in press; Sarbin, 1977), intelligence (Dittmann-Kohli & Baltes, in press; Sternberg, 1983), and cognition (Bruce, 1985; Dixon & Hertzog, in press; Hultsch & Pentz, 1980; Nilsson, 1984). Certainly, one continuing thrust has been the dissatisfaction on the part of some psychologists with what are perceived to be limitations in extant models of development, for example, mechanism and organicism (Pepper, 1970; Reese & Overton, 1970).

In the wake of these purported "paradigm clashes," a third model has become increasingly popular. This family of principles, perhaps known best as contextualism, derives in part from turn-of-the-century contextual pragmatists such as Charles S. Peirce, William James, John Dewey, George Herbert Mead, and from functional psychologists such as James Rowland Angell, Harvey Carr, James Mark Baldwin, and of course, James and Dewey (Pepper, 1970). In this section, we summarize briefly the origin and main features of this model, its application to developmental psychology, and in particular its relevance to the study of intelligence. Although there are some important differences among them, we shall use the terms contextualism, pragmatism, and functionalism somewhat interchangeably.

Contextualism – its categories and metaphors, its emphases and ramifications, its epistemology and methodologies, its history and intellectual brethren – has been reviewed sufficiently in recent years (Lerner et al., 1983; Pepper, 1970; Rosnow & Georgoudi, in press; Sarbin, 1977). These reviews indicate that, overall, contextualism emphasizes multilevel change and novelty as well as the functional interrelationship of these constantly changing multiple levels. Insofar as contextualism has been a tangible sponsor of an approach to psychology, that approach has portrayed psychological development as an active, continuing, adaptive lifelong process, related to

other "internal" or mental processes, and interacting with biological processes, external activities, and sociohistorical processes. In this way, a contextual psychology is related to (and occasionally identified with) psychologies derived from pragmatism, dialecticism, and functionalism, but it is not
entirely disjunctive with psychologies derived from mechanism and
organicism.

Some features of a functional approach

Contextualism has been said to be a post-Darwinian philosophy that has
sponsored a functional psychology in which the influence of evolutionary
thinking is unmistakable (Bawden, 1910; Ghiselin, 1969; Morris, 1970; Wiener, 1949). Clearly, the concept of function was one way in which Darwin's
theory of evolution was incorporated into turn-of-the-century American psychology (Dallenbach, 1915). The biological version of this concept suggested
that anatomical structures, shaped as they were by contextually based natural selection, functioned so as to further the survival of the organism (Ghiselin, 1969). Thus, according to Boring (1957, p. 551), a functional approach
is concerned with "success in living, with the adaptation of the organism to
its environment, and with the organism's adaptation of its environment to
itself."

Early functional psychologists such as James (1890, 1907) applied this
perspective in a rather straightforward manner. Consciousness, although
having no mechanical function, is useful in securing the survival needs of
the organism because of its presumed causal efficaciousness. Put simply,
the mind is an organ selected for its value in benefitting the adaptation of
the complex human organism to a complex environment. Consciousness is
not simply passively useful, however. Rather, it is actively useful, for one
of its most salient characteristics is its selectivity (James, 1890). In contemporary terms, James viewed consciousness as a changing, adaptive, selective
system of knowledge. Indeed, if cognition is a principal function of mind
(James, 1890, 1907), knowledge is a principal commodity of cognition.

Most functionalists favored dynamic portrayals of adaptive activity (Carr,
1925). Although used in numerous ways, the term function appears to have
been reserved by most authorities for the value or adaptiveness of activity
(Carr, 1930; Heidbreder, 1933). Consequently, the emphasis was on developing a practical psychology (Bawden, 1910; Dewey, 1908), with attention directed not only to mental contents or structures (see Titchener, 1898,
1899), but also to processes and operations that occur in actual living conditions (Angell, 1907; Brunswik, 1952; Dewey, 1910a; Heidbreder, 1933;
Petrinovich, 1979).

Another important feature of early functional psychology was its concern
with the temporality of mental and behavioral phenomena and, by impli-

cation, the relationship to early developmental approaches to psychology. It is well known that the intellectual climate surrounding (and in part inspired by) Darwinism propagated a temporal approach to the study of human social and psychological phenomena (Dewey, 1910c; Dixon & Lerner, 1985; Toulmin & Goodfield, 1965; White, 1968). In brief, this temporization of psychological phenomena led to more vigorous study of individual mental development. Indeed, many of the major contemporary models of human development can be traced to the intellectual climate of evolutionary thinking (Dixon & Lerner, 1984). Many functionalists (e.g., Angell, 1907, 1908; Baldwin, 1895; and Dewey, 1910c) were explicit in their linkage of Darwinism and the study of psychological development. Like other natural entities, Baldwin argued, the mind grows and develops. Distinguishing their enterprise from the simple description of substances or faculties of the mind, the functionalists focused on the conditions and development of mental activity. It was thought that from this genetic approach explanatory statements could be derived. Partly for this reason, Angell (1907), indeed, called for "longitudinal," rather than "transverse," methods in human developmental psychology.

One additional emphasis of some functionalists was the evanescent and fleeting nature of mental contents. The obvious empirical problems this perspective engendered did not go unrecognized. Angell (1907) argued that, as in the physical realm, in mental life it is the functions that endure. Mental contents may be evanescent but successive contents may have the same meaning, that is, they may function in the same practical way. As with biological phenomena, the functions may persist even though different structures may, under special conditions, be called upon to perform them. The transitory statelike nature of mental phenomena is an important aspect of this approach, for it is one way in which affective and cognitive processes are interrelated. That is, a given mental event is portrayed as dependent on such features of the internal conditions as moods and goals as well as on its functional relationship with selected external circumstances (Angell, 1907, 1908). As it was put in the early part of the century, one task, then, is to identify and distinguish the modus operandi of mental phenomena.

In brief, from its inception, this approach has directed attention to such current issues as the practical, everyday, and adaptive features of intellectual functioning. Furthermore, it has done so in the context of dynamic, developmental portrayals of knowledge transformation and mental activity. Let us turn now to a more specific consideration of this latter aspect.

Functions of knowledge and intelligence

Within the context of a natural selection epistemology, early pragmatists emphasized the functional nature of cognition, from its everyday usefulness to its performance as a selecting instrument of survival (Baldwin, 1909; Bruce, 1985; James, 1890, 1907; Neisser, 1976, 1978), both during ontogeny and evolution. Because past experience (which is the primary foundation for personal knowledge) is based on encounters between an active organism and a changing environment – because the learning that has occurred has been a function of the organism's continuing adaptive activities – the knowledge with which organisms face their own futures, was considered fallible (Campbell, 1974; Lewontin, 1978; Plotkin & Odling-Smee 1982; Popper, 1965, 1972; Rescher, 1980; Toulmin, 1961). The simultaneity of (1) the fallibility of knowledge, and (2) the functional character of intelligence is an issue much discussed by modern evolutionary epistemologists (Campbell, 1974; Popper, 1965, 1972). If this perspective seems somewhat self-evident today, it was not at the turn of the century. Indeed, much of the early work in developing an experimental or pragmatic theory of knowledge – a theory of knowledge as a natural function – was conducted as a response to classical rational models (e.g., Dewey, 1910b, 1910e). The functional argument was that the conditions of knowledge activation and use are practical ones, involving the interests of an active organism, and that the test of truth is the operational value of the thought, judgment, or action (Bawden, 1910; Dewey, 1910b, 1910d).

Therefore, the functionalist portrayed (1) knowledge (or knowing) as practical, (2) intelligence as instrumental, (3) reason as efficacious, and (4) experience as being future oriented. In looking back at his own use of the expression, Dewey (1939) acknowledged that the term intelligence captures much of what he meant by "thought" in some instances, and "knowledge" in others; that is, it is an instrumental process that functions to make one experience available for use in other experiences, of effecting and planning transitions of life events, of making specific adjustments of things to purposes and purposes to things (see also Dewey, 1910d, 1916; Thayer, 1973). Bawden (1910, p. 156) noted that such cognition is "man's method of managing his experience." Overall, this position may have been summarized best by Dewey (1925, p. 371):

The function of intelligence is . . . not that of copying the objects of the environment, but rather of taking account of the way in which more effective and profitable relations with these objects may be established in the future.

It is notable that Dewey (1933, 1939), in eschewing what was then termed capacity psychology, emphasized the plasticity of intelligence in the context of an argument for multidimensionality. Similarly, Allport (1939) interpreted this argument to mean that, in the absence of severe illness or physical defect, poor intellectual performance in all domains is rare; that is:

Anyone is capable of thinking and so improving his adaptations and mastery within his environment. A pupil labelled as hopeless . . . may react in a quick and lively fashion when the thing in hand seems to him worthwhile. . . . In short, individual differences in capacity are of far less consequence than is the fact that everyone can be taught to think more effectively than he does. (Allport, 1939, p. 277)

Even at this early stage, then, intelligence is viewed as multidimensional and, probably, as including that realm covered by psychometric tests. It is, however, not restricted to that realm and, for some important aspects of intelligent activity in adulthood, may not be precisely indicated by such measurement techniques. Rather, a great deal of attention is devoted to the "practical predicament of life" (Thayer, 1952, p. 33) and the efficaciousness of reason in marshaling prior experience and knowledge in the solution of practical problems. As Thayer (1973) noted, the pragmatists maintained the following point of view:

The mark of intelligent life, perhaps the root of reason, is the maintenance of life itself through continuously changing environments by evolving techniques of adaptation and control, i.e., efficacious modification and direction of existing conditions. Reason, thus portrayed in the service of life, is to be understood as a natural function with a natural history like those of breathing and digestion. (p. 221)

The pragmatists (perhaps especially James and Dewey) developed new conceptions of experience, its content and function, its biological and anthropological nature, its application to the selection and control of life consequences and outcomes, as well as its multiple forms, multiple origins, and multiple courses (Dewey, 1910a, 1929, 1939; Smith, 1978). Smith (1978) asserted that experience in the contemporary American vernacular is derived from the pragmatic formulation in two particular ways:

First, the personal undergoing, *living through*, or enduring of situations and events, and second, the *acquisition of skills* enabling one to respond in appropriate fashion to the way objects encountered will behave, persons will conduct themselves, or systems will "work." (p. 94)

One connotation of this view is especially pertinent to contemporary efforts to examine practical knowledge and skills in adulthood. The notion is that a person who is experienced in a given domain (whether painting, yachting, schoolwork, remembering jokes, automechanics, or chess) has the skill, ability, or "know-how" to perform effectively, or to accomplish given objectives, in problems pertaining to that domain. Thus, the active, transformatory aspect of experience and skill is emphasized (Charness, in press; Smith, 1978).

This rendering of intelligence focuses attention on such mental skills as those involved in the pragmatics of life, and on efforts to perform effectively in those uncertain matters pertaining to life experience and the life course (Dewey, 1908, 1939). Thus, the broadening of the concept of intelligence – to include not only psychometric intelligence, practical intelligence, logical reasoning, and practical reasoning, but also judgment, common sense, expertise, deliberation, and wisdom – was suggested.

It is, in part, on this conceptual basis that researchers in the field of intellectual aging have begun to consider the influence of experience, knowledge, and skills on processes such as cognitive performance, judgment, reasoning, and wisdom (Baltes et al., 1984; Dittmann-Kohli, 1984; Dittmann-Kohli & Baltes, in press; Salthouse, in press). It is, in part, these domains that comprise what we have called the pragmatics of intelligence and that may not suffer inevitable age-related decline (Baltes et al., 1984). Like younger adults, older adults must continually face incomplete, uncertain situations and, on the basis of both cognitive and noncognitive experiences – as well as reservoirs of truth, morality, common sense, and practical knowledge – make evaluations, judgments, or other transformations of knowledge into action (Dewey, 1939; Parodi, 1939). It is worth noting that, for Dewey, as well as other pragmatists, intelligence marked "the intersection of knowledge and wisdom" (Smith, 1978, p. 158). Although this view is partly in contrast to some traditional orientations, it is not, as we shall see below, diametrically opposed (Baltes et al., 1984; Dixon et al., 1985; Labouvie-Vief, 1985; Sternberg, 1983, 1984).

Contributions of the psychometric tradition

In the preceding subsection we introduced the functional approach to knowledge, intelligence, and experience, with some attention devoted to its possible application to the study of intellectual development throughout adulthood. It should be understood, however, that, although dating to the contextual pragmatists in the early part of this century, this approach did not foster a "tradition" of research in the community of life-span developmental psychologists. This is the case despite (or, perhaps, as Heidbreder, 1933, suggests, because of) the apparent common-sense ring of the principal propositions of functionalism. Instead, much of what we know about intellectual aging derives from the historically predominant body of psychometric research.

This is not to say that murmurings of the issues we have tentatively attached to the functional model were never heard, for on numerous occasions during the past fifty to sixty years they have indeed been raised (Dixon et al., 1985; Woodruff, 1982). This is also not to imply that we are describing, or even forecasting, a revolution in intelligence and aging research, for what we term the functional approach is continuous (i.e., it is confrontive but not insurgent) with a psychometric orientation. Indeed, there are at least two major examples of this simultaneous movement away from, and continuity with, the traditional psychometric model, viz., the contextual cognitive components viewpoint (Sternberg, 1983, 1984) and the dual-process metaphor derived from a life-span developmental perspective (Baltes et al., 1984). Before describing recent advances in the application of this approach to aging research, we devote some attention to the prepotent context of its emergence.

Understanding change in adult intellectual performance

In reviewing much of the literature pertaining to life-span intellectual development, Baltes and Willis (1979; see also Willis & Baltes, 1980) abstracted four underlying conceptions. Together, these conceptions were advanced as a useful characterization of the development of intelligence in adulthood and old age. In brief, these four conceptions are as follows:

1. *Multidimensionality*, the notion that intelligence is composed of multiple mental abilities, each with potentially distinct structural, functional, and developmental properties
2. *Multidirectionality*, signifying that there are multiple distinct change patterns associated with these abilities
3. *Interindividual variability*, a conception reflecting the observed differences in the life-course change patterns of individuals
4. *Intraindividual plasticity*, which indicates that, in general, throughout the life course individual behavioral patterns are modifiable.

That these abstractions reflect a particular interpretation of predominantly recent psychometric research on the development of intelligence is clear. That this interpretation is consonant with the bulk of the empirical research and conceptual commentaries that have accumulated over a much longer period is also possible (Dixon et al., 1985; Woodruff, 1982).

For example, both pre-Darwinian observers (e.g., Abercrombie, 1839; Quetelet, 1842; Tetens, 1777) and post-Darwinian observers (e.g., Porter, 1891) foreshadowed several aspects of this contemporary characterization of human intelligence (see Dixon et al., 1985). Similarly, even after the proliferation of mental testing – in the dawn of psychometric work – such conceptions as multidimensionality and intraindividual plasticity were present; the vigorous efforts of, for example, Binet (1909; Binet & Henri, 1895; Binet & Simon, 1911; Peterson, 1925) to advance mental orthopedics and to question atomistic representations are noteworthy in this regard. More directly relevant, however, is the question of whether those early reports that were directly addressed to issues of intellectual development in adulthood also shared in some or all of these conceptions. As we have seen elsewhere (Dixon et al., 1985), several early commentators certainly did (e.g., Hall, 1922; Hollingworth, 1927; Kirkpatrick, 1903; Sanford, 1902).

As alluded to at the outset, since the advent of empirical investigations of intellectual aging there has been a decided lack of consensus concerning whether the course of adult intelligence is typified by stabilization, progression, decrement, or some combination thereof. So many studies, both cross-sectional and longitudinal, have found a verbal-nonverbal (as well as a power-speeded) bifurcation in the pattern of life-span results that Botwinick (1977) derived an expression, the classic intellectual aging pattern, to synopsize them. This bow to multidimensionality or multidirectionality was echoed in several of the very early cross-sectional investigations (e.g., Jones & Conrad, 1933; Pressey, 1917, 1919; Weisenburg, Roe, & McBride, 1936; Willoughby, 1927) and longitudinal studies (see Bayley, 1955; Botwinick, 1967, 1977; Cunningham & Owens, 1983; Jones 1959; Owens, 1966; see also Garrett, 1946).

In addition, early observers noted the wide range of interindividual variation in intellectual aging (Bayley, 1955; Garrett, 1946; Wechsler, 1952; Weisenburg et al., 1936), as well as the apparent deleterious effects that biological aging has on "native capacity," "sheer modifiability," adaptability, or plasticity (e.g., Jones & Conrad, 1933; Marsh, 1933; Ruch, 1934; Thorndike, 1928). In accounting for aging decrements, the influence of such modern-sounding age-related performance factors as diminished familiarity, practice, interest, motivation, and sensorimotor functioning was cited (e.g., Foster & Taylor, 1920; Jones & Conrad, 1933). Furthermore, the beneficial compensatory effect of accumulated knowledge, life conditions, and experience was noted by several observers (e.g., Jones & Conrad, 1933; Miles, 1933; Miles & Miles, 1932; Nisbet, 1957; Willoughby, 1927; Yerkes, 1921, 1923).

All of this is to suggest that, despite the accumulation of a great deal of unambiguous evidence for intellectual decline, many of the early investigators did not blindly promulgate a general decline model. Rather, some marshaled arguments and conceptions that were similar to contemporary ones. With varying degrees of exactitude and cogency, they drew some attention to the evidence for multidimensionality, multidirectionality, and interindividual variability in life-span intellectual development, as well as to performance conditions that might have the effect of magnifying age-related performance deficits, and to life conditions, experience, and knowledge that may be activated or used to compensate for some of the decline that does occur.

Other reviewers of this early psychometric work have alluded to one or more of these conclusions; indeed, some have argued for the broadening of the concept of intelligence (1) to include problem solving in real-life (or ecologically relevant) problem situations, and (2) to incorporate a more global matrix of psychological functioning, including personality (or affect) and morality (or wisdom) components (i.e., Guilford, 1967; Jones, 1959; Pressey & Kuhlen, 1957; Wechsler, 1958; Weisenburg et al., 1936; Woodruff, 1983). One exception to the classic aging pattern – indeed, to the very possibility of stabilization or progression – and to the line of reasoning we have sketched, should be mentioned. When the very late years of life are considered, or when nonnormal adults are tested, firm evidence for decrements has often been found, evidence emanating from both verbal and nonverbal test results (Jarvik & Bank, 1983; Schaie, 1983; Schaie & Hertzog, 1983).

The modern era

With the surfacing of this exception, this brief overview of the contribution of the psychometric tradition to a functional interpretation of portions of the adult intelligence literature shifts to the more contemporary scene. In this setting, the contributions associated with Schaie's (1979, 1983) Seattle Longitudinal Study, Horn and Cattell's (1966; Horn, 1980, 1982) model of fluid and crystallized intelligence, and research on experiential intervention in adulthood (e.g., Baltes & Willis, 1982; Denney, 1982; Willis, 1985) are the central characters. We will not address the considerable controversy surrounding some of these research programs (see, instead, Baltes & Kliegl, 1986; Baltes, Dittmann-Kohli, & Kliegl, in press; Baltes & Schaie, 1976; Birren, Cunningham, & Yamamoto, 1982; Botwinick, 1977; Horn & Donaldson, 1976; Willis, 1985), but will focus instead on specific issues.

Cohort differences. To begin where we left off in the previous subsection, much has been made of Schaie's apparent emphasis on positive age change (or stabilization) in several intellectual functions (Botwinick, 1977; Horn & Donaldson, 1976; see also Baltes & Schaie, 1976; Schaie & Baltes, 1977). Indeed, the discord surrounding the results of Schaie's twenty-one year cohort-sequential study has been notable.

In addition to the issue of Schaie's interpretation of stability in most functions through middle age, the controversy has stemmed from the relative emphasis placed on cohort effects in the interpretation of the age/cohort relationship. That is, after each occasion of measurement, the data indicated that observed age differences across a wide range of performance tasks may be in part a function of differential cultural and historical experiences (as represented in cohort differences) and not entirely due to universal ontogenetic functions (e.g., Nesselroade, Schaie, & Baltes, 1972; Schaie, 1979, 1983; Schaie & Hertzog, 1983; Schaie & Labouvie, 1974; Schaie, Labouvie, & Buech, 1973; Schaie & Strother, 1968a; 1968b). As such, cohort differences for same-age adults are not easily accounted for in terms of genetic differences in the population; rather, the primary emphases are on treating them as environmentally or experientially based.

Overall, the interpretation was advanced that what is seen in descriptive aging research as decline may be, at least in part, a reflection of age differences in social and environmental opportunities (Baltes & Kliegl, 1986; Baltes et al., 1984). This position echoes the remarks of some of the earliest commentators (e.g., Sanford, 1902).

Indeed, it was not until the more recent Schaie and Hertzog (1983) report that decidedly clear evidence for decline on all tests was presented forcefully. Nevertheless, even here notable attention was paid to the observed interindividual performance differences, viz., that to age seventy there are still some adults who do not decline at all (see also Schaie, 1983). Furthermore, the authors remarked that the observed decrements should be seen in the context of the findings pertaining to cohort differences and to interindividual variability. They suggested that the decrements in the fifties may be small enough to be of little practical importance, whereas the decrements observed in old age (60 to 80 years) were of considerably more salience (Schaie, 1983).

A theory of multidimensionality. Another major contribution of the modern era is primarily theoretical and focuses directly on the joint occurrence of growth and decline. Horn and Cattell (1966, 1967; see also Horn, 1980, 1982), the principal proponents of this second major contemporary approach, proposed a conceptually attractive model to account for the classic aging pattern: viz, the theory of fluid and crystallized intelligence. In brief, this alternative to the classic aging pattern takes the following shape. Crystallized intelligence, because it is indexed primarily by the life-long accumulation of cultural knowledge and skills, usually increases over the adult years. Fluid intelligence, on the other hand, is thought to be more dependent on physiological functioning and especially on the support of a relatively determinate neurological base. If this neurological base, which is continually subject to change, is impaired (e.g., because of traumatic insult or biological aging) the ability to perform the associated intellectual skills is undermined.

Although the Horn–Cattell model provides a potentially fruitful rationale for the verbal–nonverbal distinction (of the classic aging pattern), there are a handful of inevitable lacunae. For example, the data base is largely cross-sectional and in need of enrichment. In addition, some details concerning the mechanics of the relationship between, for example, the neurological base and fluid intelligence on the one hand, and knowledge (and experience) and crystallized intelligence on the other, are as yet unavailable. In any event, experience, knowledge, and acculturation are important aspects in the development of one form of intelligence.

The conceptual unpacking of crystallized intelligence (e.g., through process-oriented work on the acquisition, activation and use of knowledge systems) is an important direction for future research. As we shall see in a later section, such work (proceeding parallel to work in the model of crystallized and fluid intelligence) is in progress.

Reserve capacity and plasticity. Multidimensionality and multidirectionality are two features the above two modern programs of research have in com-

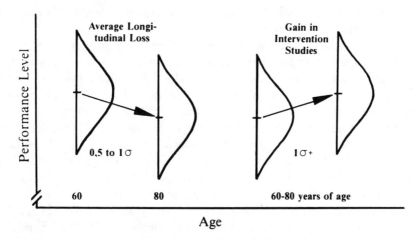

Figure 1. Average aging loss (descriptive) and magnitude of gain following training in fluid intelligence measures. *Source:* Baltes et al. 1984.

mon. In addition, a concern for interindividual variability and (at least implicitly) intraindividual plasticity is apparent in Schaie's work. The latter conception, however, has been the focus of a third line of scholarship, that devoted to intervention research (Baltes & Willis, 1982; Denney, 1979, 1982; Labouvie-Vief, 1985; Sterns & Sanders, 1980; Willis, 1985; Willis & Baltes, 1980; Woodruff, 1982). The logic of this research is as follows.

It is possible that much of the extant variation in the interpretation of the descriptive work in intellectual aging can be assigned to contrasting accounts of both the evidence for age-related decline (or stabilization) and the purported demonstrations of intraindividual plasticity as a result of both naturally occurring experiential differences and concerted efforts at intervention. There is considerable descriptive evidence for subgroup (e.g., cohort) differences in level and rate of intellectual functioning. If experiential differences (e.g., those associated with educational and work histories of cohorts) are in part responsible for observed interindividual and intertask performance differences, then the programmatic manipulation of specific experiences may have the effect of enhancing specific performances in individuals. Such manipulations may take the form of practice, modeling, education, training, or other techniques of ecological intervention.

A rationale for this approach is illustrated in Figure 1. If it is possible to show, within groups of elderly persons, positive performance changes roughly equivalent to longitudinally observed negative age differences then the arguments for the plasticity of intellectual aging are enhanced. Such findings are subject to certain constraints, for example, questions regarding sample selection, maintenance and generalization of training, whether younger adults would benefit equally from similar interventions, or whether the observed intervention benefits are restricted to average rather than maximum levels of functioning.

More specifically, suggestive results of research on short-term intraindividual variability in life-span intellectual performance have appeared. This training research has examined the modifiability, flexibility, and plasticity of intelligence in late adulthood as a function of experimental treatments such as test practice and training of ability-specific reasoning skills. That is, perhaps some of the observed age-related performance differences may be accounted for by the fact that older adults are less knowledgeable of, familiar with, and practiced at taking psychometric tests or engaging in test-related cognitive activities. In general, older adults who have practiced taking standard psychometric and cognitive tests, and especially those who have participated in training of relevant problem-solving skills, are differentiated from those who have not (Baltes & Willis, 1982; Denney, 1979, 1982; Jones, 1959; Kamin, 1957; Rabbitt, 1982; Taub, 1973).

Intraindividually, continued increments (and maintenance up to six months) in performance across multiple occasions as a function of practice with test items and ability-related reasoning skills have been found, even in such fluid intelligence measures (which are thought to be associated with inevitable age-related decline) as induction and figural relations (Baltes & Willis, 1982; Baltes, Dittmann-Kohli, & Kliegl, in press; Hofland, Willis, & Baltes, 1981; Plemons, Willis, & Baltes, 1978). Moreover, although it is impossible to compare precisely the magnitude of gain observed in these studies to the magnitude of loss observed in longitudinal studies covering the same age range (e.g. Schaie & Hertzog, 1983), it is instructive to note that the magnitudes of training gain and longitudinal loss, respectively, are similar (Baltes & Kliegl, 1986).

Despite the limitations noted above, this research has two potentially important theoretical contributions. First, it is conceivable that observed age-related decline in psychometric test performance – even in performance on dimensions predicted to decline ineluctably – is modifiable to some extent. More specifically, in late adulthood, age and cohort effects may be mitigated as a function of exposure to pertinent training. Second – and related to this – the aging effects typically observed on some standard psychometric tests are, although presumably (and by design) valid indicators of age-related performance differences, potentially invalid indicators of age-related "capacity" differences. Thus, intervention research has contributed to the recent surge of interest in reserve capacity (Baltes et al., 1984; Baltes & Willis, 1982; Kliegl & Baltes, 1985; Salthouse & Somberg, 1982). This interest, irrespective of questions concerning absolute magnitude or comparisons to that of younger adults, highlights the considerable capacity of older adults for continued learning (Willis, 1985). Such a conception is a necessary condition for some of the arguments to follow concerning the pragmatics of intelligence in late life.

Further issues

It is impossible to summarize the contributions of the psychometric tradition to the study of the functions and pragmatics of intellectual aging in so brief a format (see also Baltes et al., 1984; Botwinick, 1977; Dixon et al., 1985; Horn, 1982; Salthouse, 1982; Schaie, 1979, 1983). In concluding this section, let us simply mention two other developments that have emerged as a result of continually testing the limits of the application of psychometric tests to understanding both the academic and practical aspects of adult intellectual development. These developments are (1) the generation of age- and cohort-appropriate tests, and (2) the further consideration of the role of cognitive skills.

The issue of the appropriateness of the test for older adults pertains both to arguments within the psychometric tradition (regarding the relative suitability of power or speeded tests in the study of aging; see Birren, 1952; Botwinick, 1977; Botwinick & Storandt, 1973; Corsini & Fassett, 1953; Green, 1969; Lorge, 1936) and the debates concerning the legitimacy of applying psychometric tests designed for adolescents or young adults to aging samples (e.g., Baltes & Willis, 1979; Cornelius, 1984; Demming & Pressey, 1957; Jones, 1959; Neisser, 1976; Pressey & Kuhlen, 1957). A variation on this latter theme has been what are generally unsuccessful attempts to develop ecologically relevant, real-world problem-solving and intelligence tests and to apply them to older adults (e.g., Demming & Pressey, 1957; Gardner & Monge, 1977; Salthouse, 1982). Recent efforts in this direction have met with only moderate success (see, for example, Denney, 1982). In a variation of this approach, Cornelius (1984) demonstrated that older adults judge fluid intelligence (nonverbal) tasks to be less familiar to them (1) than crystallized intelligence (verbal) tasks, and (2) than did younger adults. This suggests that aging-sensitive tests (such as those tapping fluid intelligence) may be associated with a practice deficit in the everyday life ecology of older adults.

With regard to the role of cognitive skills in life-span intellectual development, it is imperative not only to describe interindividual or intraindividual differences in performance, but also to examine the processes presumably underlying those differences. Our discussion has emphasized the descriptive facts regarding inter- and intraindividual differences in intellectual performance. Such facts do not address, and do not allow for inferences regarding, the relative status of the cognitive processes involved in that performance.

Consequently, the processes that either support or fail to support intellectual stability throughout the adult years have not been identified.

Research on plasticity represents one effort to move in the direction of identifying relevant factors or variables involved in regulating performance. Such research may also be used to identify limits or constraints on plasticity. Indeed, methods that allow for valid inferences regarding age-related "capacity" differences could be useful supplements to the methodological armamentary of the cognitive gerontologist.

Another research strategy is to focus more directly on the cognitive processes involved in intellectual functioning. Holding special promise, perhaps, is the cognitive components approach (Berg & Sternberg, 1985; Kliegl & Baltes, 1985; Pellegrino & Glaser, 1979; Salthouse, in press; Sternberg, 1980, 1981, 1983), which attempts to decompose the tasks of intelligence tests into their component processes, and to investigate these processes via methods normally identified with experimental psychology (but see also Neisser, 1983). As applied to life-span research, one goal would be to recover the information–processing components of intelligence test performance and to identify those components associated with age-related change. Such a componential analysis may contribute to the understanding of the classic aging pattern described above; that is, it may shed light on why some dimensions of intelligence appear to decline with advancing age and why others appear to remain stable, and, furthermore, why there are substantial interindividual differences in change profiles.

In any event, whether one pursues a cognitive-components approach, applies another programmatic cognitive approach (such as that associated with Hunt, 1978, 1982, 1983; or that of Carroll & Maxwell, 1979) to the study of aging, or follows up one of the occasional nonprogrammatic efforts (e.g., Cornelius, Willis, Nesselroade, & Baltes, 1983; Dixon et al., 1984; Hultsch, Hertzog, & Dixon, 1984), the role of information-processing skills involved in intelligence test performance (and vice-versa) is a topic of considerable importance. In the long run, cross-domain information on the relationship between cognitive processes and psychometric constructs, especially with regard to their potentially changing relationship across the life span, is a necessary precursor to the understanding of intelligent behavior as functional and processual.

Some new directions: functions and pragmatics of intelligence

Two domains of intellectual functioning have as yet been underrepresented in empirical work on intellectual aging. Interest in these domains can derive from the functional approach to intellectual development, from within the psychometric tradition and from various cognitive psychology approaches. Two of the domains that seem to merit special consideration in aging research are (1) the study of mental skills, expertise, and specialization, and (2) wisdom and interpretive knowledge. In our view, both of these domains operate within the range of what has been termed the pragmatics of intelligence (Baltes et al., 1984). Furthermore, they may also be seen as prototypical aspects of intellectual functioning throughout adulthood.

Before discussing these aspects of intellectual functioning in somewhat more detail, we will first sketch the logic of our own theoretical and methodological approach. This approach rests on several recent reviews of the historical and contemporary intelligence literature, as well as consideration of selected psychological, sociological and biological literatures relevant to adult development and aging (e.g., Baltes, et al., 1984; Botwinick, 1977; Dixon et al., 1985; Labouvie-Vief, 1985; Woodruff, 1982). We begin by providing a firmament upon which a model of intellectual aging – one that heuristically distributes the province of intelligence into two interrelated categories, namely, the mechanics and pragmatics of intelligence – is based.

Aging and selective optimization with compensation

Earlier, we referred to four abstractions derived from the literature on the life-span development of intelligence. These abstractions – multidimensionality, interindividual variability, multidirectionality, and intraindividual plasticity – have been shown to represent both the extant data base (Baltes & Willis, 1979; Willis & Baltes, 1980) and to have considerable historical precedent (Dixon et al., 1985). Furthermore, we have recently formulated eight propositions that focus directly on the dynamic interplay among growth, decline, and stabilization, and, at the same time, promote further understanding of intelligence during adulthood and old age. These propositions are based on a review of a wider range of information than the original four abstractions (Baltes et al., 1984). They are designed to integrate the data base at a somewhat lower level of analysis than were the four abstractions, and at the same time to provide a more thorough foundation for the delineation of one approach to intellectual development in adulthood. A brief description of these propositions follows.

By distinguishing between capacity and performance (Baltes et al., 1984; Fries & Crapo, 1981), the first three propositions maintain as follows:

1. Stability in reserve capacity for "average" intellectual functioning is maintained until the sixties.
2. Nevertheless, some dimensions of intellectual ability may show decided decrements, particularly those in which very difficult performance situations are involved.
3. Intellectual progression may continue in some persons, at least until late adulthood, as demonstrated by some suggestive (but as yet inconclusive) evidence.

Each of the instances described by the first three propositions is characterized by marked interindividual variability in onset, rate, and patterning.

The fourth and fifth propositions (below) were derived from the more general field of the psychology of adult development and aging. From this perspective, it is important for the researcher in life-span intellectual development to recognize certain aging-related changes:

4. With aging there is often a change in the structure of life goals such that the acquisition and maintenance of school-related cognitive skills becomes deemphasized and is replaced by an accentuation of pragmatic skills (such as problem solving in social, family, personal, and professional activities).
5. Because aging is often accompanied by individualization and interindividual differentiation, general psychological and intellectual functioning may be increasingly typified by specialization.

This latter notion is supported by sociological evidence (Featherman, 1983; Kohn & Schooler, 1978, 1982; Riley, 1985) pertaining to another proposition:

6. Aging-related loss in the social-structural conditions of (and expectations for) performance seems to be associated with a general performance context for older adults that is less than optimal, with some variation across social clusters.

Two additional propositions derive from research on age-related biological functioning (e.g., Fries & Crapo, 1981):

7. Normal biological aging is characterized by increased vulnerability, reduced adaptability to environmental variation, and decreased maximum levels of performance. A psychological implication is that there may be a growing awareness on the part of aging persons that they are both psychologically and biologically at risk.
8. Nevertheless, because some important features of the biological (and psychological) status of aging persons are, in principle, modifiable, efforts to compensate for specific debilitations or vulnerabilities may result in selective optimization of functioning. Whether psychological or biological, this optimization would operate within proscriptions imposed by, among other things, these very systems (see Baltes, in press; Baltes et al., 1984).

This set of propositions could provide a foundation for theory building in several ways. The approach of interest to us has been called selective optimization with compensation (Baltes et al., 1984; Baltes & Willis, 1982). This inchoate approach proceeds from the assumption that intellectual aging displays features of growth, stabilization, and decline. It suggests that the process of "successful aging" may be typified by the person's own aptitude in "selecting" life goals and trajectories for which internal and external conditions are supportive. As long as this support is garnered, intellectual skills and realms of expertise may be maintained and, more important, may compensate for those realms that are not supported (or supportable).

A dual-process model. A first application of this approach distributes the province of intellectual functioning into two interrelated domains and, as such, has been called a dual-process conception (Baltes et al., 1984). There are many ways of carving up the conceptual space of intelligence, and all are more or less useful, especially insofar as the divisions are not reified. Thus, our model is descriptive in intent and heuristic in practice. The first domain, described as the "mechanics of intelligence," includes the content-free architecture of information processing and problem solving. It represents those tasks and abilities on which (like fluid intelligence or speeded nonverbal tests) one normally observes aging-related decline.

The second domain has been termed the "pragmatics of intelligence." It includes both pragmatic and specialized features of intelligence, as well as accumulated systems of knowledge and skills of application. This second domain may be the reservoir from which some practical compensatory or substitutive efforts are marshaled and some adaptive intellectual functioning is derived. In this way, some facets of the second domain may (like crystallized and some verbal intelligence) be associated with patterns of stabilization and even advancement in intellectual functioning through much of adulthood. Naturally, the pragmatics of intelligence cannot operate without the mechanics, and solutions to mechanics of intelligence tasks can, with only a modicum of manipulation, necessitate the use of pragmatic skills (hence the cautionary note above regarding reification). Indeed, as Bawden (1910) noted, the functional viewpoint is that each abstract member of a given theoretical distinction is true only in relation to the other; thus, the mechanics of intelligence is true only in relation to the pragmatics.

Nevertheless, in the remainder of this chapter we focus on research in generally untapped aspects of the pragmatics of intelligence, with special emphasis on the applications to the study of life-span intellectual development.

Knowledge, expertise, and specialization

This emerging emphasis in research on intellectual development in adulthood is influenced especially by current trends in cognitive psychology (Dörner, 1982, 1983; Glaser, 1981; Hoyer, 1985; Sternberg, 1982, 1984) but also, to some extent, by the extension of cognitive structuralism (Edelstein & Noam, 1982; Kuhn, Pennington, & Leadbeater, 1983; Labouvie-Vief, 1985). The strategy employed is to identify domains of knowledge and problem solving that are characteristic of aging adults and the varying conditions of their life courses.

Recent efforts to identify tasks indigenous to adulthood are more concentrated than earlier attempts (e.g., Demming & Pressey, 1957) in their attention to the components of intelligence and the associated processes of problem solving. Explicit concern with both the contents of knowledge and the component processes of intelligence leads to the specification of adaptive forms of functioning.

We shall describe briefly this strategy of research as it applies to the forms of intellectual functioning especially relevant to adulthood, namely, mental skills and expertise. The emphasis is on those strategies that exemplify the consideration of knowledge as an essential part of intelligence, a consideration that has been in the literature at least since Henmon (1921, p. 195) asserted that "intelligence is intellect *plus* knowledge."

One assumption of this approach is that much of intellectual development beyond adolescence is not related to further evolution of basic cognitive processes. Possible adult trajectories, it is argued, involve the elaboration, maintenance, and transformation of knowledge rather than basic cognitive skills (see also Edelstein & Noam, 1982; Labouvie-Vief, 1980, 1982). Thus the primary form of intellectual development during the second part of human life is not represented by further changes of the basic processing capacities and associated cognitive structures, but by the procedural and factual knowledge systems (Anderson, 1982; Brown, 1982; Chi, Glaser, & Rees, 1983) associated with education, occupational life, and other pragmatic aspects of adult development and aging. A related assumption of such a view is that further acquisition, maintenance, and transformation of intelligence can be best studied by understanding it in terms of indices of cumulative evolution of effectiveness and high levels of performance. Among the key concepts are those of expertise and specialization.

As alluded to earlier, such a cognitive psychology approach may be an alternative treatment of the notion of crystallized intelligence, which has been described as the centerpiece of intellectual growth during the second part of the life span (Horn, 1970, 1982). Work on knowledge systems and expertise would address the sufficiency of current psychometric measures of crystallized intelligence (they consist primarily of measures of vocabulary and social intelligence) as well as the direction in which the refinement and expansion of crystallized intelligence could proceed. However, cognitive science work on knowledge and expertise represents an approach that in itself deserves more attention by life-span researchers on intelligence; that is, it is not simply an elaboration of the concept of crystallized intelligence. For example, consideration of factors and mechanisms involved in the maintenance of expertise could provide a useful model of the processes we consider typical of adaptive aging, namely, those involved in selective optimization with compensation.

One concrete example of a form of intelligence that may evince further growth in adulthood is seen in the study of professional knowledge and productivity (Baltes & Kliegl, 1986; Bertram, 1981; Birren, 1969; Cole, 1979;

Featherman, 1980; Kohn & Schooler, 1978, 1982; Miller, Slomcynski, & Kohn, 1984). Occupational careers belong to the experiences of adult life that may involve maintenance and further transformation of factual and procedural knowledge. Intellectual performances of scientists as studied in the field of scientific productivity will be used here as a sample case.

From its inception, research on knowledge systems and expertise (Chi et al., 1983) has addressed such occupational and professional knowledge domains as chess, physics, and mathematics. Such work has demonstrated, not unlike cognitive training research in aging (Baltes & Willis, 1982; Denney, 1979), that older adults in good health and in supportive environments have the capacity to maintain or increase high levels of functioning in select areas. Longitudinal research on the relationship between characteristics of work environments and cognitive functioning (Kohn & Schooler, 1978, 1982) has substantiated this view in natural settings. Level and rate of intellectual development during adulthood vary as a function of cognitive complexity and demands of work environments. Such research exemplifies the notion that interindividual differences in adult cognition and the nature of intellectual aging reflect in part the socioprofessional structure of society and everyday life (Bertram, 1981).

The study of age and scientific productivity has undergone a trend similar to research on intellectual aging. Early cross-sectional studies indicated a general pattern of age-related decline in scientific productivity (Lehman, 1953). Later work, however, based, for instance, on cohort and citation analysis, failed to corroborate the incidences of such widespread decrement (Cole, 1979; Dennis, 1966). Thus, Cole (1979) found that for scientists who remain active, the dominant finding is one of stabilization in scientific performance up to the ages of 60 to 65, and not one of decline. This finding of age invariance applies to all fields studied by Cole, including physics and mathematics.

In our view, research on professional knowledge and specialization, particularly if connected to a cognitive science and life-span approach, is an important vehicle for better conceptualization of dimensions of efficacy in the domain of the pragmatics of intelligence during adulthood and old age. On the one hand, such research represents the structure and function of intelligence as a system of factual and procedural knowledge. On the other hand, it makes explicit two related major features of adult development and aging: (1) increased specialization, and (2) a dynamic interplay between selected aspects of growth and decline. We described this interplay earlier as a process of selective optimization with compensation. Finally, this research highlights the importance of representing aging in terms of adaptations to changing social and professional contexts, rather than simply comparing the performance and products of aging adults with those of young adults.

Wisdom and interpretive knowledge

Wisdom is another example of what we label the pragmatics of intelligence, one that is perhaps of particular interest to life-span researchers (Baltes et al., 1984; Baltes & Dixon, 1985; Clayton & Birren, 1980; Dittmann-Kohli & Baltes, in press). As Kekes (1983) has observed, wisdom is a kind of interpretive knowledge, combining breadth and depth, an understanding of the significance of what is descriptively or commonly known. It involves an understanding of the limits and conditions for life and living (e.g., death, developmental tasks, and age-graded and history-graded givens), the limitations and possibilities that accrue as a function of the species, the individual, and the individual's phase of life (Kekes, 1983; Meacham, 1982; Mergler & Goldstein, 1983).

Because wisdom is an amorphous concept, and because it has rarely been the object of empirical operationalization, it is important to distinguish it from other related psychological constructs. According to Kekes (1983), wisdom is not to be equated with booklearning, simple expertise, or descriptive knowledge (as the accumulation of facts). Although wisdom and knowledge are not the same thing, they are not necessarily opposed:

> A man may have knowledge of many things and not be wise, but a wise man cannot be ignorant of the things he is wise about. (Hook, 1974, p. 7)

One potentially tangible (or measurable) sign of wisdom is good or sound judgment regarding the conduct of life, the factors influencing life, and the tasks of the life course. Good judgment may be manifested within the context of decision-making in hard cases. That is, as distinct from platitudes, wisdom emerges when there is a legitimate "jurisdictional conflict" among such features of the problem as goals or ideals, when it is uncertain which ideals or goals should guide the problem-solving process (Kekes, 1983). Wisdom can be seen not only as involving good judgment, but also as action guiding, and perhaps – given the analogy of moral judgment versus moral behavior – even as action. In an action-guiding function, wisdom is corrective in that it distinguishes between the significant and trivial aspects of life (or of a given life problem) and serves as a reminder of human limitations, for example, mortality, physical capacity, health, temperament, emotional range, personal talents, social constraints, cultural givens, age-graded factors, and history-graded influences (Kekes, 1983). Kekes argued that there are two ways in which wisdom guides action:

> By differentiating between what is possible and impossible for anyone, and by drawing the same distinction for a particular person in his context. (p. 282)

Because of the apparent temporal dependency, wisdom is often associated with late adulthood, and the emergence of noetic or meditative urges, philosophic calm, impartiality, and the desire to draw moral lessons (Clayton & Birren, 1980; Hall, 1922). Hall, in fact, referred to the tendency to draw moral lessons as a task of old age, and to the urge to sum up and keep perspective as a function of old age. It is partly through disillusionment that older adults – wise older adults – are able to sift through the "shams and vanities of life," in the service of moving "toward a new and higher type of personality, evolving a new synthesis of the significant factors of life" (Hall, 1922, pp. 413–414).

Toward psychological research on wisdom. Recently, some investigators have begun to examine the concept of wisdom as a potentially progressive feature of aging and to explore its amenability to operational and empirical investigation. Following earlier suggestions on this topic (Clayton, 1975, 1982; Clayton & Birren, 1980; Hall, 1922; Meacham, 1982), Dittmann-Kohli and Baltes (in press; see also Baltes & Dixon, 1985) defined wisdom as indexed by "good judgment about important but uncertain matters of life." In addition, the task of specifying heuristic criteria by which to assess wisdom has also begun.

Accordingly, wisdom involves the following attributes:

1. Expertise (including descriptive and procedural knowledge) in the fundamental pragmatics of life
2. Interpretive and evaluative knowledge about the significance of this content domain
3. Contextual richness (breadth) of problem definition and solution
4. Uncertainty (especially, complexity and difficulty) of problem situation and definition
5. Good (sound, effective, practical, action-guiding) judgment regarding the conduct of life.

Classification of wisdom as an expertise in the pragmatics of life connotes that it is an ability associated with a highly developed form of factual and procedural knowledge and, furthermore, that its acquisition and development are enhanced by the existence of a long-term series of experiences with the human condition and its varying processes and outcomes. In this instance, then, living longer and into old age may be advantageous. That is, to return to the growth and decline theme, one might expect to observe positive age differences or age-related advances in developmental functions associated with wisdom.

Identifying and defining wisdom in this manner facilitates the tasks of specifying and expanding the psychometric concepts of verbal or crystallized intelligence. That is, it offers a distinctive research example of the pragmatics of intelligence that is not normally considered in traditional research on intellectual aging. In addition, the cognitive study of wisdom can focus on mechanisms and processes rather than on product, as might be true for much research in the psychometric orientation. It is important to note in this context that a concern with wisdom and aging does not imply that wisdom-related phenomena do not exist at earlier stages of life or that it is the only highlight of adult intellectual development. Rather, the study of wisdom is given as an example of how some forms of mental activity in adulthood may be adaptive and progressive and how ontogenetically earlier facets of intelligence (e.g., social intelligence) may be refined and transformed as adulthood progresses.

Summary

We have covered a broad range of material, some of it historical and some quite contemporary. All of it, we believe, supports the direction being taken in some recent research on life-span intellectual development. In particular, in attempting to account for, if not understand, the dynamic interplay between growth and decline in life-span intellectual performance, it is necessary to examine both the mechanics and the pragmatics of intelligence, as well as the multiple ways in which they interpenetrate.

Much research, primarily psychometric in nature, has contributed significantly to our understanding of facets of both domains. Nevertheless, our analysis suggests that, with regard to life-span questions, the lacunae in our understanding of the pragmatics of intelligence are especially notable. Specifically, our understanding of life-span intellectual development may be incomplete insofar as it is not applied, either in principle or in practice, to those functional aspects of intelligence associated with the practical demands of adult life.

Our position is that much of successful adult intellectual functioning may be typified by such conceptions as knowledge accumulation and activation, expertise, and wisdom. We have described how inchoate research in these life-span areas is being formulated.

In part, our present remarks are based on earlier summaries of a wide range of literature (Baltes et al., 1984; Dixon et al., 1985), which resulted in the formulation of one approach to research on adult intelligence, namely, selective optimization with compensation. This model suggests that the process of successful aging (including intellectual adaptation and functioning throughout life) may be related to the individual's potential for, and aptitude in, selecting everyday or life-course goals for which internal and external sources of support are available. Furthermore, the maintenance of select domains of skill and expertise may serve to compensate for those realms that are not maintained or supported. This model informs the present discussion of the current status of research in, and the identification of some future directions for, life-span research on the functions and pragmatics of intelligence.

References

Abercrombie, J. (1839). *Inquiries concerning the intellectual powers and their investigation of truth.* Boston: Otis, Broaders.

Allport, G. W. (1939). Dewey's individual and social psychology. In P. A. Schilpp (Ed.), *The philosophy of John Dewey* (pp. 263–290). Evanston: Northwestern University Press.

Anderson, J. R. (1982). Acquisition of cognitive skill. *Psychological Review, 89,* 369–406.

Angell, J. R. (1907). The province of functional psychology. *Psychological Review, 14,* 61–91.

Angell, J. R. (1908). *Psychology: An introduction to the structure and function of human consciousness* (4th ed.). New York: Holt.

Baldwin, J. M. (1895). *Mental development in the child and the race.* New York: Macmillan.

Baldwin, J. M. (1909). *Darwin and the humanities.* Baltimore: Review Publishing.

Baltes, P. B., Dittmann-Kohli, F., & Dixon, R. A. (1984). New perspectives on the development of intelligence in adulthood: Toward a dual-process conception and a model of selective optimization with compensation. In P. B. Baltes & O. G. Brim, Jr. (Eds.), *Life-span development and behavior* (Vol. 6, pp. 33–76). New York: Academic.

Baltes, P. B., Dittmann-Kohli, F., & Kliegl, R. (1985). Reserve capacity of the elderly in aging-sensitive tests of fluid intelligence. Unpublished manuscript, Max Planck Institute for Human Development and Education, Berlin.

Baltes, P. B., & Dixon, R. A. (1985). Notes on future research directions on wisdom as an exemplar of the pragmatics of intelligence. Unpublished manuscript, Max Planck Institute for Human Development and Education, Berlin.

Baltes, P. B., & Kliegl, R. (1986). On the dynamics between growth and decline in the aging of intelligence and memory. In K. Poeck, H. J. Freund, & H. Gänshirt (Eds.), *Neurology* (pp. 1–33). Heidelberg: Springer-Verlag.

Baltes, P. B., & Labouvie, G. V. (1973). Adult development of intellectual performance: Description, explanation, and modification. In C. Eisdorfer & M. P. Lawton (Eds.), *The psychology of adult development and aging* (pp. 157–219). Washington: American Psychological Association.

Baltes, P. B., & Schaie, K. W. (1976). On the plasticity of intelligence in adulthood and old age: Where Horn and Donaldson fail. *American Psychologist, 31,* 720–725.

Baltes, P. B., & Willis, S. L. (1979). The critical importance of appropriate methodology in the study of aging: The sample case of psychometric intelligence. In F. Hoffmeister & C. Miller (Eds.), *Brain function in old age* (pp. 164–187). Heidelberg: Springer-Verlag.

Baltes, P. B., & Willis, S. L. (1982). Plasticity and enhancement of intellectual functioning in old age: Penn State's Adult Development and Enrichment Project (ADEPT). In F. I. M. Craik & S. E. Trehub (Eds.), *Aging and cognitive processes* (pp. 353–389). New York: Plenum.

Bawden, H. H. (1910). *The principles of pragmatism: A philosophical interpretation of experience.* Boston: Houghton-Mifflin.

Bayley, N. (1955). On the growth of intelligence. *American Psychologist, 10,* 805–818.

Bayley, N. (1970). Development of mental abilities. In P. H. Mussen (Ed.), *Carmichael's Manual of Child Psychology* (Vol. 1, 3rd ed., pp. 1163–1209). New York: Wiley.

Beilin, H. (1984). Functionalist and structuralist research programs in developmental psychology: Incommensurability or synthesis? In H. W. Reese (Ed.), *Advances in child development and behavior* (Vol. 18, pp. 245–257). Orlando: Academic.

Berg, C. A., & Sternberg, R. J. (1985). A triarchic theory of intellectual development during adulthood. *Developmental Review, 5,* 334–370.

Bertram, H. (1981). *Sozialstruktur und Sozialisation: Zur mikrosoziologischen Analyse von Chancenungleichheit.* Darmstadt: Luchterhand.

Binet, A. (1909). *Les idées modernes sur les enfants.* Paris: Flammarion.

Binet, A., & Henri, V. (1895). La psychologie individuelle. *L'Annee Psychologique, 2,* 411–465.

Binet, A., & Simon, T. (1911). *A method of measuring the development of the intelligence of young children.* Lincoln, IL: Courier.

Birren, J. E. (1952). A factorial analysis of the Wechsler-Bellevue Scale given to an elderly population. *Journal of Consulting Psychology, 16,* 399–405.

Birren, J. E. (1969). Age and decision strategies. In A. T. Welford & J. E. Birren (Eds.), *Decision making and age: interdisciplinary topics in gerontology* (Vol. 4). Basel, Switzerland: Karger.

Birren, J. E., Cunningham, W. R., & Yamamoto, K. (1982). Psychology of adult development and aging. *Annual Review of Psychology, 34,* 543–575.

Boring, E. G. (1957). *A history of experimental psychology* (2nd ed.). Englewood Cliffs, NJ: Prentice-Hall.

Botwinick, J. (1967). *Cognitive processes in maturity and old age.* New York: Springer.

Botwinick, J. (1977). Intellectual abilities. In J. E. Birren & K. W. Schaie (Eds.), *Handbook of the psychology of aging* (pp. 580–605). New York: Van Nostrand Reinhold.

Botwinick, J., & Storandt, M. (1973). Speed functions, vocabulary ability, and age. *Perceptual and Motor Skills, 36,* 1123–1128.

Brown, A. L. (1982). Learning and development: The problem of compatibility, access and induction. *Human Development, 25,* 89–115.

Bruce, D. (1985). The how and why of ecological memory. *Journal of Experimental Psychology: General, 114,* 78–90.

Brunswik, E. (1952). *The conceptual framework of psychology.* Chicago: The University of Chicago Press.

Campbell, D. T. (1970). Natural selection as an epistemological model. In R. Naroll & R. Cohen (Eds.), *A handbook of method in cultural anthropology* (pp. 51–85). Garden City, NY: The Natural History Press.

Campbell, D. T. (1974). Evolutionary epistemology. In P. A. Schilpp (Ed.), *The philosophy of Karl Popper* (pp. 413–463). La Salle: Open Court.

Carr, H. A. (1925). *Psychology.* New York: Longmans, Green.

Carr, H. A. (1930). Functionalism. In C. Murchison (Ed.), *Psychologies of 1930* (pp. 59–78). Worcester, MA: Clark University Press.

Carroll, J. B., & Maxwell, S. E. (1979). Individual differences in cognitive abilities. *Annual Review of Psychology, 30,* 603–640.

Charness, N. (in press). Age and expertise: Responding to Talland's challenge. In L. W. Poor, D. C. Rubin, & B. A. Wilson (Eds.), *Everyday cognition in adult and late life.* New York: Cambridge University Press.

Chi, M. T. H., Glaser, R., & Rees, E. (1983). Expertise in problem solving. In R. J. Sternberg (Ed.), *Advances in the psychology of human intelligence* (Vol. 1). Hillsdale, NJ: Erlbaum.

Clayton, V. P. (1975). Erikson's theory of human development as it applies to the aged: Wisdom as contradictory cognition. *Human Development, 18,* 119–128.

Clayton, V. P. (1982). Wisdom and intelligence: The nature and function of knowledge in the later years. *International Journal of Aging and Human Development, 15,* 315–323.

Clayton, V. P., & Birren, J. E. (1980). The development of wisdom across the life span: A reexamination of an ancient topic. In P. B. Baltes & O. G. Brim, Jr. (Eds.), *Life-span development and behavior* (Vol. 3, pp. 103–135). New York: Academic.

Cole, S. (1979). Age and scientific performance. *American Journal of Sociology, 84,* 958–977.

Cornelius, S. W. (1984). Classic pattern of intellectual aging: Test familiarity, difficulty, and performance. *Journal of Gerontology, 39,* 201–206.

Cornelius, S. W., Willis, S. L., Nesselroade, J. R., & Baltes, P. B. (1983). Convergence between attention variables and factors of psychometric intelligence in older adults. *Intelligence, 7,* 253–270.

Corsini, R. J., & Fassett, K. K. (1953). Intelligence and aging. *Journal of Genetic Psychology, 83,* 249–264.

Cunningham, W. R., & Owens, W. A. Jr. (1983). The Iowa State study of the adult development of intellectual abilities. In K. W. Schaie (Ed.), *Longitudinal studies of adult psychological development* (pp. 20–39). New York: Guilford.

Dallenbach, K. M. (1915). The history and derivation of the word 'function' as a systematic term in psychology. *American Journal of Psychology, 26,* 473–484.

Demming, J. A., & Pressey, S. L. (1957). Tests indigenous to the adult and older years. *Journal of Counseling Psychology, 4,* 144–148.

Denney, N. W. (1979). Problem solving in later adulthood: Intervention research. In P. B. Baltes & O. G. Brim, Jr. (Eds.), *Life-span development and behavior* (Vol. 2, pp. 37–66). New York: Academic.

Denney, N. W. (1982). Aging and cognitive changes. In B. B. Wolman (Ed.), *Handbook of developmental psychology* (pp. 807–827). Englewood Cliffs, NJ: Prentice-Hall.

Dennis, W. (1966). Creative productivity between the ages of 20 and 80 years. *Journal of Gerontology, 21,* 1–18.

Dewey, J. (1896). The reflex arc concept in psychology. *Psychological Review, 3,* 357–370.

Dewey, J. (1908). What does pragmatism mean by practical? *The Journal of Philosophy, Psychology and Scientific Methods, 5,* 85–99.

Dewey, J. (1910a). "Consciousness" and experience. In J. Dewey, *The influence of Darwin on philosophy and other essays in contemporary thought* (pp. 242–270). New York: Holt.

Dewey, J. (1910b). The experimental theory of knowledge. In J. Dewey, *The influence of Darwin on philosophy and other essays in contemporary thought* (pp. 77–111). New York: Holt.

Dewey, J. (1910c). The influence of Darwinism on philosophy. In J. Dewey, *The influence of Darwin on philosophy and other essays in contemporary thought* (pp. 1–19). New York: Holt.

Dewey, J. (1910d). The intellectualist criterion for truth. In J. Dewey, *The influence of Darwin on philosophy and other essays in contemporary thought* (pp. 112–153). New York: Holt.

Dewey, J. (1910e). The significance of the problem of knowledge. In J. Dewey, *The influence of Darwin on philosophy and other essays in contemporary thought* (pp. 271–304). New York: Holt.

Dewey, J. (1916). *Democracy and education.* New York: Macmillan.

Dewey, J. (1925). The development of American pragmatism. In The Department of Philosophy of Columbia University (Ed.), *Studies in the history of ideas* (Vol. 2, pp. 353–377). New York: Columbia University Press.

Dewey, J. (1929). *Experience and nature* (rev. ed.). New York: Norton.

Dewey, J. (1933). *How we think* (rev. ed.). New York: Heath.

Dewey, J. (1939). Experience, knowledge and value: A rejoinder, In P. A. Schilpp (Ed.), *The philosophy of John Dewey* (pp. 515–608). Evanston: Northwestern University Press.

Dittmann-Kohli, F. (1984). Weisheit als mögliches Ergebnis der Intelligenzentwicklung im Erwachsenenalter. *Sprache und Kognition, 2,* 112–132.

Dittmann-Kohli, F., & Baltes, P. B. (in press). Toward a neofunctionalist conception of adult intellectual development: Wisdom as a prototypical case of intellectual growth. In C. Alexander & E. Langer (Eds.), *Beyond formal operations: Alternative endpoints to human development.* New York: Cambridge University Press.

Dixon, R. A., & Hertzog, C. (in press). A functional approach to memory and metamemory development in adulthood. In F. E. Weinert & M. Perlmutter (Eds.), *Memory development across the life span: Universal changes and individual differences.* Hillsdale, NJ: Erlbaum.

Dixon, R. A., Hultsch, D. F., Simon, E. W., & von Eye, A. (1984). Verbal ability and text structure effects on adult age differences in text recall. *Journal of Verbal Learning and Verbal Behavior, 23,* 569–578.

Dixon, R. A., Kramer, D. A., & Baltes, P. B. (1985). Intelligence: A life-span developmental perspective. In B. B. Wolman (Ed.), *Handbook of intelligence: Theories. measurements, and applications* (pp. 301–350). New York: Wiley.

Dixon, R. A., & Lerner, R. M. (1984). A history of systems in developmental psychology. In M. H. Bornstein & M. E. Lamb (Eds.), *Developmental psychology: An advanced textbook* (pp. 1–35). Hillsdale, NJ: Erlbaum.

Dixon, R. A., & Lerner, R. M. (1985). Darwinism and the emergence of developmental psychology. In G. Eckhardt, W. G. Bringmann, & L. Sprung (Eds.), *Contributions to a history of developmental psychology* (pp. 245–266). Berlin: Mouton.

Dörner, D. (1982). The ecological conditions of thinking. In D. R. Griffin (Ed.), *Animal mind – human mind (Dahlem Konferenzen)* (pp. 95–112). New York: Springer-Verlag.

Dörner, D. (1983). Heuristic and cognition in complex systems. In R. Groner, M. Groner, & W. F. Bischof (Eds.), *Methods of heuristics* (pp. 89–106). Hillsdale, NJ: Erlbaum.

Edelstein, W., & Noam, G. (1982). Regulatory structures of the self and "postformal" stages in adulthood. *Human Development, 6,* 407–422.

Featherman, D. L. (1980). Schooling and occupational careers: Constancy and change in worldly success. In O. G. Brim, Jr. & J. Kagan (Eds.), *Constancy and change in human development* (pp. 675–738). Cambridge, MA: Harvard University Press.

Featherman, D. L. (1983). The life-span perspective in social science research. In P. B. Baltes & O. G. Brim, Jr. (Eds.), *Life-span development and behavior* (Vol. 5, pp. 1–57). New York: Academic Press.

Flavell, J. H. (1970). Cognitive change in adulthood. In L. R. Goulet & P. B. Baltes (Eds.), *Life-span developmental psychology: Research and theory* (pp. 247–253). New York: Academic.

Foster, J. C., & Taylor, G. A. (1920). The applicability of mental tests to persons over fifty years of age. *Journal of Applied Psychology, 4,* 39–58.

Fries, J. F., & Crapo, L. M. (1981). *Vitality and aging.* San Francisco: Freeman.

Gardner, E. F., & Monge, R. H. (1977). Adult age differences in cognitive abilities and educational background. *Experimental Aging Research, 3,* 337–383.

Garrett, H. E. (1946). A developmental theory of intelligence. *American Psychologist, 1,* 372–378.

Ghiselin, M. (1969). *The triumph of the Darwinian method.* Berkeley: University of California Press.

Glaser, R. (1981). The future of testing: A research agenda for cognitive psychology and psychometrics. *American Psychologist, 36,* 923–936.

Green, R. F. (1969). Age-intelligence relationship between ages sixteen and sixty-four: A rising trend. *Developmental Psychology, 1,* 618–627.

Guilford, J. P. (1967). *The nature of human intelligence.* New York: McGraw-Hill.

Hall, G. S. (1922). *Senescence: The last half of life.* New York: Appleton.

Heidbreder, E. (1933). *Seven psychologies.* Englewood Cliffs, NJ.: Prentice-Hall.

Henmon, V. A. C. (1921). Intelligence and its measurement: A symposium. *The Journal of Educational Psychology, 12,* 195–198.

Hofland, B. F., Willis, S. L., & Baltes, P. B. (1981). Fluid intelligence performance in the elderly: Intraindividual variability and conditions of assessment. *Journal of Educational Psychology, 73,* 573–586.

Hollingworth, H. L. (1927). *Mental growth and decline: A survey of developmental psychology.* New York: Appleton.

Hook, S. (1974). *Pragmatism and the tragic sense of life.* New York: Basic.

Horn, J. L. (1970). Organization of data on life-span development of human abilities. In L. R. Goulet & P. B. Baltes (Eds.), *Life-span developmental psychology: Research and theory* (pp. 423–466). New York: Academic.

Horn, J. L. (1980). Concepts of intellect in relation to learning and adult development. *Intelligence, 4,* 285–317.

Horn, J. L. (1982). The theory of fluid and crystallized intelligence in relation to concepts of cognitive psychology and aging in adulthood. In F. I. M. Craik & S. Trehub (Eds.), *Aging and cognitive processes* (pp. 237–278). New York: Plenum.

Horn, J. L., & Cattell, R. B. (1966). Refinement and test of the theory of fluid and crystallized intelligence. *Journal of Educational Psychology, 57,* 253–270.

Horn, J. L., & Cattell, R. B. (1967). Age differences in fluid and crystallized intelligence. *Acta Psychologica, 26,* 107–129.

Horn, J. L., & Donaldson, G. (1976). On the myth of intellectual decline in adulthood. *American Psychologist, 31*, 701–719.

Hoyer, W. J. (1985). Aging and the development of expert cognition. In T. M. Schlechter & M. P. Toglia (Eds.), *New directions in cognitive science* (pp. 69–87). Norwood, NJ: Ablex.

Hultsch, D. F., Hertzog, C., & Dixon, R. A. (1984). Text recall in adulthood: The role of intellectual abilities. *Developmental Psychology, 20*, 1193–1209.

Hultsch, D. F., & Pentz, C. A. (1980). Encoding, storage, and retrieval in adult memory: The role of model assumptions. In L. W. Poon, J. L. Fozard, L. S. Cermak, D. Arenberg, & L. W. Thompson (Eds.), *New directions in memory and aging: Proceedings of the George A. Talland Memorial Conference* (pp. 73–94). Hillsdale, NJ: Erlbaum.

Hunt, E. B. (1978). Mechanics of verbal ability. *Psychological Review, 85*, 109–130.

Hunt, E. (1982). Towards new ways of assessing intelligence. *Intelligence, 6*, 231–240.

Hunt, E. (1983). On the nature of intelligence. *Science, 219*, 141–146.

James, W. (1890). *The principles of psychology* (2 vols.). New York: Dover.

James, W. (1907). The function of cognition. In W. James, *Pragmatism and four essays from The Meaning of Truth* (pp. 204–224). New York: New American Library.

Jarvik, L. F., & Bank, L. (1983). Aging twins: Longitudinal psychometric data. In K. W. Schaie (Ed.), *Longitudinal studies of adult psychological development* (pp. 40–63). New York: Guilford.

Jenkins, J. J. (1974). Remember that old theory of memory? Well, forget it! *American Psychologist, 29*, 785–795.

Jones, H. E. (1959). Intelligence and problem solving. In J. E. Birren (Ed.), *Handbook of aging and the individual: Psychological and biological aspects* (pp. 700–738). Chicago: University of Chicago Press.

Jones, H. E., & Conrad, H. S. (1933). The growth and decline of intelligence: A study of a homogeneous group between the ages of ten and sixty. *Genetic Psychology Monographs, 13*, 223–298.

Kamin, L. J. (1957). Differential changes in mental abilities in old age. *Journal of Gerontology, 12*, 66–70.

Kekes, J. (1983). Wisdom. *American Philosophical Quarterly, 20*, 277–286.

Kirkpatrick, E. A. (1903). *Fundamentals of child study: A discussion of instincts and other factors in human development with practical applications.* New York: Macmillan.

Kliegl, R., & Baltes, P. B. (1985). *Cognitive reserve capacity, expertise, and aging.* Unpublished manuscript, Max Planck Institute for Human Development and Education, Berlin.

Kohn, M. L., & Schooler, C. (1978). The reciprocal effects of the substantive complexity of work and intellectual flexibility: A longitudinal assessment. *American Journal of Sociology, 84*, 24–52.

Kohn, M. L., & Schooler, C. (1982). Job conditions and personality: A longitudinal assessment of their reciprocal effects. *American Journal of Sociology, 87*, 1257–1286.

Kuhn, D., Pennington N., & Leadbeater, B. (1983). Adult thinking in developmental perspective. In P. B. Baltes & O. G. Brim, Jr. (Eds.), *Life-span development and behavior* (Vol. 5), (pp. 157–195). New York: Academic.

Labouvie-Vief, G. (1980). Beyond formal operations: Uses and limits of pure logic in life-span development. *Human Development, 23*, 141–161.

Labouvie-Vief, G. (1982). Dynamic development and mature autonomy: A theoretical prologue. *Human Development, 25*, 161–191.

Labouvie-Vief, G. (1985). Intelligence and cognition. In J. E. Birren & K. W. Schaie (Eds.), *Handbook of the psychology of aging* (rev. ed., pp. 500–530). New York: Van Nostrand Reinhold.

Lehman, H. C. (1953). *Age and achievement.* Princeton, NJ: Princeton University Press.

Lerner, R. M., Hultsch, D. F., & Dixon, R. A. (1983). Contextualism and the character of developmental psychology in the 1970s. *Annals of the New York Academy of Sciences, 412*, 101–128.

Lerner, R. M., & Lerner, J. V. (in press). Contextualism and the study of child effects in personality and social development. In R. L. Rosnow & M. Georgoudi (Eds.), *Contextualism and understanding in behavioral research*. New York: Praeger.

Lorge, I. (1936). The influence of the test upon the nature of mental decline as a function of age. *Journal of Educational Psychology, 27*, 100–110.

McCall, R. B. (1979). The development of intellectual functioning in infancy and the prediction of later IQ. In J. D. Osofsky (Ed.), *Handbook of infant development* (pp. 707–741). New York: Wiley.

Marsh, C. J. (1933). Human adaptability as related to age. *Psychological Bulletin, 30*, 589.

Manicas, P. T., & Secord, P. F. (1983). Implications for psychology of the new philosophy of science. *American Psychologist, 38*, 399–413.

Meacham, J. A. (1982). Wisdom and the context of knowledge: Knowing that one doesn't know. In D. Kuhn & J. A. Meacham (Eds.), *On the development of developmental psychology* (pp. 111–134). Basel: Karger.

Mergler, N. L., & Goldstein, M. D. (1983). Why are there old people: Senescence as biological and cultural preparedness for the transmission of information. *Human Development, 26*, 72–90.

Miles, W. R. (1933). Age and human ability. *Psychological Review, 40*, 387–414.

Miles, C. C., & Miles, W. R. (1932). The correlation of intelligence scores and chronological age from early to late maturity. *American Journal of Psychology, 44*, 44–78.

Miller, J., Slomczynski, K. M., & Kohn, M. L. (1984). *The impact of job on intellective process in the United States and Poland: Continuity of learning-generalization throughout adult life*. Unpublished paper, National Institute of Health, Bethesda, MD.

Morris, C. (1970). *The pragmatic movement in American philosophy*. New York: Braziller.

Neisser, U. (1976). General, academic and artificial intelligence. In L. B. Resnick (Ed.), *The nature of intelligence* (pp. 135–144). Hillsdale, NJ: Erlbaum.

Neisser, U. (1978). Memory: What are the important questions? In M. M. Gruneberg, P. Morris, & R. H. Sykes (Eds.), *Practical aspects of memory* (pp. 3–24). New York: Academic.

Neisser, U. (1983). Components of intelligence or steps in routine procedures? *Cognition, 15*, 189–197.

Nesselroade, J. R., Schaie, K. W., & Baltes, P. B. (1972). Ontogenetic and generational components of structural and quantitative change in adult behavior. *Journal of Gerontology, 27*, 222–228.

Nilsson, L.-G. (1984). New functionalism in memory research. In K. M. J. Lagerspetz & P. Niemi (Eds.), *Psychology in the 1990s* (pp. 185–224). Amsterdam: North-Holland.

Nisbet, J. D. (1957). IV. Intelligence and age: Retesting with twenty-four years' interval. *British Journal of Educational Psychology, 27*, 190–198.

Owens, W. A., Jr. (1966). Age and mental abilities: A second adult follow-up. *Journal of Educational Psychology, 51*, 311–325.

Parodi, D. (1939). Knowledge and action in Dewey's philosophy. In P. A. Schilpp (Ed.), *The philosophy of John Dewey* (pp. 229–242). Evanston, IL: Northwestern University Press.

Pellegrino, J. W., & Glaser, R. (1979). Cognitive correlates and components in the analysis of individual differences. In R. J. Sternberg & D. K. Detterman (Eds.), *Human intelligence: Perspectives on its theory and measurement* (pp. 61–88). Norwood, NJ: Ablex.

Pepper, S. C. (1970). *World hypotheses*. Berkeley: University of California Press. (Original work published in 1942.)

Peterson, J. (1925). *Early conceptions and tests of intelligence*. New York: Harcourt, Brace & World.

Petrinovich, L. (1979). Probabilistic functionalism: A conception of research method. *American Psychologist, 34*, 373–390.

Plemons, J. K., Willis, S. L., & Baltes, P. B. (1978). Modifiability of fluid intelligence in aging: A short-term longitudinal training approach. *Journal of Gerontology, 33*, 224–231.

Plotkin, H. C. (1982). Evolutionary epistemology and evolutionary theory. In H. C. Plotkin (Ed.), *Learning, development, and culture* (pp. 3–13). New York: Wiley.

Popper, K. R. (1965). *Conjectures and refutations: The growth of scientific knowledge.* New York: Harper & Row.

Popper, K. R. (1972). *Objective knowledge: An evolutionary approach.* Oxford: Clarendon Press.

Porter, N. (1891). *The human intellect with an introduction upon psychology and the soul* (4th ed.). New York: Scribner.

Pressey, S. L. (1917). Distinctive features in psychological test measurements made upon dementia praecox and chronic alcoholic patients. *Journal of Abnormal Psychology, 12,* 130–139.

Pressey, S. L. (1919). Are the present psychological scales reliable for adults? *Journal of Abnormal Psychology, 14,* 314–324.

Pressey, S. L., & Kuhlen, R. G. (1957). *Psychological development through the life span.* New York: Harper.

Quetelet, A. (1842). *A treatise on man and the development of his faculties.* Edinburgh: Chambers.

Rabbitt, P. M. A. (1982). How do old people know what to do next? In F. I. M. Craik & S. Trehub (Eds.), *Aging and cognitive processes* (pp. 79–98). New York: Plenum.

Reese, H. W., & Overton, W. F. (1970). Models of development and theories of development. In L. R. Goulet & P. B. Baltes (Eds.), *Life-span developmental psychology: Research and theory* (pp. 115–145). New York: Academic.

Rescher, N. (1980). *Scepticism: A critical reappraisal.* Oxford: Blackwell.

Riley, M. W. (1985). Age strata in social systems. In R. H. Binstock & E. Shanas (Eds.), *Handbook of aging and the social sciences* (pp. 369–411). Princeton, NJ: Van Nostrand Reinhold.

Rosnow, R., & Georgoudi, M. (Eds.). (in press). *Contextualism and understanding in behavioral research.* New York: Praeger.

Ruch, F. L. (1934). The differentiated effects of age upon human learning. *Journal of General Psychology, 11,* 261–286.

Salthouse, T. A. (1982). *Adult cognition: An experimental psychology of human aging.* New York: Springer-Verlag.

Salthouse, T. A. (in press). Age, experience, and compensation. In C. Schooler & K. W. Schaie (Eds.), *Cognitive functioning and social structure over the life course.* Norwood, NJ: Ablex.

Salthouse, T. A., & Somberg, B. L. (1982). Skilled performance: Effects of adult age and experiences on elementary processes. *Journal of Experimental Psychology: General, 111,* 176–207.

Sanford, E. C. (1902). Mental growth and decay. *American Journal of Psychology, 13,* 426–449.

Sarbin, T. R. (1977). Contextualism: A world view for modern psychology. In J. K. Cole & A. W. Landfield (Eds.), *Nebraska Symposium on Motivation 1976* (Vol. 24, pp. 1–41). Lincoln: University of Nebraska Press.

Schaie, K. W. (1979). The primary mental abilities in adulthood: An exploration in the development of psychometric intelligence. In P. B. Baltes & O. G. Brim, Jr. (Eds.), *Life-span development and behavior* (Vol. 2, pp. 67–115). New York: Academic.

Schaie, K. W. (1983). The Seattle Longitudinal Study: A 21-year exploration of psychometric intelligence in adulthood. In K. W. Schaie (Ed.), *Longitudinal studies of adult psychological development* (pp. 64–135). New York: Guilford.

Schaie, K. W., & Baltes, P. B. (1977). Some faith helps to see the forest: A final comment on the Horn and Donaldson myth of the Baltes–Schaie position on adult intelligence. *American Psychologist, 32,* 1118–1120.

Schaie, K. W., & Hertzog, C. (1983). Fourteen-year cohort-sequential analyses of adult intellectual development. *Developmental Psychology, 19,* 531–543.

Schaie, K. W., & Labouvie-Vief, G. (1974). Generational vs. ontogenetic components of change in adult cognitive behavior: A fourteen-year cross-sequential study. *Developmental Psychology, 10,* 305–320.

Schaie, K. W., Labouvie, G. V., & Buech, B. U. (1973). Generational and cohort-specific differences in adult cognitive functioning: A fourteen-year study of independent samples. *Developmental Psychology, 9,* 151–166.

Schaie, K. W. & Strother, C. R. (1968a). The cross-sequential study of age changes in cognitive behavior. *Psychological Bulletin, 70,* 671–680.

Schaie, K. W., & Strother, C. R. (1968b). The effects of time and cohort differences on the interpretation of age changes in cognitive behavior. *Multivariate Behavioral Research, 3,* 259–293.

Smith, J. E. (1978). *Purpose and thought: The meaning of pragmatism.* New Haven, CT: Yale University Press.

Sternberg, R. J. (1980). Sketch of a componential subtheory of human intelligence. *Behavioral and Brain Sciences, 3,* 573–614.

Sternberg, R. J. (1981). Testing and cognitive psychology. *American Psychologist, 36,* 1181–1189.

Sternberg, R. J. (Ed.). (1982). *Handbook of human intelligence.* Cambridge: Cambridge University Press.

Sternberg, R. J. (1983). Components of human intelligence. *Cognition, 15,* 1–48.

Sternberg, R. J. (1984). Toward a triarchic theory of human intelligence. *Behavioral and Brain Sciences, 7,* 269–315.

Sterns, H. L., & Sanders, R. E. (1980). Training and education of the elderly. In R. R. Turner & H. W. Reese (Eds.), *Life-span developmental psychology: Intervention* (pp. 307–330). New York: Academic.

Taub, H. A. (1973). Memory span, practice and aging. *Journal of Gerontology, 28,* 335–358.

Tetens, J. N. (1777). *Philosophische Versuche über die menschliche Natur und ihre Entwicklung.* Leipzig: Weidmanns Erben und Reich.

Thayer, H. S. (1952). *The logic of pragmatism: An examination of John Dewey's logic.* New York: Greenwood.

Thayer, H. S. (1973). *Meaning and action: A study of American pragmatism.* Indianapolis: Bobbs-Merrill.

Thorndike, E. L. (1928). *Adult learning.* New York: Macmillan.

Titchener, E. B. (1898). Postulates of a structural psychology. *Philosophical Review, 7,* 449–465.

Titchener, E. B. (1899). Structural and functional psychology. *Philosophical Review, 8,* 290–299.

Toulmin, S. (1961). *Foresight and understanding: An inquiry into the aims of science.* New York: Harper Torchbook.

Toulmin, S., & Goodfield, J. (1965). *The discovery of time.* Chicago: The University of Chicago Press.

Wechsler, D. (1952). *The range of human capacities.* Baltimore: Williams & Wilkins.

Wechsler, D. (1958). *The measurement and appraisal of adult intelligence* (4th ed.). Baltimore: Williams & Wilkins.

Weisenburg, T., Roe, A., & McBride, K. E. (1936). *Adult intelligence: A psychological study of test performance.* London: Commonwealth Fund.

White, S. H. (1968). The learning-maturation controversy: Hall to Hull. *Merrill-Palmer Quarterly, 14,* 187–196.

Wiener, P. P. (1949). *Evolution and the founders of pragmatism.* Cambridge, MA: Harvard University Press.

Willis, S. L. (1985). Towards an educational psychology of the older adult learner: Intellectual and cognitive bases. In J. E. Birren & K. W. Schaie (Eds.), *Handbook of the psychology of aging* (rev. ed., pp. 818–847). New York: Van Nostrand Reinhold.

Willis, S. L., & Baltes, P. B. (1980). Intelligence in adulthood and aging: Contemporary issues. In L. W. Poon (Ed.), *Aging in the 1980s: Psychological issues* (pp. 260–272). Washington, DC: American Psychological Association.

Willoughby, R. R. (1927). Family similarities in mental-test abilities. *Genetic Psychology Monographs, 2,* 239–277.

Woodruff, D. S. (1982). *Age and intelligence: The history of an idea.* Unpublished manuscript, Department of Psychology, Temple University, Philadelphia.

Woodruff, D. S. (1983). A review of aging and cognitive processes. *Research on Aging, 5,* 139–153.

Yerkes, R. M. (1921). *Psychological examining in the United States Army.* Washington, DC: Government Printing Office.

Yerkes, R. M. (1923). Testing and the human mind. *Atlantic Monthly, 131,* 358–370.

11   Practical intelligence in later adulthood

Sherry L. Willis and K. Warner Schaie

Some eight decades have passed since Binet's seminal research on the assessment of human intelligence (Binet & Simon, 1905), yet discussion on the nature of intelligence and its measurement continues. During the past two decades, the volume of research on traditional or "academic" forms of intelligence has increased with the refinement of new approaches (i.e., artificial intelligence, information processing) to the study of the phenomenon. Recently, there has been considerable debate regarding the relevance of traditional conceptions of intelligence for the study of practical, everyday intellectual competence (Connolly & Brunner, 1974; McClelland, 1973; Schaie, 1978; Sternberg, 1981; Willis & Baltes, 1980). Some argue that traditional conceptions of intelligence can serve as a useful basis for studying intelligence in real-world contexts; others question their applicability to contextually relevant forms of intelligence. From a historical perspective, these criticisms seem ironic, given the very appplied concerns of Binet in developing those early psychometric measures.

The issue of the nature of practical intelligence and its relationship to traditional conceptions of cognition is particularly salient in the study of intellectual aging. The ecological relevance of traditional conceptions of intelligence has been demonstrated most clearly for the earlier portion of the lifespan, when schooling is a major developmental task. Psychometric measures have been shown to predict performance in academic settings (Anastasi, 1976). Societal changes, including the extension of schooling into the period of young adulthood and the increase in the proportion of the labor force in professional occupations, have also contributed to the sustained use of academic intelligence measures. Performance on traditional intelligence tests (Egan, 1978; Hills, 1957; Smith, 1964) has been shown to be a useful predictor of entry-level competence in a number of professions (e.g., engineering, piloting, computer programming). However, in later adulthood neither academic performance nor entry-level work-related skills are useful criterion tasks for studying practical intelligence. During that age period, intellectual functioning is reflected in social competence and in tasks of daily living.

236

Thus, the relevance of traditional forms of intelligence to everyday functioning in old age is of particular concern.

One of the ambiguities in studying practical intelligence is that there is no commonly agreed-upon definition for the term. Generally, researchers can more readily agree upon what it is *not*. For example, it is said to be different from traditional or academic intelligence. Our research has focused on real-life type tasks that may be experienced by a particular community-dwelling age cohort in the pursuit of daily living. It should be noted, however, that other researchers are studying forms of optimal cognitive functioning in adulthood that may also be considered a form of practical intelligence. In work on gerontological intelligence, numerous attempts have been made to define, assess, and study the concept of wisdom (Clayton, 1975, 1980; Dittman-Kohli & Baltes, in press; Meacham, 1982). Others are attempting to define and study stages of cognitive functioning specific to adulthood and beyond formal operations (Commons, Richards, & Armon, 1982; Labouvie-Vief, 1982; Sinnott, 1982). Sternberg's "nonentrenched tasks" may also involve the notion of optimal levels of functioning, since they are said to require new conceptual systems of thought. The relationships between traditional intelligence and these new conceptions of optimal functioning should be differential.

This chapter considers the relevance of the psychometric approach to the study of everyday intellectual functioning in later adulthood. First, we will discuss what we believe to be some of the merits of a psychometric abilities approach to the study of practical intelligence in later adulthood. Second, we will consider the specification of criterion tasks for assessing real life intelligence in old age. Third, the findings of two studies examining the relationship between psychometric abilities and everyday cognition in the elderly will be reported. The first of these studies focuses on actual performance in every day tasks; the second study examines perceptions of competence. Finally, we will discuss issues and directions for future research in this area.

Psychometric abilities and practical intelligence in old age

Mainstream cognitive psychology has studied traditional or "academic" intelligence by means of three major approaches using either psychometric, Piagetian, or information processing paradigms (Eysenck, 1982; Resnick, 1976; Sternberg, 1982). Each of these approaches, with its many variations, addresses a different set of issues regarding intellectual functioning. A primary concern of the psychometric approach is the examination of individual differences among persons on a set of mental ability factors, derived through factor analytic procedures. The study of adult intelligence from a psychometric approach has been primarily concerned with quantitative changes in the individual's level of performance across the lifespan and with age-related qualitative changes in the structural relationships of the abilities. The Piagetian perspective provides a description of stages in cognitive development during childhood and adolescence. The information processing approach is concerned with the way in which people mentally represent and process information; the focus is on developing componential or process models of how individuals process information across a variety of settings and stimuli. In contrast to the emphasis of psychometric models upon between-subject variability, the information processing perspective focuses on between-stimulus variance.

Given these three paradigms for the study of traditional intelligence, how shall we approach the study of practical intelligence in later adulthood? At what level of analysis might practical intelligence be most profitably examined? Because the three paradigms evolved in response to different issues regarding the development and nature of traditional intelligence, it appears reasonable that they may also be of differential value in the study of practical intelligence at different life stages. Within the past two decades, strong concerns have been raised regarding the limitations of the psychometric approach's focus on the products of behavior (McClelland, 1973; Sternberg, 1980; Willis & Baltes, 1980). Consequently, much recent research in cognitive psychology has either followed Piaget's quest for accurate description of the origin and transformation of cognitive structures in childhood, or has sought to apply information-processing strategies to develop fine-grained portrayals of the components and timing of effortful behavior. The strengths of the Piagetian and information processing approaches are most obvious when the focus is on the emergence or acquisition of behaviors or on optimal level of functioning under speeded conditions, most commonly occurring in early life (Hooper, Hooper, & Colbert, 1984; Sternberg, 1982). However, when we consider the nature of practical intelligence in later adulthood, the focus is then primarily not upon emergent behaviors, but on previously acquired, intact abilities and skills.

We believe that there are some inherent limitations to the application of existent Piagetian and information processes to the study of everyday functioning in later adulthood. A number of students of adult development have attempted to conceptualize further Piagetian stages that might account for qualitatively different aspects of intellectual functioning beyond young adulthood, but the question remains whether there are cognitive transformations in adulthood that lead to even near-universal stages, based on assumptions of pure logic (Commons, Richards, & Kuhn, 1982; Flavell, 1970; Labouvie-Vief, 1980, 1982). The basic problem seems to be that the Piagetian approach was conceptualized for the study of the acquisition of cognitive behaviors in childhood. Without extensive reconceptualization, it remains limited in its explanation of maintenance or decline or the reorganization of cognitive structures in adulthood (Hooper et al., 1984; Kramer, 1983; Roberts, Papalia-Finlay, Davis, Blackburn, & Dellmann, 1982).

Somewhat different limitations may exist when the information-processing approach is considered the basic measurement system for the study of practical intelligence in old age. First, many of the information-processing studies to date have examined the cognitive processes and capabilities of optimally functioning persons, such as college students. Much of the work has been concerned with response speed as the dependent variable, when studied under various instructional conditions, and with the primary requirement that subjects have reached a uniform criterion level of accuracy (Eysenck, 1982; Jensen, 1982; Sternberg, 1981). Such an approach may be problematic in work with average adults and the elderly. Many subjects may never be brought to a reasonably high criterion level. More importantly, speed of response may not be a relevant predictor for many real-life tasks wherein the range of response speed acceptable for an adaptive response may be quite wide (Cornelius, Willis, Nesselroade, & Baltes, 1983).

Second, there is the issue of whether a parsimonious set of componential processes has been identified that can be applied to a wide array of cognitive tasks (Detterman, 1980; Baron, in press). Any real-life situation would be expected to involve a wide array of componential processes; previous research suggests that any one of these components might have only a low correlation with the real-life criterion task (Egan, 1978, 1981).

In view of the above issues, we believe that there is merit in employing the psychometric approach as a basic measurement system in the study of practical intelligence in old age. The largest and richest research literature on adult intelligence has been couched within the psychometric approach (Botwinick, 1977). Virtually all longitudinal and cohort-sequential studies of adult intelligence involve the psychometric approach (Schaie, 1983). Thus, the psychometric approach provides the most complete data base on quantitative and structural developmental changes in adult intelligence, as they may apply to practical intelligence. Second, a well-defined and reliable measurement system is available for studying abilities at the construct level. A limited set of ability factors has been identified, which should be useful in accounting for as much individual difference variance in as many classes of real-life behaviors as possible (Baltes, Cornelius, Spiro, Nesselroade, & Willis, 1980; Schaie, 1983). Psychometric ability measures have been tested on and adapted for a broad spectrum of adults, including those in the old-old age range.

The criterion issue

A major issue in the study of practical intelligence is the identification of criterion tasks for assessing intelligent behavior in real-world contexts. For

Binet and those who followed there was a clear focus on the ecologically relevant criterion task of school performance. For the more basic researcher, however, the focus soon turned to theoretical issues regarding the structure of intelligence (Matarazzo, 1972). The criterion tasks became relatively pure measures of specific abstract components (i.e., mental abilities) of intelligence, rather than the complex tasks characterizing real life. A distinction emerged between competent performance on measures of these abstract "building blocks" of intellectual structure and the competencies involved in daily life (Connolly & Bruner, 1974; McClelland, 1973).

For the purposes of this chapter, we shall use the term "traditional intelligence" to denote those genotypic ability factors commonly identified with the psychometric approach to the study of structural intelligence. In contrast, practical intelligence will be viewed as the phenotypic expression of that combination of genotypic factors that, given minimally acceptable levels of motivation, will permit adaptive behavior within a specific situation or class of situations (Schaie, 1978). Since behavior in real-world contexts is of necessity complex, we assume that no single measure or genotypic factor can adequately predict performance in a specific situation, rather some composite of genotypic ability factors will best predict everyday performance in such a situation.

What, then, might be some useful parameters for defining a set of criterion tasks for assessing practical intelligence in later adulthood? Even brief reflection suggests that the criterion tasks will vary by age or life stage. With respect to childhood there appears to be considerable consensus regarding the near-universal biologically and societally defined developmental tasks, that may serve as criteria for assessing practical intelligence. Across the adult life course, however, matters are complicated by increasing individual differences in the range of environments and experiences encountered (Schaie, 1983; Willis & Baltes, 1980). There appears to be no comparable, parsimonious set of near-universal developmental tasks in adulthood that have the situational generality and the biologically and societally defined age norms characteristic of developmental tasks identified in childhood, hence, the need for identifying *multiple* criterion tasks for assessing practical intellectual competence in various stages of adulthood. The nature of the criterial tasks, moreover, will vary not only by life stage, but across cohorts for any given life stage as well. For example, although relatively few of today's elderly are computer literate, we may expect that future generations of elderly will have interacted with a computer from childhood. A few other instances of cohort-specific forms of intellectual performance have been noted in the literature (Gardner & Monge, 1977; Looft, 1970).

A second parameter focuses on whether the form of practical intelligence studied reflects previously acquired skills and knowledge or is indicative of emergent, newly developed abilities. Because our focus is on the common everyday types of practical problem solving the elderly may experience, we are primarily concerned with the older adult's competence in applying previously acquired abilities and skills to new instances of a problem involving those skills, rather than with the emergence of new forms of thought. It should be noted, however, that those who are concerned with nontraditional forms of intelligence in later adulthood focus on optimal and unique forms of intelligent behavior in old age and are thus concerned primarily with newly emerging abilities and skills (Baltes, Dittman-Kohli, & Dixon, 1984; Kramer, 1983; Labouvie-Vief, 1982).

Berg and Sternberg (1985) have discussed related issues with regard to their triadic model of intellectual development in adulthood. The two-facet subtheory of the triadic model holds that tasks are differentially valid as measures of intelligence as a function of the familiarity of these tasks to the people performing them. Tasks are considered particularly appropriate for measuring intelligence when they are either relatively novel or in the process of becoming automatized. Of the three forms of novelty discussed by Berg and Sternberg (1985), it appears that the ability to operate within new conceptual systems is most likely to be associated with the development of optimal and/or unique forms of intelligence in young adulthood. The two other forms of novelty discussed (i.e., familiar problems involving novel stimuli, or application of previously acquired cognitive operations in new contexts) may occur more frequently in the common everyday problem solving exhibited by the elderly.

A third parameter deals with the distinction between explicit versus implicit conceptions of intellectual competence. Explicit theories of intelligence are developed by behavioral scientists, based on data examining individual performance on measures of intellectual functioning. Implicit theories may involve both laypersons' conceptions of competence and their perceptions of their own intellectual competence (Sternberg, Conway, Ketron, & Bernstein, 1981); perceived competence has also been related to intellectual self-efficacy (Bandura, 1982; Lachman & Jelallian, 1983). Just as there are wide individual differences in people's performance on measures used in explicit theories of intelligence, there is considerable variability in people's perceptions of the areas in which they consider themselves intellectually competent.

How then shall we derive criterial tasks for assessing practical intelligence specific to the stage of later adulthood? Our own research has employed two distinct approaches. One approach proceeds from the assumption that certain classes of everyday activities are critical for adaptive functioning in given life situations. A major concern in old age is maintenance of independent living, and the activities in this approach focus on tasks associated with independent effective functioning. For example, inability to perform tasks, such as comprehending a medicine bottle label or utilizing information in the yellow pages of a phone directory, may lead to the curtailment of independent living for many elderly. Although no exhaustive taxonomy of real-life tasks has thus far been developed at any life stage, measures have been designed to tap substantial subsets of such a taxonomy. These real-life tasks represent categories of common problems experienced by many elderly, even though specific stimuli in the test item might not have been encountered previously. It is assumed that the person applies the same relevant cognitive skills and information to the test item that he/she would in a real-life problem. It is difficult, if not impossible, to observe directly an elderly subject's performance in many real-life situations; thus, these task items attempt to simulate the way in which an elderly person might perform in daily life. In developing prototypical problems, it is important that the items indeed represent categories of situations experienced by the elderly, as documented in the gerontological research literature, and that the problems have high face validity and appear to be meaningful and relevant to the older adult.

Our second approach to the development of criterion tasks has involved the specification of a situational taxonomy for the adequate description of the kind of settings within which older adults exhibit behavioral competence. Effective functioning in different situations may demand various combinations of intellectual abilities. Moreover, situational taxonomies must be specific to a particular life stage. In this approach, a set of situations relevant to but not necessarily peculiar to the life experiences of urban older adults was developed; these situations were classified according to a taxonomy of situational dimensions (Scheidt & Schaie, 1978). Two studies that used these two approaches to the study of practical intelligence in later adulthood are briefly summarized below.

Study I. Fluid/crystallized ability correlates of practical intelligence

The objective of this study was to examine the relationship between older adults' performance on tasks of daily living and an established structural model of psychometric intelligence. The fluid-crystallized model (G_f-G_c) of intelligence is of particular interest in later adulthood, given the differential developmental patterns predicted for the two intelligence dimensions (Cattell, 1971). Fluid intelligence is said to develop in childhood and to peak in young adulthood; a normative pattern of decline is assumed to occur through middle and later adulthood. Crystallized intelligence is thought to remain relatively stable or even to increase through much of adulthood. Seven primary mental abilities were chosen to represent the G_f-G_c dimensions. Fluid intelligence is represented by primary abilities such as figural relations and inductive reasoning. Crystallized intelligence is represented by such abilities as vocabulary and social knowledge.

The primary purpose of the research was to identify differential sets of predictors for the various real-life tasks categories. The specific abilities identified as predictors were expected to vary with the type of real-life task studied. Although most of the abilities studied were hypothesized to be significantly correlated with the real-life tasks, given the phenomenon of positive manifold, it was expected that different sets of abilities would be found to have the greatest shared variance with the various real-life tasks.

The question then arises as to the nature of the ability predictors when considered at the second-order level of fluid versus crystallized intelligence. Hypotheses were derived from the G_f-G_c theory regarding the relative importance of these two second-order dimensions in predicting performance on everyday tasks. It was hypothesized that the predominant pattern of ability predictors would be crystallized rather than fluid. Crystallized intelligence involves knowledge and skill acquired through acculturation; it is thus closely related to specific content matter and to skills (e.g., defining vocabulary words, simple mathematics) acquired in schooling. By contrast, fluid abilities are said to be relatively content free; rather, G_f focuses on the ability to identify and apply complex relationships in solving problems. As most of the real-life tasks studied involved specific types of content, required verbal ability (e.g., reading medicine bottle labels, comprehending newspaper text), and dealt with relatively common types of experiences, it was expected that the most significant predictors of real-life tasks would be crystallized in nature, although the specific G_c ability identified as a predictor was expected to vary with the content of the real-life task.

Method

Subjects. Subjects were eighty-seven (F,68; M,19) community-dwelling older adults ($\overline{X}$ age: 68.6 years; range: 60–88 years) from rural areas of Pennsylvania. Mean educational level was 11.9 years (range: 6–19 years). Subjects were recruited through community organizations and were paid ($2 per hour) for their participation.

Procedure and measures. Subjects were administered an extensive battery of psychometric ability measures and a real-life tasks measure in two testing sessions. The psychometric ability battery, shown in Table 1, was selected to represent the seven primary abilities of Figural Relations (CFR), Inductive Reasoning (I), Vocabulary (V), Verbal Analogies (CMR), Social Knowledge (EMS), Memory Span (Ms), and Perceptual Speed (Ps). A composite score was computed for each primary ability by summing the total scores for the

Table 1. *Measurement battery.*

Primary ability	Test[a]	Source
Figural Relations (CFR)	Culture Fair Test (scale 2, form A), Power Matrices (scale 3, Form A & B)	Cattell & Cattell (1957)
	ADEPT Figural Relations	Plemons et al. (1978)
	Raven's Progressive Matrices	Raven (1962)
Inductive Reasoning (I)	Induction Standard Test	Ekstrom et al. (1976); Thurstone (1962)
	ADEPT Induction Test	Blieszner et al. (1981)
Memory Span (Ms)	Visual Memory Span	Ekstrom et al. (1976)
	Auditory Number Span	Ekstrom et al. (1976)
	Auditory Number Span-Delay	After Ekstrom et al. (1976)
Verbal Analogies (CMR)	Verbal Analogies I	Guilford (1969a)
	Word Matrix	Guilford (1969b)
Social Knowledge (EMS)	Social Translations	O'Sullivan & Guilford (1965)
	Social Situations	Horn (1967)
Vocabulary (V)	Verbal Meaning (9–12)	Thurstone (1962)
	Vocabulary (V-2,V-3,V-4)	Ekstrom et al. (1976)
Perceptual Speed (Ps)	Finding A's	Ekstrom et al. (1976)
	Number Comparison	Ekstrom et al. (1976)
	Identical Pictures	Ekstrom et al. (1976)

[a] Induction and Vocabulary are composites of several subtests. Induction Standard and ADEPT Induction include subtests of Letter Sets, Letter Series, Number Series. Vocabulary includes subtests V-2, V-3, V-4 (Ekstrom et al., 1976).

tests representing that ability. Composite scores were used in the correlational and multiple regression analyses to be reported, as they provided more reliable estimates of the abilities.

Real-life task performance was assessed by the ETS Basic Skills Test (1977). This sixty-five-item measure was developed to assess real-life competencies achieved by high school seniors. However, examination of the items indicated that they dealt with tasks encountered by adults of all ages. A total score and two subscores (Literal and Inference) are typically obtained (Educational Testing Service, 1977). The split-half reliability (KR 20) of the total score is .94. Literal comprehension items involve responses based on information present in the item stem, whereas inference items require logical induction of answers from the material presented. We were also interested in whether different abilities were associated with different types of tasks (e.g., interpreting medicine bottle labels versus reading newspaper editorials). To examine this question, the sixty-five items were clustered into eight item categories on the basis of item content and format. The eight categories were understanding labels on household articles, reading a street map, understanding charts/schedules, paragraph comprehension, filling out forms, reading newspaper and phone directory ads, understanding technical documents, and comprehending newspaper text. The number of test items per category ranged from four to twelve. Correlations between category scores and total score were all above .70, except for map reading ($r = .41$).

An exemplar item from each category is given below:

> *Labels.* Subject is shown the label from a plant insecticide container and asked, "How much spray should be mixed with a gallon of water?"
> *Maps.* Subject is shown a street map and asked, "What route should you take to get to Salem College from the airport?"
> *Charts.* Subject is shown a chart of daily dietary allowances and asked, "About how many calories does a seventy-two-pound girl need each day?"
> *Paragraphs.* Subject is shown a paragraph about symptoms of a heart attack and asked, "What was the main theme of the passage?"
> *Forms.* Subject is shown a portion of an income tax form and asked, "If you are getting a refund, on which line should you write the amount you are getting back?"
> *Advertisements.* Subject is shown a page from the Yellow Pages of a telephone book and asked, "Which number could you call to buy fish for dinner?"
> *Technical documents.* Subject is shown a guarantee for a calculator and asked, "The calculator is guaranteed for (how many days)?"
> *News text.* Subject is shown two letters to the editor of a newspaper and asked, "Both writers agree on which of the following points?"

Results. The relationship between ability functioning and performance on the Basic Skills test was examined at three levels. First, the correlations among the Basic Skills scores (total, literal, inference) and ability composite scores were computed. All ability and Basic Skills scores were significantly correlated. However, the correlations ranged from .18 to .83, indicating a wide range in the magnitude of the ability – task relationships.

A second set of analyses examined the relationship between the Basic Skills total score and a preestablished structural model of intelligence. In previous research (Baltes et al., 1980; Cornelius et al., 1983), the structure of the ability battery used in the present study had been examined via confirmatory factor analysis. A four-factor model, shown in the upper part of Table 2, was identified as the most appropriate model, based on statistical and conceptual criteria. The four intelligence dimensions identified were: fluid reasoning, crystallized knowledge, memory span, and perceptual speed. The relationship of the Basic Skills test to these four ability factors was examined via extension analysis (Table 2). The Basic Skills test was found to have a primary loading on the fluid reasoning factor (.58) and a secondary loading on the crystallized knowledge factor (.29).

The third level of analysis was concerned with the abilities associated with specific real life task categories. Stepwise multiple regression analyses were performed for the Basic Skills total, literal, inference, and the eight task cat-

Table 2. *Extension analysis of four-factor G_f-G_c model and ETS basic skills test.*[a]

Variable	Factor[b] 1	2	3	4	Unique variance
Culture Fair (CFR)	0.800	0.0	0.0	0.0	.360
ADEPT Fig. Rel. (CFR)	0.827	0.0	0.0	0.0	.316
Raven's Matrices (CFR)	0.788	0.0	0.0	0.0	.378
ADEPT Induction (I)	0.885	0.0	0.0	−0.054	.294
Induction Standard (I)	0.868	0.0	0.0	0.0	.247
Verbal Analogies (CMR)	0.718	0.0	0.0	0.0	.484
Word Matrix (CMR)	0.676	0.0	0.0	0.0	.543
Social Translations (EMS)	0.592	0.0	0.0	0.0	.650
Social Situations (EMS)	0.336	0.422	0.0	0.0	.489
Verbal Meaning (V)	0.0	0.988	0.0	0.0	.024
Vocabulary (V)	0.0	0.908	0.0	0.0	.175
Visual Memory Span (Ms)	0.0	0.0	0.638	0.0	.572
Aud. Number Span (Ms)	0.0	0.0	0.668	0.0	.554
Aud. Number Span (Delay)	0.0	0.0	0.966	0.0	.066
Finding A's (Ps)	0.0	0.0	0.0	0.637	.594
Number Comparison (Ps)	0.0	0.0	0.0	0.747	.442
Identical Pictures (Ps)	0.0	0.0	−0.039	0.862	.284
ETS Basic Skills Test	0.577	0.287	−0.073	0.168	.156
1. Fluid Reasoning	1.000				
2. Crystallized Knowledge	0.773	1.000			
3. Memory Span	0.606	0.490	1.000		
4. Perceptual Speed	0.815	0.669	0.437	1.000	

[a] x^2 (248) = 315.997, p = .0008.
[b] Underscored factor loadings are significant.

egory scores. The seven ability composite scores, age, and education were the predictor variables. As expected, both fluid and crystallized abilities were found to be predictors of the total, literal, and inference scores. The most significant predictor variable for five of the eight task categories was a fluid ability.

An index of level of difficulty was also computed for the eight task categories. The mean percentage of items answered correctly in each task category was computed (mean items correct divided by total items in category). The mean percentage of items answered correctly per category was understanding labels (67%), reading maps (74%), understanding charts (66%), paragraph comprehension (63%), filling out forms (63%), reading ads (64%), technical documents (54%), news text (25%). The lower level of performance on items involving news text is attributable to the fact that most items within this cluster occurred toward the end of the Basic Skills test and were attempted by only 32% of the subjects.

A final question focused on the frequency with which subjects encountered the types of tasks included on the Basic Skills test. Subjects were presented with verbal descriptions of tasks from each of the eight task categories and asked to rate how often they did these tasks on a five-point scale (daily, weekly, monthly, rarely, never in the past year). For five of the task categories (labels, charts, ads, news text, paragraphs), subjects reported doing those types of tasks at least weekly, on average. The average frequency rating for the forms category was monthly, and for technical documents and maps the frequency rating was rarely.

Discussion. The primary focus of this study was the examination of differential ability–real-life task relationships. Given the phenomenon of positive manifold, it was expected and found that there were significant correlations among the abilities and all task categories. Research across the life-span has indicated a positive correlation among psychometric abilities (Anastasi, 1976); moreover, several studies suggest that the covariance among ability factors increases in later adulthood (Baltes et al., 1980; Cunningham, 1980; Reinert, 1970). In order to identify differential sets of ability predictors for various task categories, it was necessary to go beyond simple correlational procedures and to examine the amount of variance shared between the primary abilities and tasks, via extension and regression analyses.

In the extension analysis, the relationship between the Basic Skills total score and the preestablished intellectual dimensions (factors) of fluid reasoning, crystallized knowledge, memory span, and perceptual speed was examined. It was hypothesized that the Basic Skills test would load on both fluid and crystallized intelligence factors, given the phenomenon of positive manifold, and the fact that real-life tasks are complex and would be expected to share variance with multiple primary abilities. However, our concern was with the relative size of the loadings on the fluid and crystallized factors. We predicted that the most significant loading would be on the crystallized factor with a secondary loading on the fluid factor. Our hypothesis was not confirmed, however. The Basic Skills measure loaded primarily on the fluid reasoning factor and secondarily on the crystallized knowledge factor.

Regression analyses were conducted in order to examine the ability predictors of the eight task categories (Table 3). It was predicted that multiple abilities would be identified as predictors for each task category and also that the specific ability predictors would vary according to task category because of the differing content of categories. Moreover, we hypothesized that for most task categories, the most salient predictor ability would be crystallized, although the specific crystallized ability accounting for the most shared variance would vary across the categories depending on content.

Table 3. *Summary of multiple regression analyses: seven primary abilities, age, and education as predictor variables.*

Criterion variable	Significant predictors	F	r^2	Mult R
Total score	Figural Relations	8.43	.80	.89
	Vocabulary	7.13		
	Social Knowledge	5.06		
Literal score	Figural Relations	7.42	.74	.86
	Vocabulary	5.44		
	Perceptual Speed	4.04		
Inference score	Figural Relations	8.02	.78	.88
	Social Knowledge	6.21		
	Vocabulary	5.14		
Labels	Inductive Reasoning	9.06	.51	.71
	Verbal Analogies	3.28		
Maps	Figural Relations	5.67	.28	.52
Charts	Figural Relations	7.39	.52	.72
Paragraphs	Vocabulary	8.49	.64	.80
	Social Knowledge	7.59		
Forms	Figural Relations	8.25	.59	.77
Ads	Figural Relations	5.88	.49	.70
Tech. documents	Social Knowledge	8.10	.70	.83
	Figural Relations	6.50		
	Vocabulary	2.97		
News text	Education	11.13	.58	.77
	Perceptual Speed	8.77		
	Verbal Analogies	3.75		
	Vocabulary	3.27		

Again, our hypotheses were only partially confirmed. Multiple ability predictors were found for four of the test categories; a single ability predictor was identified for the remaining four categories. For five of the eight task categories (labels, maps, charts, forms, and ads), the most significant ability predictor was a fluid ability. Paragraph comprehension was the only task category for which only crystallized abilities were the significant predictors. The task categories of labels and technical documents included both fluid and crystallized predictors. The finding of perceptual speed as a significant predictor of the news text category is congruent with the fact that only 32% of the subjects completed the news text items that appeared toward the end of the measure.

It is noteworthy that age was not found to be a significant predictor in any of the regression analyses. Education was a significant predictor only for the news text category; this finding must be interpreted with caution, given the small percentage of subjects answering these items. Although age and education are not identified as significant predictors in most analyses, this does not indicate that these variables are uncorrelated with practical tasks. Age and education are index variables and provide little information on the specific factors or processes associated with practical intelligence; in this case they accounted for little additional variance once that associated with the primary abilities was extracted.

In summary, the data suggest strong relationships between traditional psychometric intelligence measures and performance by the elderly on a variety of practical tasks. The correlation between the Basic Skills total score and Figural Relations, a relatively "pure" G_f ability, was .83; the correlation with vocabulary was .78. The magnitude of these correlations are on the order of those found among the primary abilities; moreover, significant proportions of variance associated with practial task performance was accounted for by these abilities (Table 3). It should be noted that the correlations among abilities and between abilities and the Basic Skills test are somewhat higher than might be expected in younger age groups; these higher correlations are congruent with the greater covariances found in previous cognitive aging research.

Study II: age differences in perceived competence in everyday situations and ability correlates

The second study focused on age differences in the perception of competence in dealing with situations experienced by the elderly. Ability correlates of these perceptions of competence were also examined. In addition to focusing on implicit rather than explicit models of intelligence, this study involved a different approach to the conceptualization of criterion tasks of practical intelligence, and was rooted more directly in a contextual view of cognitive functioning. It was assumed that situations involving intellectual competence would vary with the developmental level of the individual and the idiosyncratic changes occurring across the individual's life course and roles. Given the wide individual differences in life experiences in adulthood, it was assumed that there was no one plausible criterion situation, but that the attributes of multiple situations in which intellectual competence was displayed would need to be examined. A Q-sort measure involving a taxonomy of situations commonly experienced by the elderly (Scheidt & Schaie, 1978) was used to examine age differences in a person's perceived competence in these situations.

Method

Subjects. Participants were 234 adults, divided into four age groups: young ($n = 27$, $\overline{X}$ age = 33.6 years, SD = 1.9, range: 29–36); middle-aged ($n =$

68, $\overline{X}$ age = 59.5 years, SD = 2.8, range: 53–64); young–old (n = 86, $\overline{X}$ age = 69.7, SD = 2.5, range: 65–74); and old–old (n = 53, $\overline{X}$ age = 78.2, SD = 2.7, range: 75–84). There were 110 men and 124 women. Subjects were members of a health maintenance organization in southern California. Quota sampling resulted in approximately equal representation of the membership for all groups except the oldest birth years. As expected, there was a significant difference in education among the groups given the cohort differences: young ($\overline{X}$ = 16.3 years); middle-aged ($\overline{X}$ = 14.1 years); young – old ($\overline{X}$ = 12.8 years); old – old ($\overline{X}$ = 11.3 years). There was a significant difference between the middle-aged and young sample in self-reported health; the middle-aged and the two elderly samples did not differ significantly.

Procedure and measures. Subjects were administered a battery of ability tests plus a measure of perceived situational competence in a two and one-half hour session. The seven ability tests involved in the present analyses represented four primary abilities: Spatial Orientation: PMA Space (Thurstone, 1948); Object Rotation (Krauss, Schaie, & Quayhagen, 1980; Schaie, 1985); Inductive Reasoning: PMA Letter Series (Thurstone, 1948); Word Series (Schaie, Gonda, & Quayhagen, 1981; Schaie, 1985); Vocabulary: PMA Verbal Meaning (Thurstone, 1984); Memory: Immediate Recognition Recall, Delayed Recognition Recall; Delayed Free Recall. Composite scores (sum of scores on marker tests) were formed for the Induction, Space, and Memory abilities to represent more stable markers of performance on these abilities.

Scheidt and Schaie (1978) developed a taxonomy of competency-requiring situations of daily living for a sample of community dwelling elderly. From interviews with more than 100 elderly subjects in a large metropolitan area, 300 situations of daily living were identified. Elderly judges rated each situation according to a set of situational attributes derived from the social–psychological literature. Four reliable attribute dimensions were identified: social–non social, active–passive, common–uncommon (for older persons), and supportive–depriving. A Q-sort instrument was then developed and validated that contains eighty prototypical situations, five for each of the sixteen possible attribute classes.

Examples of situations from eight of the sixteen attribute classes are given below:

> *Social–active–common–supportive:* being visited by son or daughter and grandchildren
> *Social–active–common–depriving:* pressured by a salesperson to buy merchandise
> *Nonsocial–active–common–supportive:* gardening
> *Nonsocial–active–common–depriving;* climbing steps to building entrance

Social–passive–common–supportive: seeking advice/aid from a friend
Social–passive–common–depriving: hearing from a friend that she or he is ill
Nonsocial–passive–common–supportive: browsing through family photo album
Nonsocial–passive–common–depriving: worrying about financial expenses

Subjects completed the Q-sort measure of perceived competency individually. They were instructed to rate each of the eighty situations as to how competent they would be to handle that situation. Situations were first sorted into the categories of most competence and least competence and in between. Situations were then subsorted into an eleven-point quasinormal distribution from least to most competent.

Results. First, we will discuss findings regarding age and gender-based differences in perceived competence on the situational dimensions studied. Second, we will examine ability correlates of perceived situational competencies. For the total sample, subjects perceived themselves to be somewhat more competent in Nonsocial, Common, and Supportive situations than in Social, Uncommon, or Depriving situations. Across the four major dimensions, the young and middle-aged groups reported greatest competence in Supportive situations and least competence in Depriving situations. The young–old and old–old groups reported greatest competence in Common situations and least competence in Uncommon situations.

Age differences in perceived competence. Age differences in perceived competence will be reported for the four main situational dimensions and for the two-way interactions. Significant age differences were found for all four of the main dimensions (Fig. 1). Significant positive age effects were found for the Social and Common dimensions. Significant negative age effects were found for the Active and Supportive dimensions. Given that ratings on one end of a dimension are the inverse of ratings on the opposite end of that dimension, it follows that there are positive age trends for the Passive and Depriving dimensions and negative age trends for the Nonsocial and Uncommon dimensions. When differences between successive age groups are examined, significant age differences between the young and middle-aged and the middle-aged and young–old are found for the Active –Passive and Common–Uncommon dimensions. The young and middle-aged differ on the Supportive–Depriving dimension. The young–old and old–old differ significantly on the Social–Nonsocial dimensions.

Turning now to the two-way dimension interactions, we found significant age differences on fourteen of the twenty-four possible two-way interactions (Table 4). For seven of these interactions, there is a positive age effect. The older age groups perceived themselves to have greater competence than did the young in Social–Common, Passive–Common, Passive–Depriving,

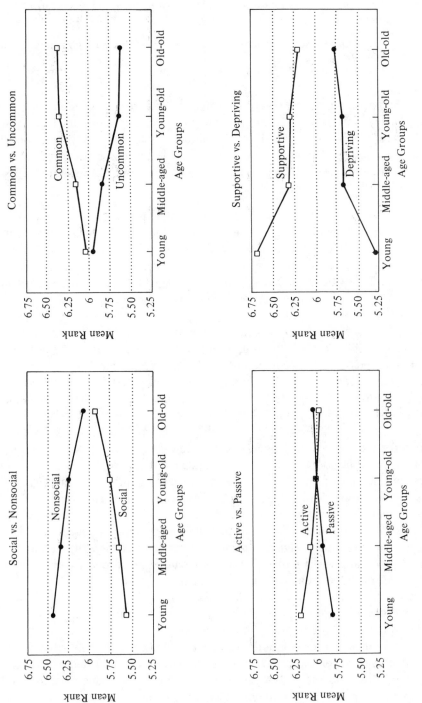

Figure 1. Age effects for main situational dimensions.

Table 4. *Significant age differences on two-way situational dimensions of perceived competence.*

Situational dimension	Young adult	Middle-aged	Young-old	Old-old	F ratio	p value
		Mean values				
Social–Passive	5.41	5.58	5.88	5.98	11.48	<.001
Nonsocial–Active	6.66	6.40	6.29	6.09	5.70	.001
Social–Common	5.43	5.77	6.05	6.29	20.28	<.001
Nonsocial–Uncommon	6.27	6.19	5.92	5.80	6.05	<.001
Social–Depriving	4.90	5.33	5.43	5.78	11.62	<.001
Nonsocial–Supportive	7.19	6.63	6.53	6.36	8.16	<.001
Active–Uncommon	6.10	5.86	5.57	5.56	10.62	<.001
Passive–Common	5.80	6.03	6.19	6.34	6.82	<.001
Active–Supportive	6.64	6.24	6.18	6.00	7.00	<.001
Passive–Supportive	6.76	6.36	6.43	6.38	2.64	.05
Passive–Depriving	4.89	5.52	5.57	5.70	9.35	<.001
Common–Depriving	5.53	5.84	5.91	6.06	5.64	.001
Uncommon–Supportive	6.88	6.15	5.98	5.74	19.28	<.001
Uncommon–Depriving	5.07	5.56	5.40	5.56	3.38	.02

Uncommon–Depriving, Social–Passive, and Social–Depriving situations. The younger age groups perceived themselves to have greater competence than did the old in Nonsocial–Uncommon, Active–Uncommon, Nonsocial–Active, Active–Supportive, Passive–Supportive, Uncommon–Supportive, and Nonsocial–Supportive situations. Figure 2 graphically presents two of these significant interactions.

Gender-based differences in perceived competence. Across all dimensions, men perceived themselves most competent in Nonsocial situations and least competent in Social situations, and women perceived themselves most competent in Supportive situations and least competent in Depriving situations. Gender-based differences were found for three of the four major dimensions. As would be expected, women perceived themselves more competent than did the men in Social, Common, and Supportive situations; men rated themselves more competent than did the women in Nonsocial, Uncommon, and Depriving situations. Significant gender-based differences were found for seventeen of the twenty-four possible two-way interactions (Table 5). Females perceived themselves to be more competent in Social–Common, Social–Uncommon, Passive–Common, Active–Supportive, Passive–Supportive, Common–Supportive, Social–Active, Social–Passive, and Social–Supportive. Age × gender interactions appear to be relatively minimal. The same pattern of significant gender-based differences (for the four major dimensions and the seventeen two-way dimensions) was found for persons over 60 years of age as for the total sample.

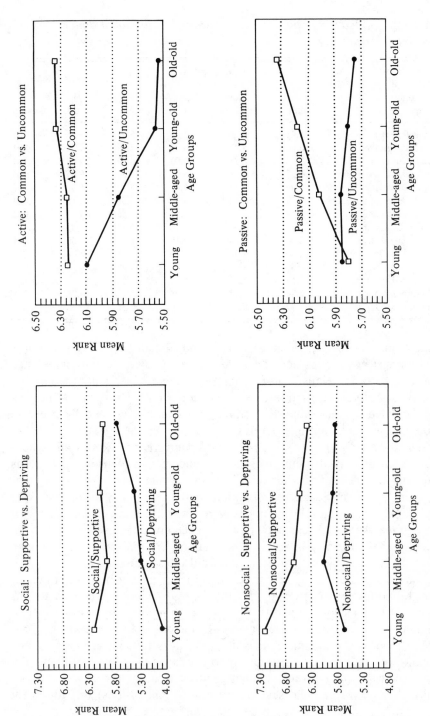

Figure 2. Age effects for two-way situational dimensions.

Table 5. *Significant gender-based differences on two-way situational dimensions of perceived competence.*

Situational dimension	Mean value		t ratio	p value
	Males	Females		
Social–Active	5.62	5.78	6.91	.009
Social–Passive	5.59	5.91	20.05	<.001
Nonsocial–Active	6.42	6.23	5.04	.02
Nonsocial–Passive	6.30	6.08	12.26	<.001
Social–Common	5.81	6.08	13.87	<.001
Social–Uncommon	5.41	5.61	10.24	.002
Nonsocial–Uncommon	6.30	5.75	51.50	<.001
Social–Supportive	5.86	6.22	20.61	<.001
Nonsocial–Depriving	6.16	5.67	28.02	<.001
Passive–Common	5.96	6.29	20.03	<.001
Passive–Uncommon	5.94	5.70	14.26	<.001
Active–Supportive	6.12	6.29	4.60	.03
Passive–Supportive	6.30	6.56	9.75	.002
Active–Depriving	5.92	5.72	6.82	.009
Passive–Depriving	5.60	5.42	3.78	.05
Common–Supportive	6.39	6.72	13.93	<.001
Uncommon–Depriving	5.69	5.23	23.25	<.001

Ability correlates of perceived competence. The ability predictors of perceived competence were examined via a series of stepwise multiple regression analyses (Table 6). In all the regression analyses, four ability predictor variables were employed (PMA Verbal Meaning, Induction composite, Space composite, and Memory composite). The criterion variables were scores of perceived competence on the four major situational dimensions and the twenty-four two-way dimensions.

Significant predictors were found for the major dimensions of Social–Nonsocial and Active–Passive. Spatial ability was found to be the most significant predictor of perceived competence on these dimensions. Spatial ability is a positive predictor of competence in Nonsocial situations and a negative predictor of perceived competence in Social situations. That is, a low performance on Spatial ability is a significant predictor of perceived competence in Social situations. Spatial and Inductive Reasoning abilities are positive predictors of competence in Active situations; Verbal ability is a significant negative predictor of competence in Active situations. Conversely, Verbal ability is a positive predictor of competence in Passive situations, and Spatial and Reasoning abilities are negative predictors of competence in passive situations.

Significant predictors were identified for thirteen of the twenty-four two-way dimensions (Table 6). Spatial ability and Inductive Reasoning were each

Table 6. *Summary of multiple regression analyses: four primary abilities predictor variables.*

Criterion variable	Predictors	β	F ratio	r^2	Multi R
	Major dimensions				
Social	Vocabulary	.043	.31	.08	.27
	Induction	−.037	.16		
	Space	−.237	8.96		
	Memory	−.055	.48		
Active	Vocabulary	−.237	9.40	.12	.34
	Induction	.171	3.63		
	Space	.261	11.30		
	Memory	−.048	.38		
	Two-way dimensions				
Social–Common	Vocabulary	.060	.61	.09	.30
	Induction	−.148	2.67		
	Space	−.161	4.22		
	Memory	−.088	1.26		
Nonsocial–Uncommon	Vocabulary	−.012	.02	.07	.26
	Induction	.000	.00		
	Space	.275	11.96		
	Memory	−.059	.55		
Passive–Common	Vocabulary	−.017	.05	.05	.22
	Induction	−.085	.83		
	Space	−.190	5.58		
	Memory	−.122	2.29		
Active–Uncommon	Vocabulary	−.247	10.66	.11	.33
	Induction	.128	2.03		
	Space	.231	8.82		
	Memory	.090	1.39		
Active–Supportive	Vocabulary	−.142	3.33	.05	.23
	Induction	.231	6.16		
	Space	.064	.63		
	Memory	−.015	.03		
Passive–Uncommon	Vocabulary	.258	10.94	.05	.23
	Induction	−.060	.42		
	Space	−.064	.64		
	Memory	−.120	2.22		
Passive–Depriving	Vocabulary	.074	.91	.06	.24
	Induction	−.227	6.00		
	Space	−.058	.53		
	Memory	.000	.00		
Uncommon–Supportive	Vocabulary	−.015	.04	.08	.28
	Induction	.269	8.57		
	Space	−.012	.02		
	Memory	.047	.35		
Social–Passive	Vocabulary	.166	4.94	.13	.36
	Induction	−.207	5.37		
	Space	−.265	11.77		
	Memory	.060	.60		

Table 6. (*continued*)

Criterion variable	Predictors	β	F ratio	r^2	Multi R
Nonsocial–Active	Vocabulary	− .108	2.00	.09	.30
	Induction	.086	.88		
	Space	.256	10.59		
	Memory	.028	.13		
Social–Depriving	Vocabulary	.012	.03	.08	.29
	Induction	− .122	1.79		
	Space	− .197	6.22		
	Memory	− .017	.05		
Nonsocial–Supportive	Vocabulary	− .063	.65	.05	.22
	Induction	.247	7.06		
	Space	− .203	.08		
	Memory	.017	.05		
Nonsocial–Depriving	Vocabulary	.010	.02	.04	.20
	Induction	− .135	2.08		
	Space	.249	9.54		
	Memory	− .025	.09		

found to be significant predictors in eight situations. Verbal ability was a significant predictor in four situations, and Memory was a significant predictor in two situations. Spatial ability was found to be the most significant predictor in seven situations, Induction in four situations, and Verbal ability in two situations.

The question arises of whether there are age differences in the pattern of ability predictors for various situational dimensions. That is, do ability predictors of perceived competence vary by age/cohorts? Given the limited number of subjects in each of the four age groups, it was not possible to run separate regression analyses by age group. However, regression analyses on the subject sample over 60 years were computed and compared with findings for the total sample. Given the smaller number of subjects, there were fewer significant predictors found for the 60 + years sample. Where significant predictors were found, however, the pattern of predictors for the total and the older sample was quite similar.

Discussion

A primary purpose of this study was to examine age/cohort and gender-based differences in perceived competence on eighty situations of daily living, classified according to a taxonomy of situational dimensions. A secondary purpose of the study was to identify ability predictors of perceived competence for these situational dimensions.

Significant age differences in perceived competence were found for the four major situational dimensions and for fourteen of the two-way situational categories. With regard to the four major dimensions, significant positive age/cohort differences were found in perceived competence for Social, Common, Passive, and Depriving situations and negative age effects for the inverse dimensions of Nonsocial, Uncommon, Active, and Supportive. The onset of these effects across successive age/cohorts is also of interest, given that the timing of occurence differs by situational dimension. Since the findings on age differences for the two-way categories generally support the findings for the four major dimensions, our discussion will focus primarily on age differences for the four major dimensions.

The finding of the greater perceived adeptness of the elderly in social settings, when compared with other age/cohorts, is in agreement with the literature on the relevance and importance of social competence for the aged (Dittman-Kohli & Baltes, in press). Studies of self-efficacy (Lachman & Jelalian, 1984) have found the elderly to report greater perceived competence on tests of verbal ability, critical in social situations, than on tests of abstract fluid reasoning.

It should be further noted that the greatest difference in perceived competence between Social and Nonsocial situations occurs for the young sample. Young subjects perceive themselves to be significantly more competent in Nonsocial situations than in Social situations. The difference in ratings of perceived competence in Social and Nonsocial situations decreases with age. Many individuals spend greater amounts of time in solitary activity with increasing age (Gordon, Gaitz, & Scott, 1976); while valuing social competence they may perceive themselves to be equally competent in nonsocial situations.

Likewise, the finding that older age groups perceive themselves to be more competent in "common" situations is congruent with previous findings in the gerontological intelligence literature. A number of studies have reported little or no age differences in problem-solving or memory tasks involving content or skills familiar or commonplace to the elderly (Botwinick & Storandt, 1980; Hanley-Dunn & McIntosh, 1984). The strongest negative age effects occur on problem-solving tasks involving novel and abstract content. Pairwise comparisons of perceived competence between successive age groups indicate that the only significant difference occurs between the middle-aged and young–old samples. Restriction in the lifespace and increased routinization of daily activities attributable to retirement or to debilitating health occur with greater frequency during the transition from middle age to old age and may be associated with a decrease in perceived competence in Uncommon situations.

The negative age effect for perceived competence in Active situations is of particular interest because of its early occurrence. Note in Figure 1 that the difference in perceived competence between Active versus Passive situations occurs only in young adulthood. There is little difference in ratings of perceived competence in middle or old age for Active versus Passive situations.

An unexpected finding was that older adult cohorts perceived themselves to be more competent in Depriving situations, compared with results among the younger cohorts. Again, note that this age difference occurs early, primarily between young adulthood and middle age. Having assumed increasing responsibilities across the life course and having encountered more of life's "hard knocks," middle-aged and older adults may perceive themselves as having become more competent to cope with depriving situations. For example, some of the literature on coping styles (Vaillant, 1977; McCrae, 1982) suggests that the coping strategies used by older adults may become increasingly more effective and less distorting of reality.

The findings on gender-based differences in situations of perceived competence are quite congruent with those from the traditional sex-role literature. Women reported greater perceived competence in Social, Common, and Supportive situations. A substantial literature indicates the female's concern for social competence, for acquiring the approval of others, and for avoiding competitive conflict situations. The data also support the traditional sex-role findings for males with regard to instrumental behaviors; men reported greater perceived competence in Nonsocial, Uncommon, and Depriving situations. There appear to be few age by sex interactions, suggesting that these gender-based differences are not significantly moderated by cohort differences in sex-role attributions.

We turn now to the data on ability predictors of perceived competence in various situational dimensions. Multiple ability predictors were found for the major dimension of Active–Passive and for about one-half of the two-way dimensions with significant predictors. In a number of instances, low ability performance is a significant predictor. Fluid abilities (i.e., Spatial Orientation, Inductive Reasoning) were found to be the most significant predictors for eleven of the two-way situational dimensions (Table 6). High fluid ability performance was found to be a significant predictor of perceived competence in Nonsocial, Uncommon, and/or Depriving situations, whereas low fluid ability was shown to be a significant predictor in Social, Common, and Passive situations. Findings are less clear with regard to the nature of Verbal ability as a predictor of perceived competence. Vocabulary was found to be a significant predictor of perceived competence in four situational types. High verbal ability performance is a significant predictor of perceived competence in Passive–Uncommon situations, whereas low verbal ability is a significant predictor of perceived competence in Active contexts (i.e., Nonsocial–Active, Active–Supportive, and Active–Uncommon situations).

Some concluding remarks

Ability correlates of practical intelligence

A major issue in the study of practical intelligence is the magnitude and nature of the relationship with traditional conceptions of intelligence. The range of individual differences increases with age for many traditional abilities (Schaie, 1983; Willis, 1985); however, it is an unanswered question as to how much of the variance in practical intelligence can be accounted for by variability in traditional intelligence measures. The studies presented in this chapter provide some relevant data. Significant ability correlates were identified for both explicit (i.e., Basic Skills test) and implicit (i.e., perceived competence) conceptions of practical intelligence. However, the traditional ability measures accounted for much more variance when actual performance in practical tasks was used as the criterion variable than when perceived competence was the criterion. The lower correlation between abilities and attributions is congruent with the personality literature (Lachman et al., 1982; Mischel, 1977). The amount of variance accounted for by psychometric abilities is impressive; 80% of the variance on the Basic Skills test was accounted for by the three primary abilities of Figural Relations, Vocabulary, and Social Knowledge (see Table 3). The multiple correlations in Table 3 are comparable to the magnitude of relationships found among primary abilities.

Our concern was not only to establish the presence of a relationship between traditional and practical intelligence, but to examine the nature of these relationships. Specifically, we wished to identify differential patterns of ability predictors for various categories of practical tasks. We were interested in examining ability–task relationships not only at the primary ability level, but with regard to hierarchical models of intelligence, such as the G_f-G_c model as well.

Multiple ability predictors were identified that included both fluid and crystallized abilities. In study I, fluid abilities were the significant predictors of performance on practical tasks of comprehending labels, reading maps, interpreting charts, completing forms, reading advertisements, and understanding technical documents. Crystallized ability predictors were found for paragraph comprehension, understanding technical documents, and reading news text. In study II both fluid and crystallized abilities were predictors of perceived competence on the Active–Passive dimension, and the fluid ability of Space was a significant predictor for the Social–Nonsocial dimension.

What surprised us, however, was the saliency of the fluid predictors. We had hypothesized that crystallized abilities would be particularly significant in the study of practical intelligence. The solution of real-life tasks would seem to require knowledge and skills acquired through sociocultural experiences. In both studies, however, fluid abilities (i.e., Figural Relations, Induction, Space) were found to be the more frequent and significant ability predictors.

Cattell (1971) has drawn the following conceptual distinctions between fluid and crystallized intelligence:

Crystallized ability (G_c) expressions operate in areas where the judgments have been taught systematically or experienced before. The differences between the words . . . "definite" and "definitive" in a synonyms test, or in a mechanical knowledge primary test, between using an ordinary wrench or a box spanner on part of one's automobile, requires intelligence for the initial perception and learning of the discrimination (therefore some never will learn it). But thereafter it becomes a crystallized skill, relatively automatically applied....Fluid ability, by contrast, appears to operate whenever the sheer perception of complex relations is involved. It thus shows up in tests where borrowing from stored, crystallized skills brings no advantage. As far as logic is concerned, it seems to spread over all kinds of relationships . . . In short, fluid intelligence is an expression of the level of complexity of relationships which an individual can perceive and act upon when he does not have recourse to answers to such complex issues already stored in memory. (pp. 98–99)

Although the content involved in the practical problems studied is crystallized in nature, these problems cannot be solved simply by automatized retrieval of previously acquired knowledge. Rather, the subject must identify the relationships among the variables in the task and must determine an appropriate strategy for solving the problem. These operations represent fluid aspects of the tasks. Practical intelligence often involves several complex forms of relationships, as evidenced by the multiple ability predictors identified. The particular types of fluid relationships that must be called upon to solve problems successfully (e.g., part–whole, causal relations, inductive reasoning, spatial relations) will vary by task.

In a similar vein, Sternberg (1981) has suggested that intelligence may better be assessed by "nonentrenched" tasks, requiring new conceptual systems. In his triadic model of intelligence, Sternberg suggests that appropriate measures of intelligence should involve a degree of novelty and tasks that are only in the process of becoming automatized. How might the concepts of automatization and novelty relate to the study of practical intelligence? Automatization implies that the knowledge to be retrieved is content bound and that the organization of the knowledge is relatively static. Previously acquired information is applied in a routinized manner to a variety of problem situations. As noted above, the solution of many practical tasks involves more than the retrieval of static information. Herein may lie part of the difficulty experienced by older adults in solving practical tasks. Since the content or type of task appears familiar, the older person recalls previous experiences with this type of content or task and applies the recalled information in a predetermined manner. The content of the practical task, however, does not dictate the types of relationships and strategies to be applied in problem solution. The relationships and strategies are "fluid" and thus may be applied to a variety of different content areas. Moreover, various instances of a task may involve different fluid relations. For example, one instance of the task, "comprehending medicine labels," may require sequential relations (e.g., the order of steps in taking a medication), whereas another instance of the task may involve inferential reasoning (e.g., if only the adult dosage is stated, what would be the appropriate child dosage).

The "novelty" involved in each instance of a seemingly familiar task lies in the need to determine the appropriate set of fluid relations and strategies. The concept of novelty has often been used to indicate unfamiliar content/ stimuli or to denote qualitatively new forms of conceptual systems. Given the large proportion of variance accounted for by traditional psychometric measures, it appears to us that practical intelligence may involve not so much the acquisition of "new" conceptual systems, but facility in identifying and utilizing multiple logical relationships. A second type of difficulty for the older adult may be related to the multiplicity of relations or strategies involved in solving a task. Whether in solving practical problems, these multiple relations are applied simultaneously or sequentially remains a topic for future research. However, research on working memory suggests there may be age-related decremental changes in the facility with which one can simultaneously deal with multiple bits of information (Hartley, Harker, & Walsh, 1980).

The logical consistency of the relationships between psychometric abilities and judgment of perceived competence found in Study II suggests that older adults may be much more proficient in accurately appraising their ability to handle the intellectual load of behavioral situations than they are often given credit for. Additional support for this inference is provided by recent work on intellectual self-efficacy (Lachman & Jelallian, 1984). It seems reasonable to speculate from these findings that the observed average age differences in perceived competence may well be a direct consequence of the congruent age differences in those abilities that provide the basic resources for solving the cognitive aspects of a given situation. A direct test of this proposition would be to examine whether training interventions that have been shown to reverse intellectual decline, of the type used by us in other contexts (Schaie & Willis, in press; Willis, Blieszner, & Baltes, 1981), would also lead to a reversal of the observed age differences in perceived competence.

Methodological issues. Both of the studies summarized in this chapter involve the examination of practical intelligence in relation to a broad ability battery with known factorial structure. We argue for the importance of this methodological approach for two reasons. First, ability–task relationships need to be studied at the *construct* level, rather than at the level of individual measures. In much of the previous research employing only a very limited number of measures of an ability or cognitive process, it has been impossible to differentiate test-specific variance from variance common to the ability construct. Thus, the relationship between a single ability measure and a single example of a real-life task may reflect communality of content or stimuli, rather than a significant relationship at the construct level. The importance of knowing the factorial structure of the independent variables and of examining ability–task relationship at the construct level is not restricted to the psychometric approach but should be an essential feature of any rigorous examination of the relationship between intellectual functioning and real-life tasks, whatever cognitive framework is chosen. Second, the examination of ability–task relationships within a structural framework permits identification of differential patterns of relationships. As we noted earlier in our discussion of Study I, most practical tasks were significantly correlated with all the primary abilities because of positive manifold and the increasing covariances among abilities noted in intellectual aging. Where all ability–task relationships are statistically significant, differential patterns of relationships can best be examined within a structural measurement framework.

Ecological validity and criterion tasks. When practical intelligence focuses, as in our research, on real-life tasks of daily living, there is the question of the extent to which the criterion tasks are indeed ecologically valid. How representative of everyday experiences of the target population are the items/ problems on the criterion tasks? The age and possibly the cohort of the target population must be considered. However, there are wide individual differences in today's elderly cohort, and many of these individual differences are only moderately correlated with age. No one set of criterion tasks will be equally representative for all elderly persons. In our own research we have attempted to define a normative set of criterion tasks critical to independent living in our society and cutting across a wide variety of situational contexts. In some instances, however, particularly if policy decisions or intervention procedures are to be derived, criterion tasks specific to a particular subpopulation of the age/cohort will need to be developed.

There is also the issue of the similarity between the cognitive demands and characteristics of the criterion tasks and the actual tasks of daily living experienced by the elderly. For example, the items on the Basic Skills measure involve one "right" answer, and thus are largely limited to problems involving linear thinking. Virtually no research has been done to determine the proportion of daily living tasks that involve primarily linear thinking. Likewise, for many of the Basic Skills items the relevant reference materials (e.g., maps, news text) are available to the subjects as they solve the problem. Thus, the memory demands for the tasks may be quite low, as suggested by the nonsignificant loading on the memory span factor in the extension analysis and the absence of memory span as a significant predictor in the regression analyses. The specific memory demands of most daily living tasks remains to be investigated. In addition, the paper-and-pencil nature of the Basic Skills measure limits its assessment of socially oriented tasks, an important competence area for the elderly.

Summary

This chapter has examined issues related to practical intelligence in later adulthood. Practical intelligence has been defined as real-life tasks of daily living experienced by a specific age/cohort. A major focus of this chapter is on the relationship between practical intelligence and traditional forms of intelligence. The types of practical tasks we have studied would seem to involve previously acquired knowledge and skills, rather than truly novel or recently developed forms of cognition. Psychometric intelligence involving the "products" of behavior may be particularly applicable. Moreover, because much of the previous longitudinal work on adult intelligence has been conducted within the psychometric approach, links with previous research can be drawn more easily.

Two studies examining the relationship between selected aspects of practical intelligence and psychometric abilities have been reported. The first study examined the relationship between fluid/crystallized intelligence and performance on eight categories of real-life tasks. Significant correlations were found between these tasks and both fluid and crystallized abilities. Extension analyses and multiple regression analyses suggest that more variance was accounted for by fluid abilities than by crystallized abilities. This differential pattern of relationships was found across a wide variety of real-life tasks varying in content. The second study examined perceived competence along a number of situational dimensions with regard to age and gender-based differences and ability correlates. The Thurstonian primary abilities studied were Verbal, Space, Number, Memory, and Inductive Reasoning. Significant age- and gender-related differences were found. Positive age effects were found for Social, Common, Passive, and Depriving situations. Negative age trends were found for Nonsocial, Uncommon, Active, and Supportive dimensions. Verbal, Space, and Inductive Reasoning have been identified as significant predictors of perceived competence for various situational dimensions. Similar to the findings in the first study, fluid abilities were found to account for more variance in perceived competence than were nonfluid abilities.

Traditional/academic forms of intelligence were originally developed with regard to critical developmental tasks of the early portion of the lifespan, such as schooling. But academic achievement is not a salient developmental task throughout much of the adult life course, particularly in old age. Nevertheless, these traditional intelligence measures have dominated research on cognition across the life course; much of our scientific knowledge about adult intellectual ability is thus based on these traditional conceptions of intelligence. The examination of relationships between traditional and practical forms of intelligence and the possible identification of new forms of cognitive functioning remain critical research themes for the coming decade.

Notes

The research reported in this chapter was supported by grants AG00133 and AG00405 from the National Institute on Aging. Preparation of this chapter was supported by grants AG03544 and AG04770, also from the National Institute of Aging.
Requests for reprints should be sent to Sherry L. Willis, S-110 Human Development Building, The Pennsylvania State University, University Park, PA 16802.
An adapted version of the Basic Skills test is now marketed by CTB McGraw-Hill.

References

Anastasi, A. (1976). *Psychological testing* (4th ed.). New York: Macmillan.
Baltes, P. B., Cornelius, S. W., Spiro, A., Nesselroade, J. R., & Willis, S. L. (1980). Integration vs differentiation of fluid-crystallized intelligence in old age. *Developmental Psychology, 16*, 625–635.
Baltes, P. B., Dittman-Kohli, F., & Dixon, R. A. (1984). New perspectives on the development of intelligence in adulthood: Toward a dual-process conception and a model of selective optimization with compensation. In P. B. Baltes & O. G. Brim, Jr. (Eds.), *Life-span development and behavior* (Vol. 6, pp. 34–76). New York: Academic.
Bandura, A. (1982). Self-efficacy mechanism in human agency. *American Psychologist, 37*, 122–147.
Baron, J. (in press). What kinds of intelligence components are fundamental? In S. Chipman, J. Segal & R. Glaser (Eds.). *Thinking and learning skills: Current research and open questions.* Hillsdale, NJ: Erlbaum.
Berg, C. A., & Sternberg, R. J. (in press). A triadic theory of intellectual development during adulthood. *Developmental Review.*
Binet, A., & Simon, T. (1905). Methodes nouvelles pour le diagnostic du niveau intellectual des anormaux. *L'Année Psychologique, 11*, 191–244.
Botwinick, J. (1977). Intellectual abilities. In J. E. Birren & K. W. Schaie (Eds.), *Handbook of the psychology of aging.* New York: Van Nostrand Reinhold.
Botwinick, J., & Storandt, M. (1970). Recall and recognition of old information in relation to age and sex. *Journal of Gerontology, 35*, 70–76.
Capon, N., & Kuhn, D. (1977). Logical reasoning in the supermarket: Adult females' use of a proportional reasoning strategy in an everyday context. *Developmental Psychology, 15*, 450–452.
Cattell, R. B. (1971). *Abilities: Their structure, growth, and action.* Boston, MA: Houghton-Mifflin.
Cattell, R. B., & Cattell, A. K. S. (1957). *Test of g: Culture fair (Scale 2, Form A).* Champaign, IL: Institute for Personality and Ability Testing.
Clayton, V. (1975). Wisdom and intelligence: The nature and function of knowledge in the later years. *International Journal of Aging and Development, 15*, 315–323.
Clayton, V., & Birren, J. (1980). The development of wisdom across the life span: A reexamination of an ancient topic. In P. B. Baltes & O. G. Brim (Eds.), *Life-span development and behavior* (Vol. 3, pp. 104–137). New York: Academic.

Commons, M. L., Richards, F., & Armon, G. (1982). *Beyond formal operations: Late adolescence and adult cognitive development.* New York: Praeger.

Commons, M. L., Richards, F., & Kuhn, D. (1982). Metasystematic reasoning: A case for a level of systematic reasoning beyond Piaget's stage of formal operations. *Child Development, 53,* 1058–1069.

Connolly, K., & Bruner, J. (Eds). (1974). *The growth of competence.* New York: Academic.

Cornelius, S. W., Willis, S. L., Nesselroade, J. R., & Baltes, P. B. (1983). Convergence between attention variables and factors of psychometric intelligence in older adults. *Intelligence, 7,* 253–269.

Cunningham, W. R. (1980). Age comparative factor analysis of ability variables in adulthood and old age. *Intelligence, 4,* 133–149.

Detterman, D. K. (1980). Understand cognitive components before postulating metacomponents. *Behavioral and Brain Sciences, 3,* 589.

Dittman-Kohli, F., & Baltes, P. B. (in press). Toward a neofunctionalist conception of adult intellectual development: Wisdom as a prototypical case of intellectual growth. In C. Alexander and E. Langer (Eds.), *Beyond formal operations: Alternative endpoints to human development.*

Educational Testing Service. (1977). *Basic Skills Assessment Test: Reading.* Princeton, NJ: Educational Testing Service.

Egan, D. E. (1978). *Characterizing spatial ability: Different mental processes reflected in accuracy and latency scores.* NAMRL-1250. Pensacola, FL: Naval Aerospace Medical Research Laboratory.

Egan, D. E. (1981). An analysis of spatial orientation test performance. *Intelligence, 5,* 85–100.

Ekstrom, R. B., French, J. W., Harman, H., & Derman, D. (1976). *Kit of factor-referenced cognitive tests* (rev. ed.). Princeton, NJ: Educational Testing Service.

Eysenck, H. J. (1982). *A model for intelligence.* New York: Springer-Verlag.

Flavell, J. H. (1970). Cognitive changes in adulthood. In L. R. Goulet & P. B. Baltes (Eds.). *Life-span developmental psychology: Research and theory* (pp. 248–257). New York: Academic.

Garner, E. G., & Monge, R. H. (1977). Adult age differences in cognitive abilities and educational background. *Experimental Aging Research, 3,* 337–383.

Gonda, J. N., Schaie, K. W., & Quayhagen, M. (1981). Education, task meaningfulness and cognitive performance in young–old and old–old adults. *Educational Gerontology, 7,* 151–158.

Gordon, C., Gaitz, C. M., & Scott, J., Jr. (1976). Leisure and lives: Personal expressivity across the life span. In R. H. Binstock & E. Shanas (Eds.) *Handbook of aging and the social sciences* (pp. 310–341). New York: Van Nostrand-Reinhold.

Guilford, J. P. (1969a). *Verbal analogies test. I.* Beverly Hills, CA: Sheridan Psychological Services.

Guilford, J. P. (1969b). *Word matrix test.* Beverly Hills, CA: Sheridan Psychological Services.

Guilford, J. P., & Lacey, J. I. (1947). Printed classification tests. A.A.F. (Aviation Psychological Progress Research Report No. 5). Washington, DC: U. S. Government Printing Office.

Hanley-Dunn, P., & McIntosh, J. L. (1984). Meaningfulness and recall of names by young and old adults. *Journal of Gerontology, 39,* 583–585.

Hartley, J. T., Harker, J. O., & Walsh, D. A. (1980). Contemporary issues and new directions in adult development of learning and memory. In L. Poon (Ed.), *Aging in the 1980's* (pp. 239–252). Washington, DC: American Psychological Association.

Hills, J. R. (1957). Factor analyzed abilities and success in college mathematics. *Educational Psychological Measurement, 17,* 615–622.

Hooper, F. H., Hooper, J. O., & Colbert, K. K. (1984). *Personality and memory correlates of intellectual functioning: Young adulthood to old age.* Basel: Karger.

Horn, J. L. (1967). *Social situation—EP03A.* Unpublished test, Department of Psychology, University of Denver.

Jensen, A. R. (1982). Reaction time and psychometric g. In H. J. Eysenck (Ed.), *A model for intelligence*. New York: Springer-Verlag.

Kramer, D. A. (1983). Post-formal operations? A need for further conceptualization. *Human Development, 26*, 91–105.

Krauss, I. K., Quayhagen, M., & Schaie, K. W. (1980). Spatial rotation in the elderly: Performance factors. *Journal of Gerontology, 35*, 199–206.

Labouvie-Vief, G. (1980). Beyond formal operations: Uses and limits of pure logic in life-span development. *Human Development, 23*, 141–161.

Labouvie-Vief, G. (1982). Dynamic development and mature autonomy: A theoretical prologue. *Human Development, 25*, 161–191.

Lachman, M. E., & Jelallian, E. (1984). Self-efficacy and attributions for intellectual performance in young and elderly adults. *Journal of Gerontology, 39*, 577–582.

Looft, W. R. (1970). Note on WAIS Vocabulary performance by young and old adults. *Psychological Reports, 26*, 943–946.

Matarazzo, J. D. (1972). *Wechsler's measurement and appraisal of adult intelligence* (5th ed.). Baltimore: Williams & Wilkins.

McClelland, D. C. (1973). Testing for competence rather than for "Intelligence." *American Psychologist, 28*, 1–14.

McCrae, R. R. (1982). Age differences in the use of coping mechanisms. *Journal of Gerontology, 37*, 454–460.

Meacham, J. A. (1982). Wisdom and the context of knowledge: Knowing that one doesn't know. In D. Kuhn & J. A. Meacham (Eds.), *On the development of developmental psychology* (pp. 111–134). Basel: Karger.

Mischel, W. (1977). On the future of personality measurement. *American Psychologist, 32*, 246–254.

O'Sullivan, M., & Guilford, J. P. (1965). *Social translations. Form A*. Beverly Hills, CA: Sheridan Psychological Services.

O'Sullivan, M., Guilford, J. P., & de Mille, R. (1965). *Measurement of social intelligence* (Tech. Rep. No. 34). Los Angeles, CA: University of Southern California Psychology Laboratory.

Plemons, J., Willis, S. L., & Baltes, P. B. (1978). Modifiability of fluid intelligence in aging: A short-term longitudinal training approach. *Journal of Gerontology, 33*, 224–231.

Raven, J. C. (1962). *Standard progressive matrices, Set II* (1962 rev.). London: Lewis.

Reinert, G. (1970). Comparative factor analytic studies of intelligence throughout the human life span. In L. R. Goulet & P. B. Baltes (Eds.), *Life-span developmental psychology: Research and theory* (pp. 468–485). New York: Academic.

Resnick, L. B. (Ed.). (1976). *The nature of intelligence*. Hillsdale, NJ: Erlbaum.

Roberts, P., Papalia-Finlay, D., Davis, E. S., Blackburn, J., & Dellmann, M. (1982). No two fields ever grow grass the same way: Assessment of conservation abilities in the elderly. *International Journal of Aging and Human Development, 15*, 185–194.

Schaie, K. W. (1978). External validity in the assessment of intellectual performance in adulthood. *Journal of Gerontology, 33*, 695–701.

Schaie, K. W. (Ed.). (1983). *Longitudinal studies of adult psychological development*. New York: Guilford.

Schaie, K. W. (1985). *Manual for the Schaie–Thurstone adult mental abilities test (STAMAT)*. Palo Alto, CA: Consulting Psychological Press.

Schaie, K. W., Gonda, J. N., & Quayhagen, M. (1981). The relationship between intellectual performance and perception of everyday competence in middle-aged, young–old, and old–old adults. *Proceedings of the XXIInd International Congress of Psychology* (pp. 233–243). Leipzig: International Union of Psychological Sciences.

Schaie, K. W., & Willis, S. L. (in press). Can decline in adult intellectual functioning be reversed? *Developmental Psychology*.

Scheidt, R. J., & Schaie, K. W. (1978). A taxonomy of situations for the elderly population: Generating situational criteria. *Journal of Gerontology, 33*, 848–857.

Sinnott, J. D. (1982). Post-formal reasoning: The relativistic stage. In M. L. Commons, F.

Richards, & G. Armon (Eds.), *Beyond formal operations: Late adolescence and adult cognitive development* (pp. 288–315). New York: Praeger.

Smith, I. M. (1964). *Spatial ability: Its educational and social significance*. London: University of London.

Sternberg, R. J. (1980). Factor theories of intelligence are all right almost. *Educational Researcher, 9*, 6–13, 18.

Sternberg, R. J. (1981). Intelligence and nonentrenchment. *Journal of Educational Psychology, 73*, 1–16.

Sternberg, R. J. (Ed.). (1982). *Advances in the psychology of human intelligence* (Vol. 1). Hillsdale, NJ: Erlbaum.

Sternberg, R. J. (1985). *Beyond IQ: A triarchic theory of human intelligence*. London: Cambridge University Press.

Sternberg, R. J., Conway, B. E., Ketron, J. L., & Bernstein, M. (1981). People's conceptions of intelligence. *Journal of Personality and Social Psychology, 41*, 37–55.

Thurstone, L. L. (1948). *Primary mental abilities*. Chicago: University of Chicago Press.

Thurstone, T. G. (1962). *Primary mental abilities for Grades 9–12* (rev. ed.). Chicago: Science Research Associates.

Vaillant, G. E. (1977). *Adaptation to life*. Boston, MA: Little Brown.

Willis, S. L. (1985). Towards an educational psychology of the adult learner: Cognitive and intellectual bases. In J. E. Birren & K. W. Schaie (Eds.), *Handbook of the psychology of aging* (2nd ed.). New York: Van Nostrand Reinhold.

Willis, S. L., & Baltes, P. B. (1980). Intelligence in adulthood and aging: Contemporary issues. In L. W. Poon (Ed.), *Aging in the 1980's: Psychological issues* (pp. 260–272). Washington, DC: American Psychological Association.

Part IV

Cross-cultural approaches to practical intelligence

12   Bricolage: savages do it daily

J. W. Berry and S. H. Irvine

The purpose of this chapter is to examine the domain of cognitive competence from the perspective of cross-cultural psychology. It is not intended to be a general commentary (many of these exist, among them Berry 1984; Irvine, 1979; LCHC, 1979, 1982); rather, it focuses on those cognitive behaviours that may be observed in day-to-day life, and that may be assessed by psychological procedures (observation or testing).[1] However, relationships between these practical aspects and more academic cognitive behaviours will be included where such a consideration may shed some light on our central concern.

A theoretical approach is outlined first that discusses the notion of *bricolage*, and the relevance of understanding daily activities in their cultural contexts. A description of this approach is followed by a selective review of a variety of empirical studies in anthropology and psychology, including collective and individual phenomena that reveal the nature and extent of cognitive competence in a variety of cultures. This chapter concludes with an attempt to expand current Western-based notions of cognitive competence to include the new aspects presented in the review, as well as a discussion of problems of their assessment. The central arguments presented are that among the world's peoples, practical knowledge and abilities really are well developed and that such cognitive activity is of the highest possible quality because it meets the highest possible relevant standard – continuing adaptation and survival of the group in the ecological setting in which its members find themselves. The task of cross-cultural cognitive psychology is to document these abilities as they are developed and displayed in everyday life and then to reflect on what this new information means for the psychology of cognition more generally.

Conceptual issues

An obscure title deserves some explanation. The key term *bricolage* was employed by Levi-Strauss (1962/1966) to refer to work of an odd-job sort. The worker (*bricoleur*) is defined as "someone who works with his hands

271

and uses devious means compared to those of the craftsman" (Levi-Strauss, 1966, pp. 16–17). To expand further, the translator adds that the term *bricoleur* has no precise equivalent in English. He is a man who undertakes odd jobs and is a Jack of all trades, or a kind of professional do-it-yourself man, but, as the text makes clear, he is of a different standing from, for instance, the English "odd job man or handy man" (Levi-Srauss, 1966, p. 17). The term was introduced as an analogy to highlight a contrast between "the savage mind" and contemporary scientific thinking; for example, "cash-crop agriculture is hardly to be confused with the science of the botanist" (Levi-Strauss, 1966, p. 3). In elucidating the contrast, one commentator (Gardner, 1973) made the following observation:

Faced with the task, say, of repairing a faulty machine, he [the bricoleur] looks over the materials at hand and improvises a solution. If the materials available do not suffice, he may try to modify them in some way; but he is unlikely to seek new tools or to redefine the problem. In contrast, the scientist or engineer will not even bother to determine what tools are available until a much later stage. Instead, he will refresh his knowledge of how the machine is supposed to work, drawing a diagram or even consulting a manual. Then, still proceeding on the plane of thought, he will specify the points at which something could have gone wrong and the set of possible repairs. Only at this point will he inventory the tools that are at hand; and if the appropriate ones are missing, he will secure them, or if necessary, even invent them. As Levi-Strauss puts it, the *bricoleur* begins with the event – the broken machine and the tools available – and attempts to build a structure – a set of operations with the tools which will repair the damage. The scientist begins with the structure – his knowledge of the intact apparatus, his deductions about possible flaws – and then gradually converges upon the event – the specific tools and actions needed to repair the damage. (Gardner, 1973, pp. 139–140)

While promoting this contrast in cognitive life, Levi-Strauss nevertheless affirmed the psychic unity of cognitive activity: Magic and science are "two parallel modes of acquiring knowledge," both requiring "the same sort of mental operations and they differ not so much in kind as in the different types of phenomena to which they are applied" (Levi-Strauss, 1966, p. 13). In his commentary, Gardner (1973, p. 134) asserted that Levi-Strauss's goal in this work was "to demonstrate that the mind of a so-called 'primitive' is no different qualitatively from that of a member of an advanced Western culture."

To complete the explanation of the title, we are concerned with the day-to-day cognitive performances of those peoples formerly referred to as *savages*; the intent of the term is to provide a little shock treatment for the inevitable residue of ethnocentrism that plagues research and interpretation in the cross-cultural study of cognition. We do not employ the term uncritically, nor do we subscribe to similar archaic terms such as *primitive* and *barbarous*.

A parallel set of ideas may be discerned in the work of Vernon (1969). With respect to developed intelligence, he argued that

We should expect people like the Eskimos or Australian aboriginals to be handi-capped in using the symbols, or acquiring the mental skills, which western culture has evolved. On the other hand we should not claim that they are intelligent in a different way just because they are better than us at survival in the snows or in the desert. These are traditional, lower-level skills, built up over generations and pos-sessing little transferability. (Vernon, 1969, p. 23)

To both Levi-Strauss and Vernon, then, cognitive activity is viewed as a shared, species-wide characteristic (a psychological universal) but one that is used in differing ways and for different purposes across groups. It is im-possible to avoid the conclusion that they value the cognitive operations of some groups less than others; the "concrete," "magical," "traditional," "lower-level" cognitive activity of some groups is clearly being valued less highly than the "scientific," "symbolic," and "transferrable" abilities of other groups. What is the basis of such a view? Is it possible to substantiate? Does it represent a "scientific" approach, or is it based on ethnocentrism?

The approach taken in this chapter is that, indeed, cognitive processes are very likely to be universal (a view now widely espoused in crosscultural psychology, and one based on a considerable amount of research) but that these day-to-day "lower-level," "concrete," survival skills are not to be so lightly dismissed. Rather, they are the very stuff on which we may be able to build a more culturally relevant, more comprehensive, and less ethno-centric conception of human cognitive functioning.

We do not know what this more comprehensive view of cognitive life will be like. For this reason, we are deliberately avoiding the term "intelligence" here, preferring instead the less loaded notion of "cognitive competence." Moreover, one of us (JWB) has serious reservations (both theoretical and empirical) about the possibility of eventually finding cross-culturally a com-mon underlying factor such as general intelligence (Berry, 1972, 1981), pre-ferring the more flexible notion of "cognitive style" to conceptualize the variable patterns of performance to be found across groups. By contrast, Irvine (1980) has been critical of the "cognitive style" notion, wherein no proof of differential operationalization has been offered, preferring the more established term "intelligence." Thus, for this second reason as well, we shall speak generically about "cognitive competence."

A final conceptual issue is to clarify just how we distinguish among cog-nitive process, competence, and performance. In one sense, these three terms parallel the distinctions made by Hebb (1949) and Vernon (1969) among intelligences A, B, and C. Only performances are overt, hence mea-surable; they are the expressions of cognitive life in natural settings as well as during assessment (cf. intelligence C, the measured intelligence). Cog-nitive competence is the developed ability to carry out a performance (cf. intelligence B, the phenotype). It does not constantly erupt into performance and, when it does, is likely to be guided by situational (including cultural) constraints. Cognitive processes are those mechanisms that are biologically rooted (cf. intelligence A, the inherited substrate) but that need some experiential (cultural) input in order to develop into competence; these processes underlie all cognitive activity. Two points should be apparent from this brief statement. First, cognitive competences and processes can only be inferred from cognitive performances. Second, all three are linked to cultural variables in important ways: Processes develop into particular competences when directed and nurtured in culturally valued ways, and competences become performances at culturally appropriate times and in culturally appropriate ways.

Empirical evidence

Three kinds of studies are available as a means to provide evidence for the nature and distribution of cognitive activity across cultures; one involves collective phenomena, and two constitute individual phenomena (i.e., observed versus tested). At the collective level (culturally shared knowledge and beliefs), substantial evidence has been provided concerning the cultural life of a group of people. Although providing a valuable historical and ethnographic context for our enquiry into individual cognitive life, we agree with Jahoda (1982, p. 219) that "collective representations such as myths cannot serve as the basis for inferences[2] about the characteristics of cognitive processes." Moreover, although displaying some collective cognitive features (such as forms of logic used), it is also the case, as Jahoda (1982, p. 230) has pointed out, that most ethnographic reports have concentrated on social and affective life (*ethos*), while paying little attention to the cognitive domain (*eidos*). Thus, our interest in collective phenomena is largely contextual and will not be used to gain direct access to individual cognitive activity. At the individual level, the two domains of evidence are rooted in the respective traditions of observing individuals in natural settings and psychological testing in artificial settings.

Collective phenomena

Within this category of evidence there are many traditions. An important historical tradition is exemplified by early researchers such as Wundt (1916) and Levy-Bruhl (1910/1926); without fieldwork experience (in which direct observations had been carried out), secondary materials were employed to produce grand characterizations of peoples of different "types" or "levels." To a great extent, we owe to these investigators our earliest phrasings of the questions surrounding relationships between culture and cognition, but they also served to perpetuate ethnocentric ideas of the "prelogical," "concrete," and "childlike" character of cognitive life beyond the "civilized" borders of Europe. Even those with direct field experience, such as Rivers (1901) and Boas (1911), occasionally subscribed to the idea that cognitive life was of a lesser sort than among Europeans; in particular, Rivers (1901) espoused the view that the well-developed sensory abilities (which are concrete qualities) of savage peoples are likely to be an impediment to the development of higher cognitive (abstract) abilities. Our most appropriate lesson from these researchers might be to be wary of affective intrusions into our thinking about other people's cognitive life – the very error attributed by Levy-Bruhl to primitive mentality.

A second tradition is represented by the formal, structural analysis of myth, social structure, and other collective achievements. We have already noted in our brief look at the work of Levi-Strauss (1966) that common panhuman cognitive processes are usually discerned as underlying these collective products. The analyses of myth into component parts and the examination of "relations" among parts (particularly in terms of contradictions and oppositions) form the basis of this structuralist approach.

A third collective tradition is that of cognitive anthropology (e.g., Tyler, 1969), in which linguistic (and other) data are analyzed in an attempt to answer two questions: "What material phenomena are significant for the people of some culture?" and "How do they organize these phenomena?" (Tyler, 1969, p. 3). The goal is to ascertain the culture's own (local or *emic*) distinctions and classifications of natural phenomena in order to grasp their understanding. In the view of Frake (1962),

The analysis of a culture's terminological systems will not, of course, exhaustively reveal the cognitive world of its members, but it will certainly tap a central portion of it. Culturally significant cognitive features must be communicable between persons in one of the standard symbolic systems of the culture. A major share of these features will undoubtedly be codable in a society's most flexible and productive communication device, its language. (p. 75)

Many cultural domains have been studied in this way; in particular, kinship terms (e.g., Romney and D'Andrade, 1964) have been well attended to.

To illustrate this approach to studying cognitive phenomena, we take the domain of wisdom itself. The value-laden and affective context of traditional wisdom was a theme first explored empirically by Irvine (1969b, 1970), who used the oral traditions of the Shona of Zimbabwe as his data base. Some expansion and refinement of that analysis is offered now. The Shona words for wisdom (Hannan, 1974, p. 933) distinguish between *uchenjeri* and *ungwaru*. The first is practical, the second is either endowed or acquired wisdom. Tracing the root, *-chenjera* first reveals the idea of caution, in the sense of taking heed. It is transferrable to animals acquiring skills (e.g., *Imbwa yako yakachenjere kwazvo*: "your dog is very clever"). It survives in this context as well (e.g., *Mwana wenyu akachenjeresa*: "your child has no manners"). The central idea is of instrumentally learned action of a socially useful kind. Even dogs have their day, if children are to be seen and not heard. The second root, -*ngwara*, itself derives from -*ngwa*, which conveys the idea of pricking up one's ears, attending, being alert. A fundamental physiology is at work here. It has secondary meanings of intelligence, wisdom, and prudence, as Hannan points out, either endowed or achieved (e.g., *Munhu akangwara haafambi rwendo asina mbuva*: "a prudent person does not go on a journey without provisions"). This proverb warns that any enterprise has its foreseeable consequences, for which responsibility must be assumed.

Clearly, both roots come to earth in the construct of learning, although instrumental learning is perceived as qualitatively different from higher-order actions that are self-initiated. Nevertheless, it would take a deep understanding of context to distinguish their consistent usage. Rather than attempt detailed analysis at this stage, we prefer to use Irvine's structural theory (Irvine, 1979) to characterize the first root as having interhominem qualities. Practical intelligence is model induced and instrumental. The second is clearly intrahominem, being an attentional state, characteristic of man as an organism. What is learned from others presupposes a primary receptiveness within the brain itself.

None of this will be strange to students of societies for whom word of mouth is the dominant force. The distinction between dispositional intelligence (that is a legacy of processes limited by brain architecture) and the knowledge, strategies, and feelings that guide the dimensionality and direction of its products is a common-sense universal. The key to understanding intelligent action that is taught to new generations in oral societies, apart from skill acquired by modeling and repetition, exists in the proverbs and lore common to the community as a whole. The difficulty of analyzing oral tradition is lessened when collections of traditional proverbs emerge in the literature. Since Irvine's original analysis of an unpublished collection of 113 proverbs provided by Hannan, a comprehensive edition of 1,595 proverbs has appeared (Hamutyeni & Plangger, 1974). The range is great, but the editors classify 104 as dealing directly with wisdom and foolishness (*ungwaru-noudununu*). Using a computer, a content analysis of these proverbs was performed to discover the positive and negative poles of each, to judge whether the proverb was direct or oblique, and to find out by what form of analogy or imagery the message was conveyed. The technique is simple and was used by Du Preez (1972), who analyzed the proceedings of parliament to determine the positive and negative poles of the universe of discourse. Irvine constructed the data-base framework and analyzed each proverb. No reliability study was attempted, but the work proved simple to carry out after practice; we predict that the study could be replicated with accuracy by independent observers.

Although the detailed presentation of the data base awaits the availability of more space (Irvine & Berry, 1986), a summary of the findings leads to some precise conclusions. The proverbs can be conceptualized parsimoniously and a "dictionary" formed using three basic notions already outlined. The first is of *alertness*, pricking up one's ears. The next is the notion that experience is the firm data base. The third distinguishes kinds of experience – observations, inferences, explanations, and prescriptions – which constitute the stuff of learning to enable survival, the prime goal of a subsistence economy among agriculturalists. Two other central observations about the proverbs are necessary. Only one-quarter of those analyzed were direct, in the sense that their message was clear from simple translation. The remainder were oblique and allusive and required metaphoric interpretation. Second, the proverbs are always sharply empirical, reinforced by down-to-earth images. The positive poles of such images are normality, food, warmth, light, shelter, and old age. The negative poles are idiosyncrasy, hunger, cold and rain, darkness, exposure, and youth. Animals and objects are given dispositional qualities based on observation of their habits or functions.

This latest study seems to provide some confirmation of Irvine's earlier (1969b) essay in the analysis of proverbs that dealt almost exclusively with prohibitions and prescriptions. In retrospect, these focused on causation and only implicitly dealt with intelligence. The present work emphasizes the acute empiricism of Shona thinking and suggests that a highly sophisticated way of ensuring survival is enshrined in an oral learning system. Its essential obliqueness recognizes intelligence in the learner and presupposes a large body of common observations and experience. The 25% tally of direct statements may be a lower bound limit for the survival of the slow learner. The vast majority (75%) require higher-order comprehension on an overlearned and accessible knowledge base. Their understanding by an outsider is impossible if only a literal translation is available.

One is left with the impression of astuteness, knowledge, and a highly developed use of spoken language to convey ideas. Rhyme, for example, is frequently employed, presumably as a mnemonic. In the proverbs themselves, the distinction between power to process information (pricking up the ears) and the correct strategies for its purposive use is clear. The Shona are well aware of individual differences in capability – that is, *Kushaya mano kwendiro/kupakurirwa isingadyi*: "as for brains, a plate has none; it is given food but does not eat!" Opportunities are missed by those who are dispositionally incapable of recognizing and using them.

The key to understanding the limits of these notions, and above all the limits of their means of measurement, is forged in studies of traditional wisdom. Shona proverbs reveal all the qualities necessary for subsistence survival in tight communities. They commend alertness, observation, vigilance, and correct inference from environmental cues. Without books, radio, or television, accumulated life experience is the foundation of all knowledge.

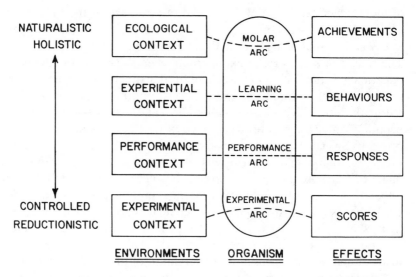

Figure 1. Multi-level arc model relating ecological contexts to cognitive performances.

Decision making requires carefulness and foresight on the one hand and opportunism on the other. Social realism dictates actions that are calculated to succeed. Toward that end, due attention must be given to the status of those affected by actions, including the spirits of the ancestors. Actions are also commendable if they enhance self-esteem based on status, honesty, humility, impartial use of authority, respect for elders, and self-criticism.

By contrast, the psychometric studies conducted on the Shona by Irvine during the past two decades exhibit a structure of intellect that can be accounted for parsimoniously by the constructs used by psychologists. Notions of intelligence; verbal, mechanical, and spatial ability; number skills; and information-processing skills do not do injustice to the Shona or indeed to any other cultural group. These constructs, and their persistence in spite of human and ecological variation, are the admittedly crude attempts of psychology to come to terms with psychic unity by measuring it.

To complete this discussion, we refer to an approach termed *ecological analysis*. Here the question is: What sorts of knowledge and abilities are needed in order to carry on life in this part of the world? Within the field of anthropology, the ecological approach has grown in recent years, so that it is now common to find explanations of cultural phenomena in terms of their interrelationships with natural phenomena within a particular ecosystem. Examples of this approach include the classic work of Forde (1934) and more recent analyses of Rappoport (1968).

Within the field of psychology, ecological analysis was stimulated by the observations by Ferguson (1956, p. 121) that "cultural factors prescribe what shall be learned and at what age; consequently different cultural environments lead to the development of different patterns of ability." Expanding this notion, one can seek and discover (in the terms of Berry, 1966), the "ecological demands" made on people living in a particular ecosystem, as well as the "cultural aids" available that permit the transmission and learning of particular abilities. This approach is also implicit in Bruner's (1966) notion of "cultural amplifiers" and in the subsequent work reported by Berland (1982, 1983) with them; that is, "every ecocultural system has a curriculum of basic experiences and attending skills provided through a variety of life-long socialization strategies" (Berland 1982, p. 50).

A model proposing four levels of ecological analyses has been developed by Berry (1980). Figure 1 illustrates four environmental (ecological and cultural) contexts and four effects related through a human organism. The structure of the diagram places the various contexts at the left and the various effects at the right. Toward the top are natural and holistic contexts and effects, while at the bottom are more controlled and reductionistic contexts and effects.

Let us examine the environmental contexts:

1. *Ecological context*: This is the "natural–cultural habitat" described by Brunswik. It consists of all the relatively permanent characteristics that provide the context for human action. Nested in this ecological context are two levels of the "life space" or "psychological world" of Lewin.
2. *Experiential context*: That pattern of recurrent experiences that provides a basis for learning, it is essentially a set of independent variables that cross-cultural psychology tries to spot as being operative in a particular habitat in the development of behavioral characteristics.
3. *Performance context:* This limited set of environmental circumstances may be observed to account for particular behaviors. These are immediate in space and time.
4. *Experimental context:* This context represents those environmental characteristics designed by the psychologist to elicit a particular response or test score. The experimental context may or may not be nested in the first three contexts; the degree to which it is nested represents the ecological validity of the task.

Paralleling these four contexts are four effects:

1. *Achievements:* This effect refers to the complex, long-standing, and developed behavior patterns that are in place as an adaptive response to the ecological context. It includes established and shared patterns of behavior that can be discovered in an individual or are distributed in a cultural group.
2. *Behaviors:* These are the molar behaviors learned over time in the recurrent experiential context. Included are the abilities and traits and attitudes that have been nurtured in particular roles or acquired by specific training or education, whether formal or informal.
3. *Responses:* These effects involve performances that appear in response to immediate stimulation or experience. In contrast to behaviors, they are not a function of role experience or long-term training but appear in fleeting reply to immediate experiences.

4. *Scores:* These effects comprise behaviors that are observed, measured, and
   recorded during psychological experiments or testing. If the experimental
   context is nested in the other contexts, the scores may be representative
   of the responses, behaviors, and achievements of the organism. If the experiment has ecological validity, the scores will have behavioral validity.

Relationships can be traced between the elements across the model:

1. *Molar arc:* The "E–O–E arc," in Brunswik's terms, operates across the
   top of the model. It is concerned with the life situation (in physical environmental and cultural terms) of an organism and its accomplishments.
2. *Learning arc:* This level is concerned with tying together recurrent independent variables in the experience of an individual with his characteristic
   behaviors.
3. *Performance arc:* This level involves more specific acts as a function of
   immediate and current experience.
4. *Experimental arc:* This element relates to the laboratory or other systematic
   study of relationships between experimental problems and test scores.
   These latter relationships are known to be variable, depending on the other
   contexts in the model (e.g., see Irvine, 1983).

A recurrent problem for general experimental psychology, in these terms,
is to say anything of value about causal relationships (at the two middle
levels) while working almost exclusively with the experimental arc. And to
this Brunswik would add the further problem of saying anything meaningful
on this basis about the molar arc as well. The problem facing cross-cultural
psychology tends to be the reverse. Rather than failing to ascend the
reductionistic–holistic dimension in order to achieve ecological validity,
cross-cultural psychology has failed to descend the dimension to achieve a
specification of experiential, performance, and experimental context variables
responsible for task performance and behavioral variation across natural hab-
itats. In Campbell's (1957) terms, insufficient concern has been shown in
these two branches of psychology for "external" and "internal" validity,
respectively.

Whether from anthropological or psychological sources, the essence of
this ecological approach (Berry 1975, 1980) is one that views cognitive (and
other psychological) functioning as being situated in an ecological and cultural context. The task is to specify the general life requirements for the
group as a whole and then to identify how they are communicated to the
developing individual. We have considered the ecological approach in this
(collective) section because work of this sort should be accomplished before
beginning individual assessment – basically making sure that we know how
the stage is set before the play begins.

Observed individual phenomena

This category of interest concerns what individual people actually do in daily
life and thereby exhibit their cognitive functioning for others to see. This

approach is shared by anthropological, ecological, and psychological field workers and, although it goes beyond descriptions of collective activity (which, as we noted, are often gained by working with secondary information), it does not always yield "scores" for cognitive performances that may be attached to individual performers.

This method of working demands that researchers live in the field with a group, observing, asking about, and seeking explanations for daily behavior. The domain of activity can vary from botanical and pharmaceutical knowledge (e.g., Motte, 1979), to hunting techniques (e.g., Bahuchet, 1978), to animal behavior (e.g., Blurton Jones & Konner, 1976), to map making (e.g., Bagrow, 1948), and to navigation techniques (e.g., Gladwin, 1970). The common denominator is an attempt to register the wealth of information and explanation about natural phenomena as well as the cognitive organization of it, which is clearly present among all peoples. Sometimes such work precedes individual assessment (i.e., sets the stage further for studies to be reported in the next section), but there is self-evident merit in this approach to studying everyday practical cognition. To illustrate this style of research, we have selected three reports that cover the areas of animal behavior, navigation techniques, and land tenure from among the many available studies.

During the previous century it was widely reported and believed that savages possessed an extraordinary relationship with nature, including a detailed knowledge of those aspects that were essential for their welfare; abilities, based on this knowledge, were also viewed as extremely well developed. It was these very beliefs that sent Rivers and his colleagues off to measure various sensory and perceptual functions in the Torres Straits Islands and Papua. As we have already noted, Rivers himself considered that such concrete activity might stifle more abstract development: "Minute distinctions of this sort are only possible if the attention is predominantly devoted to objects of sense, and I think there can be little doubt that such exclusive attention is a distinct hinderance to higher mental development" (Rivers, 1901, p. 44). Similarly, the metaphor of the *bricoleur* (in contrast to the scientist), created by Levi-Strauss, and the charge of "lower-level skills," purported by Vernon, both conform to the view that the savage has a certain cognitive life but one that is substandard when viewed from the norms of Western industrialized society.

We begin now to document the real extent of such practical knowledge in these populations. Peoples' knowledge of plants and animals, including similiarities, differences, uses, structure, habitat, and behavior, all have extensive documentation in the literature. For example, Motte (1979), working with the forest-dwelling Biaka Pygmy people in the Central African Republic, has documented more than 300 plant uses (leaves, stalks, and roots) in indigenous Biaka medicine; she has further discovered their conceptual organization, which reveals a highly structured and systematic set of relationships that is generally understood by the Biaka.

In their study of !Kung knowledge of animal behavior (which they subtitle "the proper study of mankind is animals"), Blurton Jones and Konner (1976) set out to discover how much is actually known by the Bushmen, how they came to know it, and how they explain it; a supplementary purpose was to check it all against the knowledge of Western science. Their technique was to hold seminars with groups of five or six !Kung men in a number of locations, each lasting two to three hours. Questions were posed, but discussion about animal behavior in general was less formal than an interview. This procedure was made difficult because "the !Kung appear to know a good deal more about many subjects than do the scientists" (p. 328), making probes and cross-questioning an essential means of getting at the information. These workers provided three sets of materials: one concerned with the "objectivity" of !Kung knowledge, another with its explanation, and a third with its purpose.

The !Kung appear to separate data carefully from theory (the original good scientist!) and to discriminate observed data from second-hand information. However, tracks and other traces are used as original data, and from these they are willing to deduce behavior. Blurton Jones and Konner (1976, p. 329) base these assertions on a number of points: (1) ignorance is readily admitted, with little evidence of guessing or filling in; (2) the !Kung dispute generalizations from minimal data; (3) they are often skeptical of each other's assertions; and (4) respondents are rarely defensive when pressed for more details. These workers concluded that the procedures of the !Kung "resemble the methods of modern-day Western ethology as regards (1) attention to detail, (2) distinguishing data from hearsay, and (3) displaying a general freedom from inference. In these respects their observations are superior to those of naturalists such as Gilbert White and Aristotle and very sophisticated indeed when compared with the legions of animal behaviorists among Western hunters, gamekeepers, and pet owners" (p. 333).

With respect to !Kung explanations of animal behavior, Blurton Jones and Konner (1976) gained the impression that they are "not particularly interested in explanations about behavior or theories about behavior" (p. 333) but noted that their questioning did focus on actual behavioral data, which may have influenced the nature of the responses. When the !Kung do make explanatory statements, they seem to be of an anthropomorphic kind, similar to those made by laymen elsewhere. Blurton Jones and Konner conclude that "although the !Kung have no clear idea about the evolution or survival value of behavior, they are not as far behind some of their post-Darwinian contemporaries in this field as one might have expected" (pp. 335–336).

Why such peoples study animal behavior is usually explained in terms of the survival value of this knowledge for hunter-gatherers; this appears to be of fundamental importance among the !Kung. Beyond this, Blurton Jones and Konner noted that "they sometimes observe animals more than is necessary for the purpose of the hunt in which they are involved" (pp. 337–338).

Finally, Blurton Jones and Konner (1976) offered a fourth line of evidence about the reasons for knowledge of behavior:

This is the immense amount of detail that they remember and, therefore, see when they are watching an animal. . . . The amount of detail observed and remembered and the evident delight in recounting these observations suggested to us that natural selection has arranged for a greater interest in animal behavior than that aroused by the practicalities of any specific hunt. This provides a system in which a large store of information is accumulated and communicated, and which may or may not turn out to be of use in hunting. . . . This indirect adult communication of important information seems comparable to the indirect way young men acquire information about animals and technology, which appears to be quite simply a matter of watching and listening to other people and then trying for one's self. There is almost no direct teaching. (p. 338).

Thus, although undoubtedly animal behavior is studied for survival reasons, there is also substantial evidence of what might be termed intellectual curiosity about natural phenomena beyond their immediate function. Whether this is true in domains other than animal behavior cannot be concluded on the basis of the Blurton Jones and Konner report. One can easily surmise, however, that it may also be true in other domains of fundamental importance to the !Kung, such as hydrology, botany, and meteorology.

Our second example, that of navigation, is also rooted in the historical observations about the abilities of nomadic peoples to range widely over large territories without disorientation or becoming lost. An adjunct to navigation, map making, has also been frequently reported on. For example,

[Galton (quoted in Werner, 1948)] remarks on the almost geographical memory of an Eskimo whose feats were directly observed by a Captain Hall. With no aid except his memory, this Eskimo drew a map of a territory whose shores he had but once explored in his kayak. The strip of country was 1100 miles long as the crow flies, but the coast line was at least six times this distance. A comparison of the Eskimo's rude map with an Admiralty chart printed in 1870 revealed a most unexpected agreement (p. 147).

Similar skill was noted by Carpenter (1955), who asked some present-day Inuit to "make sketches of the world as they conceived it," with results that proved astonishingly accurate. Moreover, Bagrow (1948) reported that the Inuit are capable of making depressions and elevations on their maps to represent the third dimension. The Inuit themselves consider the relief maps more valuable, as providing a more accurate representation. The area is rugged, intersected by fiords and glaciers, making relief maps helpful to the nomadic Inurt in surveying and identifying a given locality. Some of these maps have been estimated to cover areas as large as 250,000 square miles

(Irwin, 1981); anecdote has it that British Admiralty charts were occasionally corrected on the basis of information contained in them. Obviously, we are not dealing here with a rudimentary knowledge or ability, but with a highly developed conceptualization of space and a sophisticated representation of this knowledge.

Actual studies of navigation techniques have demonstrated a number of important features. One study (Gladwin, 1970) of navigation in Micronesia (that in its broadest sense includes map making and specialized sailing canoe design), reports on three phases to each inter-island voyage. The first phase is the development of the sailing plan and the setting of the initial course. This is accomplished by selecting an island destination (from the mass of information every navigator possesses about the archipelago), by noting such gross factors as weather, wind, and season, and then by employing back-sights (a line taken on established points on the island of departure that are known to indicate the direction to the island of destination) to start the canoe in the correct direction.

Second, during the bulk of the voyage, the navigator must maintain the course en route. This is done partly by dead reckoning, a process based on integrating knowledge about distance already traveled and the direction taken since the last known location. This information on direction and distance is obtained through the use of a Western-type compass, by stars (at night) and sun (by day), by wind and wave patterns, and by *etak*. This last concept is a system that conceptually divides the journey into sectors based on extensions of imaginary lines between a reference island (an island known to be to one side of the path of the journey and about halfway along it) and a series of star positions above the reference island. These reference islands cannot be seen, so their positions must be known before the journey. In addition to dead reckoning, certain signs may be encountered along the way. These include other islands and reefs of known position and shape. This information is often sought out, for example, by following the outline of a reef to ascertain its identity, as a check on the dead reckoning process.

Third, toward the end of the voyage, special techniques are employed for locating the island of destination. One of these involves the observation of birds that head for land at dusk, as well as any odors, sounds, and lee effects (used at night when islands cannot be easily seen). Throughout the last phase, however, there is a built-in island-locating mechanism in their style of tacking. This zig-zag pattern (needed to work one's way upwind) in fact constitutes a search pattern, as it is guided by the *etak* procedure.

These three phases, as described by Gladwin, are part of an overall system that can be represented by a cognitive map shared by the navigators. Knowledge of the system, and the recounting of voyages within the system, is readily recalled, indicating that it is not simply a rote-learned and concrete set of data. It is an abstract understanding, based on a view that the islands are moving. This view is valid, according to their experience of being in canoes for long periods and observing a constant relationship between themselves and an overhead sky. Within this framework, the islands are considered to be moving by or toward them.

Commenting on these activities, Gladwin (1970) moves from treating navigation only as a technology to viewing it as "a sample of purposeful thinking in another culture" (p. 214). He notes that there is likely to be a contrast between the high level of conceptualization and practical achievement of the island peoples and their performance on standard academic intelligence tests. He further argues that this contrast parallels that found among the poor and subjugated peoples in industrialized nations between their daily competence and their academic achievement. Thus, by treating this navigational achievement as intellectual activity, Gladwin hopes to call attention not only to the cognitive qualities of the savage, but also to those that are likely to be found among other populations who do things other than excelling at academic work.

For Gladwin,

Puluwat navigation is unquestionably intelligent behavior, but Puluwatans do not necessarily think of it this way. It is an obvious feat of intellect to travel far across the ocean and arrive at a tiny island through the use of nothing but one's mind and senses. We in the Western world value intelligence highly. For this reason we respect the Puluwat navigator. Puluwatans also respect their navigators, but not primarily because they are intelligent. They respect them because they can navigate, because they can guide a canoe safely from one island to another. There is, it is true, a Puluwat word one can translate as "intelligent," and in these terms navigators are considered intelligent, but etymologically it refers only to having a good memory. There are furthermore many useful ways to use one's mind in addition to remembering technical information. A Puluwatan who is asked to identify people who think well or use their minds effectively is likely to select those whose decisions are wise, who are moderate and statesmanlike in discussion, not the technicians. This does not mean that the statesman is more important than the navigator. On Puluwat nothing is more important that navigation. It means that, whereas *we* can recognize and respect navigation as a pre-eminently intelligent activity, this is not its significant quality for the Puluwatan. Because navigation is in our terms intelligent, it can provide useful perspectives on intelligence in our own culture. (Gladwin, 1970, p. 219)

Two qualities enable us to characterize their navigation as logical, rather than only technological, activity; "it is comprised of a system of explicit theory . . . and works with a limited array of predetermined alternatives of acceptable input and output" (Gladwin, 1970, p. 220). Furthermore,

Puluwat navigation (and canoe design) can be said to be cast in theoretical terms because it is explicitly taught and conceptualized as a set of principles governing relationships between phenomena. The phenomena are sometimes directly observed but at other times are only inferred, as in the case of star-compass bearings when the course star is not in position to be directly observed. These relationships and these inferences are unquestionably abstractions. Some, for example *etak*, are abstractions of a rather high order. The concept in *etak* of a specified but invisible island moving under often invisible navigation stars is not only an abstraction. It is also a purposefully devised logical construct by the use of which data inputs (rate and time) can be processed to yield a useful output, proportion of the journey completed. Abstract thinking is therefore a pervasive characteristic of Puluwat navigation. (Gladwin, 1970, p. 220)

However, concrete thinking is involved among the Puluwat as well:

Each observation a navigator makes of waves, stars, or birds is related directly without any logical reordering or interpretation to a conclusion about position, direction, or weather. Each such conclusion in turn permits of only one or at most two or three clearly defined alternative responses. Some of the observations are based on perceptions we (but not the Puluwatans) would consider extraordinarily acute, and some of the responses are complex, but once the initial observation has been made the steps which follow upon it are unequivocal. Is this concrete thinking? Few psychologists would argue otherwise. Not only is it concrete but direct pathways of this sort between observation and response comprise the principal operational mode of the entire navigation system. In other words, Puluwat navigation is a system which simultaneously employs fairly high orders of abstraction and yet is pervaded by concrete thinking. (Gladwin, 1970, p. 222)

What might be concluded from this detailed study? We are once again confronted with a cognitive enterprise that is based on a broad and specific knowledge, on which both logical and abstract operations are carried out, and from which practical action is taken. This latter is of two types, one leading to the development of various cultural artifacts such as maps, canoes, and sails, and the other to the actual successful completion of voyages. Clearly, these competencies represent major cognitive accomplishments that cannot be dismissed as "lower level."

A third domain to be examined is that of systems of land tenure, of which the work of Hutchins (1980) provides an example. In explaining why he worked on this topic, Hutchins indicated that "this whole endeavour rested on the conviction that a careful analysis of real-world skilled behaviour can yield scientific data about cognitive processes involved in the production of . . . behaviour" (1980, p. vii). And, like Gladwin (1970), Hutchins found a major discrepancy: "Like so many field-workers before me, I was impressed by the intelligence, resourcefulness, and wisdom of the people with whom I lived. Yet there was a striking discontinuity between the work I was doing and the life I was living. Whereas my daily interactions with people told me that they were quite capable of elaborate reasoning strategies, the battery of intelligence tests we administered showed the unschooled village adults to be performing at a level appropriate for an elementary school child in our society" (Hutchins, 1980, p. vii).

The study itself used naturalistic observation of relationships between people and the land they own and of the disputes (litigation in public courts) that arise between people in this land use. The specific focus of the analyses of these data was on the inferences displayed in arguments used during three cases of land litigation. Each court transcript is broken down into segments and episodes (all in the Trobriand language) and is then examined for examples of inferential reasoning. It is important to note that although based on linguistic analysis (as in some studies from cognitive anthropology), there are two important differences between cognitive anthropology and Hutchins's method: (1) these are actual utterances, the real-life behavior, of individual actors in a social interaction; and (2) the verbal evidence is set in a local land tenure context, which was studied ethnographically, as a supplement to studying the litigation.

In commenting on a fragment of one litigation case, Hutchins argued:

Understanding this brief fragment of discourse requires a total of twelve inferences. Six are weak plausible inferences and six are strong deductive inferences. All of the inferences are based on the simplified major premises of land tenure defined earlier in terms of causal and temporal relations among abstract classes of events. The act of either understanding or producing this bit of discourse requires (1) the ability to treat concrete instances as members of abstract event classes, (2) a comprehension of the nature of causal and temporal relations between abstract event classes, and (3) the ability to determine the truth values of hypothetical concepts in accordance with their logical relations to other concepts whose truth values have already been established. (Hutchins, 1980, p. 16)

And, more generally, he concluded:

The analysis of litigation has shown that a model of folk logic developed from purely western sources is quite adequate as an account of the spontaneous reasoning of Trobriand Islanders. . . . The clear difference between cultures with respect to reasoning is in the representation of the world which is thought about rather than in the processes employed in doing the thinking. It is clear that Trobrianders cut the world into a different set of categories from those we entertain, and that those categories are linked together in unfamiliar structures. But the same types of logical relations underlie the connections of propositions in our conceptions and theirs, and the inferences that are apparent in their reasoning appear to be the same as the inferences we make. (Hutchins, 1980, pp. 127–128)

Tested individual phenomena

More familiar to most psychologists will be evidence based on standard tests and interviews that lead to some sort of individually based score. One way to begin would be to find testing counterparts to each of the three practical areas surveyed in the last section; actual testing studies of these are rare, however. Instead, we will review studies that are in related areas and will turn to other studies that attempt to assess cognitive functioning related to daily behavior.

Knowledge of animal behavior and of navigation is prerequisite for successful hunting (and fishing), whereas navigation and botanical knowledge are of importance for successful gathering. Analyses of these activities (e.g., by Laughlin, 1968) point out that tracking, finding, and returning are essential abilities. Although such ecological analyses are compelling and, as we have seen, discussions with hunters reveal a sophisticated knowledge, the question remains, Can we actually tap these cognitive activities with psychological tests?

One study (Berry, 1966) made an assessment of the "ecological demands" on hunting peoples. These included the need for "the ability to isolate slight variation in visual stimulation from a relatively featureless array . . . and to organize these small details into a spatial awareness" (Berry, 1966, p. 212). Tasks of visual discrimination, visual disembedding, and visual spatial ability were selected and employed with samples of Canadian Inuit hunters and nonhunting African Temne, who were equated on degree of exposure to Western culture. Results indicated that, indeed, the Inuit were better equipped to carry out these tests than were the Temne and were generally no different in performing these tasks from a group of educated Scots. In this study then, psychological tests were able to "pick up" the ecologically functional ability patterns. More generally (Berry, 1971, 1976), this initial finding has been shown to be valid across a broader range of hunting and nonhunting samples in Australia, New Guinea, and northern Canada.

Extensions of this general strategy have been carried out by Annis (1980) and van de Koppel (1983) as part of an interdisciplinary study of human adaptation and development in Central Africa (see Berry et al., 1986). Employing a variety of discrimination and disembedding tests (in the visual and in the auditory and tactile sensory domains) with a group of hunter-gatherers (Biaka Pygmy) and agriculturalists (Bangandu villagers), a number of findings relevant to this issue were obtained. First, it became apparent that acculturation (in two senses) provided ecological and cultural experiences that were not part of the original Pygmy or village life-styles: In one form of acculturation, the villagers had partially entered into the hunter-gatherer life-style, giving them some of the knowledge and experience that could lead to the development of discrimination and disembedding skills; in the other form, European influences (particularly in terms of formal schooling) had penetrated the region but had done so differentially, such that the villagers had experienced more exposure than the Pygmy. Thus, a simple prediction of more developed abilities in the Pygmy group than in the village group had to be tempered by these two acculturative changes. When European acculturation was statistically controlled for (by covariance analysis), and when a nearby third cultural group was added (to represent an agricultural life-style without any hunter-gatherer experience), discrimination and disembedding abilities in visual and auditory domains (but not tactile) showed a tendency to vary across groups in the predicted way. Indeed, in one test (the portable rod and frame test, which involves visual and proprioceptive orientation ability), European acculturation had little effect and the obtained scores indicated substantial differences across the three groups, with the

Biaka Pygmy scoring rather dramatically toward the more accurate end of the scale.

Another study of a similar range of abilities was conducted by Kearins (1976) with desert dwelling Australian Aboriginal children. She argued that basic survival would require the development of visual acuity for finding game and plants and of visual memory for patterns for retaining such information. A group of Aboriginal children (who were attending rural schools) was tested, as was a group of children of European descent (who had little desert experience). On the visual discrimination task, Aboriginal children outperformed the European children, and this was attributed either to "a finer sensory acuity, or to differences in sensory mechanism" (Kearins, 1976, p. 211). Similarly, the Aboriginal children demonstrated clearly better performance on the visual memory task, a fact interpreted as support for the view that ecological engagement and experience can lead to differential ability development.

Taken together, these various testing studies of hunter-gatherer populations (across a wide regional spectrum from the Arctic to Central Africa to Central Australia) suggest that psychological testing is indeed able to "pick up" individual and group variations in practical abilities that are ecologically functional for them. They correspond to the observational and ethnographic material already available, and together these findings provide an empirical basis for the argument that abilities important in carrying on one's daily life may be the very stuff of cognitive life. Just because they appear to us as *bricolage* is not sufficient reason to set them aside (or even down) as lower-level abilities unworthy of being considered important cognitive competencies in their own right.

The work that comes closest to testing logic and inference (as a counterpart to Hutchins's 1980 analysis) is that of Cole and his colleagues (e.g., Cole et al., 1971; Scribner & Cole, 1981). These studies also adopt an ecological or contextual perspective; in a recent overview of this research project (LCHC, 1982), Cole and colleagues articulated "a formulation that retains the basic eco-cultural framework, but [that] rejects the central processor assumption as the organizing metaphor for culture's effect on cognition. Instead . . . we will assume that learning is *context-specific*, so that context-specific intellectual achievements are the *primary* basis for cognitive development" (LCHC, 1982, p. 674).

What contexts and what achievements have been attended to in this research? With respect to logical reasoning, we can take as an example the verbal logical problems posed in two sets of studies in Liberia, one with the Kpelle and the other with the Vai peoples. The first (see Cole & Scribner, 1974, pp. 160–168, for overview), presented verbal syllogisms of two types, one involving information relevant to everyday life, and the other type quite unfamiliar (cf. the report by Luria, 1971, on Soviet peasants). Most of the first type of syllogism were solved correctly; however, answers were usually supported by appealing to the facts of experience rather than by appealing to logical relations. In the words of Cole and Scribner (1974, p. 162), "There is clearly involved here a process of active reasoning – but one proceeding from evidence that is real and experiential, rather than from the theoretical evidence incorporated in the problem."

By contrast, those of the second type of syllogism were less frequently solved. These workers made the following general conclusion from their Kpelle work:

Among people in traditional societies is a refusal to remain within the boundaries of the problem presented by the experimenter. In the case of the more standard experimental material [syllogistic reasoning], the terms of the problem were often not accepted or were modified; additional information was supplied in order to bring the statements and their implications into closer conformity with the factual world of experience. In the folk-tale problem, subjects tended to reject the restricted set of possible solutions if the outcome violated some standard of social truth. We know, too, that when traditional people have some schooling [as in our studies in Liberia] or become involved in complex acts of social planning [Luria's data], verbal problems of this kind are accepted, and reasoning is constrained by the structure of the problem. Why this switchover occurs is a challenging problem for investigation. And equally challenging is the task of adapting traditional procedures so that they yield a detailed account of how, in fact, traditional people do reason when they are presented with hypothetical verbal problems. (Cole and Scribner, 1974, p. 168)

In their more recent work, on the effects of literacy among the Vai people, Scribner & Cole (1981) again presented verbal syllogisms, with correctness and reasons both scored as before. The major factor affecting the score was experience of schooling (which included English literacy); no effects were found for literacy without schooling (i.e., literacy in the Arabic or Vai scripts). This suggested that they might be dealing with a language understanding rather than a purely logical factor. To check this, Scribner and Cole presented a "fantasy" version of the syllogism (e.g., "All stones on the moon are blue/The man who went to the moon saw a stone/Was the stone he saw blue?"). For this version, both correct answers and explanations were relatively frequent. In general, Scribner & Cole (1981, p. 156) concluded that variability in solutions was largely attributable to variations in materials, procedures, and experimenters or, in other words, to variations in experimental contexts. Such differences as could be observed were externally induced; they did not support the hypothesis of a culturally determined shift in the internal representation of the stimulus. These studies (and others similar to them) clearly indicate that logical thinking is available to nonliterate and nonschooled people (as it obviously was among the Trobriand litigants in Hutchin's study) but that its use depends on context. Under day-to-day conditions of living, logical thinking is purposefully linked to the solution of practical problems (as it is for most folk in Western industrialized societies) but, when this link is not present, thinking can resemble the abstract forms that appear so important for us.

A variety of other practical abilities has been studied in the field. Perhaps the best known are the studies carried out by Bartlett (1932) on memory among Swazi cowherders in southern Africa. On the assumptions that records of cattle ownership and transactions are of great practical importance among herdsmen, and that among nonliterate peoples these records would of necessity be in memory, he sought details about cattle from herdsmen. In one case, a remarkable stream of information followed, on nine different animals, including type, color, markings, price, and with whom a trade had taken place. The obvious question is whether this differs in essence from any other complex store of information entailed in any other practical and important domain of activity; even after twenty-five years, one of us can still remember all the mold numbers of beer and wine bottles (for which he had production responsibility in a glass factory) and can today still recognize these on the table.

Another classic study, one that has led to a series of follow-up projects, is that conducted by Price-Williams (1962) in Nigeria. His interest lay in the claim by Levy-Bruhl (1910/1926) that concrete thinking was the typical (even sole) mode among preliterates, abstract thinking being unknown to them. By the time of Price-William's study, a number of field reports had claimed to provide support for this view, although in one study (Jahoda, 1956) an attempt was made to assess the degree of abstract thinking in a Ghanaian sample instead of viewing the issue as a dichotomy.

The task involved classification and sorting of objects familiar to Nigerian schoolchildren and nonschoolchildren, including toy animals (e.g., cocks, hens, horses, goats, rats) and local plant materials (e.g., guinea-corn, cassava, yams). The specific instruction was to put together in rows those objects that "belong together." Scores were assigned based on the number of alternative ways of classifying employed by each subject and on the reasons for them. Purely concrete sorting (based on sensory qualities, such as color, shape, or size) was assigned a 0, abstract sorting (e.g., edibility vs. inedibility) was scored 2, and intermediate responses were scored 1. The results indicated considerable evidence (up to 80%) of abstract sorts in both the schooled and unschooled samples. Price-Williams (1962) argued that these results probably reflect the use of familiar local materials that the children had had an opportunity to use in early life, as opposed to earlier assertions about the concrete thinking of savages based on the use of nonindigenous materials that could not provide an adequate opportunity for abstract thought to manifest itself during testing.

Taking this theme further, Price-Williams, Gordon, and Ramirez (1969) sought out a group that had a particular learning experience by virtue of its carrying out a specific economic role and compared this group to one that had had no experience in that role. Sons of potters in Mexico, matched for age, schooling, and social class with boys who had had no experience with pottery making, were tested on a series of Piagetian conservation tasks (number, quantity, weight, volume, and substance). The expectation that pottery experience would lead to earlier conservation on substance was borne out; there were no significant differences on the other tasks.

Similarly, Dasen (1975) predicted that children from hunter-gatherer groups (Australian Aborigine and Canadian Inuit) should show a different sequence of achievement on Piagetian concrete operational tasks from that shown by a farming group (Ivory Coast Africans). Children (ages 6 to 14) were presented with three spatial tasks (order, rotation, horizontality) and three conservation tasks (quantity, weight, and volume). The sequence of development within the stage (*horizontal décalage*) showed that spatial operations were achieved earlier in the two hunting-gathering samples compared with the agricultural sample, whereas the achievement of conservation was better in the agricultural sample (at the older ages only, however). Dasen interpreted this two-way difference as demonstration of the importance of ecological and cultural factors in Piagetian development and as support for the general ecocultural model proposed by Berry (1975). However, recent criticism of the reliability and generalizability of Piagetian type tasks given to small samples (Irvine, 1983; Dasen, 1984) may yet limit the claims that can be advanced for this type of research.

Although not in the Piagetian mode, the study by Cole, Gay, and Glick (1968) on Kpelle quantitative behavior makes a similar point. Arguing that in the Kpelle culture certain measurements are of importance (such as quantities of rice, sold at the market in bulk and measured by cups), these workers devised a rice-quantity estimation task. Four samples (Kpelle and American, adults and children) were asked to estimate how many cups were in bowls containing different amounts of rice. Relative error (ratio of estimated to actual number of cups) was greatest for the American adults and least for Kpelle adults, and children of both cultures had results close to the Kpelle adults. A possible interpretation of these data is that the functional significance of even small quantities of rice in Kpelle culture as well as the daily experience of making such transactions on the market equip the Kpelle with greater ability to perform the task accurately. (However, the accuracy of the American children cannot be accounted for on this basis.)

In this same vein, Serpell (1979) addressed the question of pattern reproduction in African children. As we have seen earlier in this chapter, there is evidence that spatial abilities may not be as well developed in agricultural societies as among hunter-gatherers. Serpell proposed that if the assessment were to be made using a daily play form, African children would excel over British children; conversely, using drawing as the medium of assessment, he proposed that British children would excel. The play technique used was the making of wire models, something commonly done to make toy cars and so forth by Zambian children. The task was to reproduce various geometric patterns (e.g., a square with diagonals), both by drawing and by wire modeling. As predicted, the Zambian children outscored the British in the wire-modeling condition, whereas the British outperformed the Zambian in the drawing condition. (It is interesting to note, in anticipation of a later discussion, that even with a limited number of subjects performing both tasks, the correlation between the tasks in the Zambian samples was above .8.) These results clearly show the importance of familiarity with the medium of performance in average level of performance and provide an important cautionary note for those who too easily claim poorer performance of groups assessed with standard tasks.

Finally, in this series, is a report by Childs and Greenfield (1980) of a research project involving Mexican weavers. The basic questions were: Does knowing how to weave a given pattern affect the weavers' mental representation or concept of that pattern?, and Can a specific skill like weaving promote a general ability to represent abstract linear patterns? (Childs and Greenfield, 1980, p. 269). This phrasing addresses the two aspects of the issue raised by Ferguson (1954, 1956): To what extent does practice in functionally important aspects of one's culture promote ability in those domains? and Can such practical ability transfer or generalize to a broader range of abilities?

The weaving of traditional striped patterns is a highly valued skill in Zinacantecan (Mayan) life; almost all clothing is made from this cloth, and girls (but not boys) are taught the necessary skills early in life. By puberty a girl is able to weave without adult supervision, and all Zinacantecan women attain proficiency, some becoming highly skilled. Learning (as in many traditional societies) is primarily by observing and doing, rather than by being told verbally.

The first experimental task involved placing wooden sticks of different colors into a frame to make representations of the two traditional Mayan cloth patterns, the test that is closest to what is already familiar to the subjects. A second less familiar test involved the representation of nontraditional patterns (varying in color and pattern). Samples included unschooled Zinacantecan female adolescents who were weavers, a similar group of boys who were not weavers, a group of schooled male nonweavers, and a small group of American female college students.

The results indicated that formal schooling does have an effect. Schooled boys (without weaving experience) represented the two traditional patterns more like the female weavers than like the unschooled boys. Analytical and abstract representations were made by more than half the female weavers and by all the American students but few of the unschooled boys. On the unfamiliar tasks, which assess the generalizability of the skill, there was little evidence "that knowing how to weave would in itself, promote a general skill in pattern representation" (Childs and Greenfield, 1980, p. 281). One possible reason offered by Childs and Greenfield is as follows:

The girls did not weave enough for their skills to become generalized; but the fact that the weavers actually performed more poorly on pattern continuations than the comparable non-weavers belies any interpretation based simply on the amount of weaving experience. The crucial factor may be that Zinacanteco culture develops general problem-solving skills more in males than in females, particularly the skills useful in carrying out economic transactions. Perhaps, then, concrete practical experience develops specific component cognitive skills . . . whereas other cultural influences, economic problem-solving for instance, develop generalized cognitive performance. . . . (1980, p. 282)

Another possible reason, they suggest, is that generalization of a cognitive skill may not occur when it would violate traditional practice, as in the case of making the representations of novel patterns. Furthermore, the very use of these research methods may be self-contradictory

if the goal is to assess the development of skills valued by a traditional non-industrial culture. We reasoned as follows. Any experiment or test, by its very nature, requires the use, in a novel situation, of skills acquired in some other situation. Hence an experiment requires cognitive innovation, often called generalization, a term which leaves the innovative aspect implicit rather than explicit. For Americans, and, to varying degrees, other Westerners, generalization is important because innovation has positive value: it allows us to adapt to constant change and to solve the ever-novel problems that come our way. But in a traditional society which both values and has stability, the reverse is true. Innovation and hence generalization, has a negative value; it constitutes a threat to tradition. Therefore, any experiment carried out in such a society requests people to use a cognitive skill – innovation – that is not valued and therefore not fostered by their own educational practices and processes (1980, p. 285).

As a general conclusion on the use of psychological tests, we may claim that test results have added important information to the debate over and above that available from the two other research strategies. In particular, it is apparent that when we attempt to assess practical abilities that may be nurtured in daily life, we need to consider the context, not only as an ecological setting or habitat for development, but also as a setting for the display of the ability in question. When we do, it becomes clear *what* is typically performed and what is not; more importantly, though, we gain some insight into the *why* of the performance. Clearly, it is not easy to claim incompetence on the basis of nonperformance; it is more likely that the ability is either not developed in our way (because it has no function) or it is not displayed (because we have not learned how to tap it with psychological tests).

Implications for cognitive theory

Given the wide-ranging display of practical abilities presented here, what are the implications for a more general theory of cognitive functioning? Three key issues need attention: context, generality, and universality. First, it is clear that no behavior (cognitive or otherwise) can be understood cross-culturally if it is not viewed in functional context (ecological setting) in which it naturally occurs; to view it otherwise is to risk ethnocentric (and hence erroneous) judgments. The second issue asks whether specific performances are linked together into patterns of cognitive activity (i.e., into more general abilities) and, if so, whether the "patterns of ability" (to use Ferguson's phrase) are constant or variable across cultural contexts. This latter question raises the third issue, that is, with such a parade of diverse daily behaviors, each understood in context, how can any general (even culturally universal) view of cognitive functioning ever be attained? These questions are appearing increasingly in the literature on cognitive functioning as cross-cultural ideas and findings begin to work their way into general psychology (e.g., Sternberg, 1984).

Context

A number of approaches to working with context have been made in cross-cultural psychology. As we have seen, Berry (1975, 1980) and colleagues have advocated an "ecological" approach to cross-cultural psychology, and Cole and colleagues have advocated a "situational" view of human behavior. With respect to cognition specifically, these workers expressed the view early on that "cultural differences in cognition reside more in the situations to which particular cognitive processes are applied than in the existence of a process in one cultural group and its absence in another" (Cole, Gay, Glick, & Sharp, 1971, p. 233). More recently (Scribner & Cole, 1981), they have demonstrated the context-specific nature of behavior as well as the importance of context in explaining variations in performance. The focus in this research project has been on accounting for specific abilities in relationship to context rather than on relationships among abilities. Most recently, Cole and colleagues (LCHC, 1982, p. 674) emphasized the value of an ecocultural framework; their primary interest remains in understanding the link between specific contexts and specific performances, while their secondary interest is in the "intercontextual generality" of behavior (i.e., relationships or links among performances).

Generality

For those of us who have roots in differential psychology, this second issue (that of how various performances may be related) has equal importance with the first. It is possible to consider them simultaneously, and Figure 2 attempts to illustrate schematically such a joint consideration. The diagram is based upon Figure 2 in Berry (1981) and Figure 11.3 in LCHC (1982). In essence, it depicts a set of ecocultural contexts on the left, a set of cog-

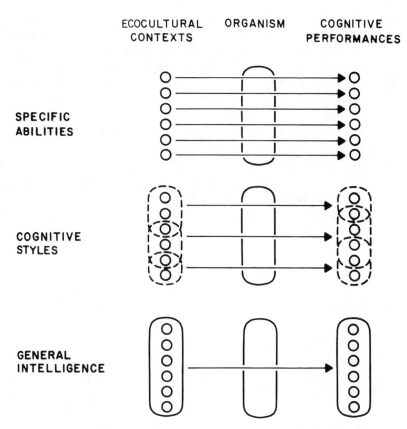

Figure 2. Three conceptions of cognitive abilities and their relationships with cultural contexts.

nitive performances on the right, and a "black box" organism in the middle. Linkages from context to performance are drawn as horizontal arrows, whereas patterns (if present) are drawn as vertical ovals. The diagram depicts three different levels of generality: specific abilities (with no test–test linkages or patterns illustrated) at the top, general intelligence (with a single a priori and invariant pattern) at the bottom, and cognitive styles (with limited and perhaps variable patterns) in the middle.

With the help of this diagram, a number of ideas can be elaborated. First, the idea is suggested that specific contexts (small circles on the left) themselves can be patterned; indeed, cultures are frequently defined as integrated sets of experiences that are shared by the group and are not just a series of unrelated inputs.

Second, relationships among tests (small circles on the right) can be discovered, varying from none (in the specific abilities approach, in which they are not usually sought) to a complete single preconceived general ability (in the general intelligence approach), through an intermediate conceptualization, in which variable patterns (cognitive styles) are sought and discovered.

Third, the organism is conceptualized variably, ranging from a set of discrete cognitive operators (in the specific abilities approach) to a single central processor (in the general intelligence approach), through a partially integrated model, in which different styles may depend on varying cognitive operations.

Fourth, the linkages across the model (the horizontal arrows) attempt to illustrate what for some is the major issue: causal linkages between context and performance. In the least general view (specific abilities approach), a set of discrete 1:1 causal relations is sought, whereas in the most general (general intelligence approach), a single cultural package (sometimes ethnocentrically conceived of as ranging from "enriched" through to "disadvantaged") is considered a causal factor in general intelligence (which is conceived of in terms of a dimension of "smart" to "stupid"). In the intermediate position, the diagram illustrates a set of causal links such that a certain range of interrelated ecocultural experiences affects a limited range of interrelated test performances; independently of these ranges, other styles may or may not exist along with them.

The purpose of presenting this diagram is threefold. At the most basic level, it presents a schematic overview of what currently appear to be the three main competing conceptualizations of culture–cognition relationships. It also serves to illustrate the point that context and generality issues can be conceived of as interrelated. And third, it points up the need to consider the patterning of elements in ecocultural contexts and not to treat the issue of generality solely in terms of intertest relationships.

The question naturally arises, Can we actually place the varied empirical observations reviewed in this chapter into such a set of alternative views of the culture–cognition relationship? In our view, this is not only possible but would be useful. The work of Cole and colleagues (including Berland and Serpell) clearly represents the specific abilities approach. The central question is one of effects of specific contextual factors on a cognitive performance, although there is a recent indication of some interest in "intercontextual generality" (LCHC, 1982). Also, Serpell (1979) has produced correlations among some of his performance measures. The cognitive-style approach is illustrated by the work of Berry (1976), Annis (1980), and van de Koppel (1983), who have searched for test–test and context–context relationships, as well as establishing context–performance links in a particular domain (that of the field-dependent–independent cognitive style). And the general intelligence model fits the work of Vernon (1969) and Irvine (1979); factor analyses have usually generated single cognitive factors, which are interpreted as general ability or intelligence. In the former case, a single packaged cultural input seems to be postulated, whereas Irvine (1983) has sought details of more specific contextual experiences to account for variations in general ability.

The choice among these models may be easier than appears, as there are signs of convergence. Some intercontextual generality is now being sought by those whose primary interests are in specific abilities, whereas some specific contextual influences are being isolated by researchers within the general intelligence tradition. This is not to say that the convergence is all toward the cognitive style view (and certainly not toward one particular cognitive style), but it is to suggest that what may eventually emerge is a cognitive parallel to the adage, "In some respects every person is like all other persons, like some other persons, and like no other person." In our view, it is not unlikely that there may be some unique (culture-specific), some partially shared, and some very general aspects to cognitive functioning cross-culturally. Such a view would parallel the hierarchical factor model proposed by Vernon (1969), without the a priori and culture-bound (ethnocentric) features it now appears to incorporate.

Universality

The issue here is how we might eventually discover cognitive universals. This chapter has surveyed the practical abilities of a variety of peoples and has argued that these are the very stuff of cognitive life, not to be ignored, but to be taken seriously as indicators of what people are capable of doing cognitively. Or, to return to the title of the chapter, *bricolage is basic* and *savages are everywhere*. If such fundamental activity is ignored, how could a picture of what people can do ever be constructed? To reverse the question, if only those performances that are related to Western academic or scientific cognitive activity are included, how could we avoid discovering only what people cannot do?

In addition to *bricolage*, there is another basic source of information – the conceptions of cognitive competence held by various cultural groups. A recent review (Berry, 1984) showed that such conceptions vary widely across cultures and do not usually resemble the "quick-analytic-abstract" complex that characterizes the Western idea of an intelligent person. Clearly, the kinds of behavior we include in any attempt at a universal framework for describing cognitive functioning should include cognitive behaviors that match indigenous conceptions of cognitive competence.

A third source of materials might be based on the concept of *adaptability* (Biesheuvel, 1972); here, the argument is that the ability to handle novel problems, and not just familiar daily problems, would be a useful index of cognitive competence. Acculturation and other forms of social change are

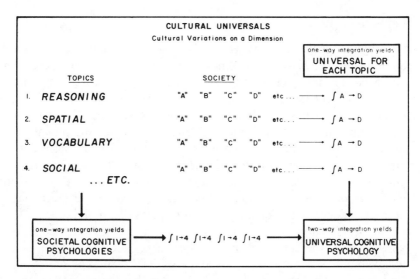

Figure 3. Framework for pursuing a universal psychology of cognitive competence.

ubiquitous. Thus it would not be inappropriate to include in the framework cognitive tasks that lie outside a group's *bricolage* or conceptions of competence, provided they are done reciprocally (e.g., tasks assessing tracking skills for a university professor).

Such a framework has been proposed (Berry, 1984), as illustrated in Figure 3. Down the left are listed areas of cognitive functioning suggested by an ecocultural analysis of *bricolage*, by indigenous conceptions, and by including some novel cognitive activities. Across the top is a broad range of cultures selected to represent the range of human societies and in which one might carry out cognitive research. Integrating information down a column (across topics within a society), we develop a local *societal psychology*. Integrating information across a row (over societies within a topic), we develop a *universal* for that particular cognitive function. And integrating both, in principle, will eventually achieve a *universal cognitive psychology*.

We have perhaps achieved a societal psychology in a few (mainly Western) cultures, and we may have achieved some degree of comprehensive knowledge about a few areas of cognitive functioning across a range of cultures (a universal for that cognitive function), but we are clearly not about to achieve a fully universal cognitive psychology. This will be particularly true if we persist in ignoring both the *bricolage* and the indigenous conceptions, remaining fixated on tests based on our *bricolage* to assess their cognitive functioning.

Implications for cognitive assessment

Although ostensive definitions are the starting point for construct validity, the existence of *bricolage* or know-how merely points to where it may be observed. The intuitive certainty of a construct such as *bricolage*, and indeed our everyday observations of it in action, does not provide evidence for its precise relationship to other forms of intellectual activity. The scientific struggle lies in the identification of *bricolage* outside the realms of the anthropological anecdote, affirmative or veto. One part of that is, as the empirical evidence demonstrates, the specific issue of how measures of practical know-how, adapted to the cultural setting, relate to other conventional measures of achievement and ability. The question of structure may be addressed independently of the question of ostensive definition.

The use of information in an overarching theory of knowledge, or world view, defines the construct of *bricolage* in yet another fashion, neither ostensively nor structurally but, in Miles's (1957) taxonomy of definitions, as "a key to understanding." We would assert that the keys to understanding *bricolage* may be found in its epistemological and social contexts. Empirical studies (Irvine, 1970) have determined that the use of practical know-how is not sanction free. A social levy is exacted for its application, in Harare as much as in Detroit.

Given the problem of two quite distinct kinds of definition, it is sensible to address it in two parts, one dealing with traditional modes, the other with structure. Oblique, if not covert, attempts by outsiders to assess practical know-how in industrial societies can be witnessed in the so-called mechanical information and aptitude tests constructed by occupational psychologists. Test results can provide structural definitions, but only if used correctly. Here, the use of tests of mechanical information with African subjects is the data base. Some of these tests have survived metamorphosis in exotic contexts, as the pioneering work of Schwarz (1964) demonstrates. The adaptation and construction of mechanical information, or rather, simple cause-and-effect tasks and items of a pictorial kind, was a goal set by Schwarz and his team in Nigeria. Like so many of us in the field at that time, Schwarz learned that these tests could not survive transposition to another culture without radical changes in the kinds of items used. As Irvine (1983) has observed, the preservation of stimulus identity ensures neither valid nor reliable measures of a construct across cultures. The context of knowing how is an intervening variable. To remove the intervening variable, all items had to be made relevant to the local environment, and pictorial items had accurately to represent it. Another intervening variable, more troublesome to testers, is the verbal comprehension of the pictorial item itself. Unable to eradicate it completely, Schwarz introduced oral instructions in a group context, because reading skills among his subjects were much less secure and much more variable than were listening skills. The subjects listened to a story about each item represented to them on the printed sheet and then chose the picture that showed the correct cause.

The tests devised by Schwarz were made available to Irvine and his co-workers (MacArthur, Irvine, & Brimble, 1964; Irvine, 1966, 1969a, 1969b, 1981, 1983). Consequently, they received construct validation of a structural nature in Central Africa. The results of this empiricism are available in the published sources; three other studies have been carried out since then that allow comparison. They address only the question of the relationship of knowledge of cause and effect in the intermediate environment to other cognitive capacities. Is this know-how, or *bricolage*, a separate frame of mind? Certainly, Gardner (1983) would have us believe so, but Irvine (1984) asserts that the question of "apartheid" in mental functions cannot be re-solved on the restricted and highly tendentious evidence assembled by Gardner.

Since 1962, the Schwarz tests of cause and effect, involving practical knowledge of the immediate environment in Africa, have been used in seven different studies that accepted correlational analysis as a method of construct validation. The studies have the historical advantage, and accident, of dif-ferential education levels independent of age. Consequently, the construct of practical intelligence can be observed under different treatments, where the quasiindependent variable between groups is the number of years of schooling completed. Moreover, dispositional and environmental correlates of test performance were recorded. Of particular interest are studies in which gender-based differences may be apparent.

Table 1 summarizes the data base for the stated conclusions. Essentially, the correlational studies that involve tests of cause-and-effect relationships in the environment are consistent. Each study shows that tests of *bricolage* involve both general intelligence and the use of more specialized skills. The acquisition of one set of problem-solving skills is likely to transfer to the other set, because the test factors are not independent of each other. Lest objections be raised about the essentially bookish context of the tasks in use, the semiliterate groups provided clear evidence of families of tests that were not dependent on literacy for their execution. In that respect, they confirm the thesis proposed by Scribner and Cole (1981), who claim no special status for literacy in the execution of intelligent actions. Such tests included the Schwarz measures of understanding cause and effect. In the worker groups, vernacular instructions and translations were standard.

Irvine (1983) points out that the correlation of test scores (which are gross products of mental process) with environmental and dispositional variables calls for caution in inference about the nature of intelligence. Often, though, scores can yield some evidence about the distinctiveness of tests from each other, using the logic that like measures will correlate in like fashion with

Table 1. *Psychometric test factors among East and Central African groups.*

Country	Year	Number of subjects	Sex	Years of education	Tests	Factors	Correlated factors or not
Zimbabwe	1975	97	M	3–6	15	v:ed2/MSpan/ps.	Y
Zimbabwe	1975	74	M	3–6	025	v:ed2/g/mech.	Y
Zambia	1964	72	M	6–8	11	g/v:ed2/n/p.	Y
Zambia	1964	442	M + F	10	22	g/v2/n/m.k*/v:ed2*	Y
Kenya	1963	185	M	12	14	g/v2/n/p.	Y
Zimbabwe	1966	339	M + F	12	10	v2*/p**/v:ed2*	Y

Factor labels are as follows: v:ed2: second language verbal/educational aptitude; MSpan: memory span; p(s): perceptual (speed); g: general intelligence; mech.: mechanical information; n: numerical; m.k: mechanical-spatial; v2: second language vocabulary.
Male high:*
Female high:**

the same set of nontest variables. In work with elite groups of Shona subjects, involving males and females, nontest variables differentiate the tests only when the gender of the subject is employed as a correlate. The tests themselves distinguish two latent variables. One is concerned with encoding speeds for symbols, characterized by superior female performance. This result is now becoming a familiar cross-cultural phenomenon (MacArthur, Irvine, & Brimble, 1964; Irvine, 1969, 1983; Irvine & Reuning, 1981; Bali, Drenth, van der Flier, & Young, 1984; Drenth, van der Flier, & Omari, 1983). As the result is a standard one in Euro-American research that has been given theoretical impetus by Estes (1971), one characteristic of intelligent behavior survives the crudities of cross-cultural use of tests. Here gender is the critical marker variable. We are not unaware of the theoretical significance of this finding, as it provides a process-anchored basis for investigating performance differences.

The other dimension, which includes the figural test of concealed shapes, tests of cause and effect, science and world knowledge, is parsimoniously interpreted as general educational aptitude, as performance is second-language mediated. Performance in that area favors males when knowledge is required, suggesting wider second-language vocabularies more speedily accessed. None of the family-background variables successfully differentiates either school, practical, or perceptually based measures of the markers for intelligence. The Tanzanian study by Drenth comes to the same conclusion, but in neighboring Kenya the environmental correlates far more resemble European results than they do those of Tanzania, Zambia, or Zimbabwe.

Although the research from all of East and Central Africa favors more than one product of intelligent action, it would be a mistake to consider them structurally independent. Indeed, this work confirms Irvine's (1979) conclusions in his essay on structural approaches to cross-cultural cognition. Despite evidence of the distinctiveness of groups of skills and abilities, these are always parsimoniously accounted for within the concept of generalized and transferrable intelligence. One suspects that successful *bricoleurs* learn other skills quickly. Empirical studies of the use of Aboriginal knowledge involving cause and effect are scarce. As Western systems of causality take root, indigenous systems either wither or, if one will allow the expression, go underground. Good studies of the coexistence of indigenous and Western systems of causality are even scarcer. The best is Jahoda's (1970) work on Ghanaian University students revealing a strong belief in witchcraft, side by side with Western ideas of cause and effect. Valuable as that is, it does not help us directly to understand the reasons for using one system over another; nor does it illuminate the role of thinking in traditional modes in the development of what Western psychologists understand to be intelligent action. That may be the central issue.

We would contend that careful studies of structure reveal *bricolage* as one valid but not necessarily uncorrelated and separate manifestation of human intelligence, that structural constructs used to define this intelligence are consistent in their meaning in all cultures, that these consistencies are process determined, and that the products of these processes are ecologically induced and language mediated. Product-oriented empiricism lacking the means to relate product to process is found in the uncritical use of group tests or individual tasks of intelligence. Savages are indeed everywhere, whenever we become psychological *bricoleurs* by chance or by design. Psychological *bricolage* cannot persist as a means to structural clarity and offers no hope of further scientific advance.

Notes

1 This concern with day-to-day cognitive functioning may be viewed as parallel to the growing interest in "social cognition" (e.g., see Forgas, 1981).
2 Jahoda (1982, pp. 224–236) goes to great pains to point out the inappropriate conclusions that are drawn when such inferences are attempted, as in the case of Hallpike (1979).

References

Annis, R. C. (1980). *Bantu and Pygmy perceptual patterns: An eco-cultural study*. Unpublished doctoral dissertation, University of Strathclyde, Glasgow.
Bagrow, L. (1948). Eskimo maps. *Imago Mundi, 5*, 92–93.
Bahuchet, S. (1978). Contraintes ecologiques en forêt tropicale humide: l'exemple des Pygmées Aka de la Lobaye. *Journal d'Agriculture Tropicale et Botanique Appliquée, 25*, 257–285.

Bali, S. K., Drenth, P. J. D., van der Flier, H., & Young, W. C. E. (1984). *Contribution of aptitude tests to the prediction of school performance in Kenya: A longitudinal study*, Lisse, Netherlands: Swets and Zeitlinger.

Bartlett, F. C. (1932). *Remembering: A study in experimental and social psychology.* Cambridge: Cambridge University Press.

Berland, J. (1982). *No five fingers are alike: Cognitive amplifiers in social context.* Cambridge: Harvard University Press.

Berland, J. (1983). Dress rehearsals for psychological performance. In S. H. Irvine & J. W. Berry (Eds.), *Human assessment and cultural factors* (pp. 139–154). New York: Plenum.

Berry, J. W. (1966). Temne and Eskimo perceptual skills. *International Journal of Psychology, 1,* 207–229.

Berry, J. W. (1971). Ecological and cultural factors in spatial perceptual development. *Canadian Journal of Behavioural Science, 3,* 324–326.

Berry, J. W. (1972). Radical cultural relativism and the concept of intelligence. In L. J. Cronbach & P. Drenth (Eds.) *Mental tests and cultural adaptation* (pp. 77–78). Mouton: The Hague.

Berry, J. W. (1975). An ecological approach to cross-cultural psychology. *Nederlands Tijdschrift voor de Psychologie, 30,* 51–84.

Berry, J. W. (1976). *Human ecology and cognitive style: Comparative studies in cultural and psychological adaptation.* New York: Sage/Halsted.

Berry, J. W. (1980). Ecological analyses for cross-cultural psychology. In N. Warren (Ed.), *Studies in cross-cultural psychology,* (Vol. 2, pp. 157–189). London: Academic.

Berry, J. W. (1981). Cultural systems and cognitive styles. In M. P. Friedman, J. P. Das, & N. O'Connor (Eds.), *Intelligence and learning* (pp. 395–405). New York: Plenum.

Berry, J. W. (1984). Towards a universal psychology of cognitive competence. *International Journal of Psychology, 19,* 335–361.

Berry, J. W., van de Koppel, J., Sénéchal, C., Annis, R., Bahuchet, S., Cavalli-Sforza, L. L., & Witkin, H. A. (1986). *On the edge of the forest: Cultural adaptation and cognitive development in Central Africa.* Lisse: Swets and Zeitlinger.

Biesheuvel, S. (1972). Adaptability: its measurement and determinants. In Cronbach, L. J. & Drenth, P. J. D. (Eds.), *Mental tests and cultural adaptation* (pp. 47–62). The Hague: Mouton.

Berlin, B., Breedlove, D., & Raven, P. (1966). Folk taxonomies and biological classification. *Science 154,* 273–275.

Blurton Jones, N., & Konner, M. (1976). !Kung knowledge of animal behavior. In Lee, R. B., & DeVore, I. (Eds.), *Kalahari hunter-gatherers* (pp. 326–348). Cambridge: Harvard University Press.

Boas, F. (1911). *The mind of primitive man.* New York: Macmillan.

Bruner, J. S. (1966). On cognitive growth. In Bruner, J. S., Olver, R., & Greenfield, P. M. (Eds.), *Studies in cognitive growth* (pp. 1–67). New York: Wiley.

Carpenter, E. S. (1955). Space concepts of the Aivilik Eskimo. *Explorations, 5,* 131–145.

Childs, C., & Greenfield, P. M. (1980). Informal modes of learning and teaching: the case of Zinacanteco weaving. In N. Warren (Ed.), *Studies in cross-cultural psychology* (Vol. 2, pp. 269–316). London: Academic.

Cole, M., Gay, J., & Glick, J. (1968). Some experimental studies of Kpelle quantitative behavior. *Psychonomic Monograph Supplements, 2,* no. 10, (Whole no. 26).

Cole, M., Gay, J., Glick, J., & Sharp, D. (1971). *The cultural context of learning and thinking.* New York: Basic.

Cole, M. and Scribner, S. (1974). *Culture and thought.* New York: Wiley.

Cooper, D. E. (1975). Alternate logic in "primitive" thought. *Man, 10,* 238–256.

Dasen, P. R. (1975). Concrete operational development in three cultures. *Journal of Cross-Cultural Psychology, 6,* 156–172.

Dasen, P. R. (1984). The cross-cultural study of intelligence: Piaget and the Baoulé. *International Journal of Psychology, 19,* 107–134.

Drenth, P. J. D., van der Flier, H., & Omari, I. M. (1983). Educational selection in Tanzania, *Evaluation in Education, 7*, 93–217.

du Preez, P. (1972). The construction of alternatives in political debate: Psychological theory and political analysis, *South African Journal of Psychology, 2*, 23–40.

Estes, W. K. (1974). Learning theory and intelligence, *American Psychologist, 29*, 740–749.

Ferguson, G. A. (1954). On learning and human ability. *Canadian Journal of Psychology, 8*, 95–112.

Ferguson, G. A. (1956). On transfer and the abilities of man. *Canadian Journal of Psychology, 10*, 121–131.

Forde, D. (1934). *Habitat, economy and society*. London: Methuen.

Forgas, J. (Ed.) (1981). *Social cognition: Perspectives on everyday understanding*. London: Academic.

Frake, C. O. (1962). The ethnographic study of cognitive systems. *Anthropology and Human Behavior*. Washington, DC: Anthropological Society of Washington.

Gardner, H. (1973). *The quest for mind*. New York: Knopf.

Gardner, H. (1984). *Frames of mind*. London: Heinemann.

Gladwin, T. (1970). *East is a big bird: Navigation and logic on Puluwat atoll*. Cambridge, MA: Harvard University Press.

Hallpike, C. R. (1979). *The foundations of primitive thought*. Oxford: Oxford University Press.

Hamutyeni, M. A., & Plangger, A. B. (1974). *Tsumo-shumo: Shona proverbial lore and wisdom*. Gwelo, Zimbabwe: Mambo.

Hannan, M. (1974). *Standard Shona dictionary* (2nd ed.), Harare, Zimbabwe, Zimbabwe (formerly Rhodesia) Literature Bureau.

Hebb, D. O. (1949). *The organization of behavior*. New York: Wiley.

Hutchins, E. (1980). *Culture and inference: A Trobriand case study*. Cambridge, MA: Harvard University Press.

Irvine, S. H. (1966). Towards a rationale for testing attainments and abilities in Africa. *British Journal of Educational Psychology, 36*, 24–32.

Irvine, S. H. (1969a). Factor analysis of African abilities and attainments. *Psychological Bulletin, 71*, 20–32.

Irvine, S. H. (1969b). Contributions of ability and attainment testing in Africa to a general theory of intellect. *Journal of Biosocial Science, 1*, 91–102.

Irvine, S. H. (1970). Affect and construct: A cross-cultural check on theories of ability. *Journal of Social Psychology, 80*, 91–102.

Irvine, S. H. (1979). The place of factor analysis in cross-cultural methodology and its contribution to cognitive theory. In L. Eckensberger, Y. Poortinga & W. Lonner (Eds.), *Cross-cultural contributions to psychology* (pp. 300–341). Amsterdam: Swets and Zeitlinger.

Irvine, S. H. (1981). Culture, cognitive tests and cognitive models: Pursuing cognitive universals by testing across cultures. In M. Friedman, J. P. Das, and N. O'Connor (Eds.), *Intelligence and learning* (pp. 407–426). New York: Plenum.

Irvine, S. H. (1983). Testing in Africa and America: the search for routes. In S. H. Irvine and J. W. Berry (Eds.), *Human assessment and cultural factors* (pp. 45–58). New York: Plenum.

Irvine, S. H. (1983). Cross-cultural conservation studies at the asymtote: striking out against the curve? In S. Modgil (Ed.), *Jean Piaget: An interdiscriplinary critique* (pp. 42–57). London: Routledge & Kegan Paul.

Irvine, S. H. (1984). In pursuit of diversity. *New Scientist, 103*, 36.

Irvine, S. H., & Berry, J. W. (1986). *Human abilities in cultural context*. London: Wiley.

Irvine, S. H., & Carroll, W. K. (1980). Testing and assessment across cultures: Issues in methodology and theory. In H. C. Triandis and J. W. Berry (Eds.), *Handbook of cross-cultural psychology: Vol. 2. Methodology* (pp. 181–244). Boston: Allyn and Bacon.

Irvine, S. H., & Reuning, H. (1981). "Perceptual speed" and cognitive controls. *Journal of Cross-Cultural Psychology, 12*, 425–444.

Irwin, C. (1981). *Inuit navigation*. Unpublished paper. Syracuse, NY: Syracuse University.

Jahoda, G. (1956). Assessment of abstract behaviour in a non-western culture. *Journal of Abnormal and Social Psychology, 53*, 237–243.

Jahoda, G. (1970). Supernatural beliefs and changing cognitive structures among Ghanaian university students. *Journal of Cross-Cultural Psychology, 1*, 115–130.

Jahoda, G. (1982). *Psychology and anthropology: A psychological perspective*. London: Academic Press.

Kearins, J. (1976). Skills of desert Aboriginal children. In G. E. Kearney & D. W. McElwain (Eds.), *Aboriginal cognition: Retrospect and prospect* (pp. 199–212). Canberra: Australian Institute of Aboriginal Studies.

Laboratory of Comparative Human Cognition. (1982). Culture and intelligence. In R. Sternberg (Ed.), *Handbook of human intelligence* (pp. 642–719). New York: Cambridge University Press.

Laughlin, W. S. (1968). Hunting: An integrating biobehavior system and its evolutionary importance. In R. B. Lee & I. DeVore (Eds.), *Man the hunter* (pp. 304–320). Chicago, Aldine.

Levi-Strauss, C. (1962/1966). *The savage mind*. London: Weidenfeld & Nicholson.

Levy-Bruhl, L. (1910/1926). *How natives think*. London: Allen & Unwin.

Luria, A. R. (1971). Towards the problem of the historical nature of psychological processes. *International Journal of Psychology, 6*, 259–272.

MacArthur, R. S., Irvine, S. H., & Brimble, A. R. (1964). *The Northern Rhodesia mental ability survey*. Lusaka, Zambia: Rhodes-Livingstone Institute.

Miles, R. T. (1957). Contributions to intelligence testing and the theory of intelligence. 1. On defining intelligence, *British Journal of Educational Psychology, 27*, 153–165.

Motte, E. (1979). Thérapeutique chez les Pygmées Aka de Mongoumba. In Bahuchet, S. (Ed.), *Pygmées de Centrafrique* (pp. 77–108). Paris: Société d'Études Linguistiques et Anthropologiques de France.

Piaget, J. (1951). *Play, dreams and imitation in childhood*. New York: Norton.

Price-Williams, D. (1962). Abstract and concrete modes of classification in Nigeria. *British Journal of Educational Psychology, 32*, 50–61.

Price-Williams, D., Gordon, W., & Ramirez, W. (1969). Skill and conservation: a study of pottery-making children. *Developmental Psychology, 1*, 769.

Rappoport, R. (1968). *Pigs for the ancestors: ritual in the ecology of a New Guinea people*. New Haven: Yale University Press.

Rivers, W. H. K. (1901). Introduction and vision. In Haddon, A. C. (Ed.), *Report of the Cambridge Anthropological Expedition to the Torres Straits* (pp. 1–140). Cambridge: Cambridge University Press.

Romney, K., & D'Andrade, K. (1964). Cognitive aspects of English kinship terms. *American Anthropologist, 66*, 146–170.

Schwarz, P. A. (1964). Adapting tests to the cultural setting, *Educational and Psychological Measurement, 23*, 673–686.

Scribner, S., & Cole, M. (1981). *The psychology of literacy*. Cambridge, MA: Harvard University Press.

Serpell, R. (1979). How specific are perceptual skills? A cross-cultural study of pattern reproduction. *British Journal of Psychology, 70*, 365–380.

Sternberg, R. J. (1984). Toward a triarchic theory of human intelligence. *Behavioral and Brain Sciences, 7*, 269–315.

Tyler, S. (Ed.) (1969). *Cognitive anthropology*, New York: Holt Rinehart and Winston.

van de Koppel, J. (1983). *A developmental study of Biaka Pygmies and the Bangandu*. Lisse: Swets and Zeitlinger.

Vernon, P. E. (1969). *Intelligence and cultural environment*. London: Methuen.

Werner, H. (1948). *Comparative psychology of mental development*. (rev. ed.). Chicago: Follet.

Wundt, W. (1916). *Elements of folk psychology*. London: Allen & Unwin.

13 The development of practical intelligence in cross-cultural perspective

Jane R. Mercer, Margarita Gomez-Palacio and
Eligio Padilla

There have been two major approaches to conceptualizing the nature of intelligence: the academic approach and the social-behavioral approach. The academic approach concentrates on the internal world of the individual and understanding and measuring the cognitive processes and structures used to manipulate the symbolic systems of the culture, to solve mathematical and logical problems, to create higher-order concepts and operate at higher levels of abstraction, to process and retain information in short-term and long-term memory, and so forth. Academic intelligence is nurtured in academic settings; persons from academically sophisticated environments tend to excel on tests that measure such academic cognitive skills. Traditional intelligence tests are validated against academic performance and provide reasonably good predictions of school functioning level and, as such, we shall refer to them as measures of academic intelligence.

The social-behavioral approach to conceptualizing intelligence has focused on the individual's ability to deal with the external world of social structures and social interactions, to play a variety of roles in various social systems, to establish and maintain interpersonal relationships and ties, to interpret the intentions and meanings of the acts of others accurately, and so forth. Various terms have been used to describe such competencies. The contributors to this book use the term "practical intelligence." Earlier scholars, such as Itard and Haslan, Sequin, Voisin, Howe, and Goddard used such terms as "social competency," "skills training," "social norms," "the power of fending for oneself in life," "adaptability to the environment," and "efficiency of social value" (Lambert, Windmiller, Cole, & Figueroa, 1975). More recent authorities write of "social maturity" (Doll, 1953), "social competence" (Cain, Levine, & Friedman, 1963), and "adaptive behavior" (Gesell & Amatruda, 1941; Leland, Nihira, Foster, & Shellhaas, 1967; Heber, 1962; Robbins, Mercer, & Meyers, 1967; Mercer, 1965, 1970, 1973, 1979; Nihara, Foster, Shellhaus, & Leland, 1969; Coulter & Morrow, 1978; Grossman, 1983).

In our discussion, academic intelligence and social-behavioral intelligence are conceptualized as two relatively distinct dimensions (Sternberg, 1981,

307

1982). We present data contrasting measures of the two components of intelligence cross-culturally. Nevertheless, we recognize that there is some overlap, especially in infancy, when the two cannot be differentiated empirically. "Intelligence" tests for very young children contain many items relating to social behaviors, such as smiling, recognizing the mother's face, and recognizing a stranger. As the child develops, social-behavioral intelligence and academic intelligence gradually become differentiated, and traditional "intelligence" tests progressively eliminate items involving social competencies as the age of the subject increases. By school age, traditional tests focus almost exclusively on academic intelligence.

The relative emphasis given to social-behavioral intelligence as compared with academic intelligence has varied historically and also varies by discipline. Before the development of "intelligence" tests, legal and lay definitions of competence rested on evaluations of social role performance. Even today, legal codes still emphasize social intelligence when the courts conduct competency hearings.

Psychological definitions began to focus almost exclusively on academic intelligence after the invention of standardized "intelligence" testing (Binet & Simon, 1905). Binet was asked to identify those students who would not benefit from the regular school program and who should be placed in special programs. The validation criterion for his and subsequent tests centered on predicting academic performance in the school rather than social competence in a broader sense. When "intelligence" testing was imported to the United States, the narrow definition of intelligence that focused primarily on academic intelligence was also imported as one of the implicit assumptions of "intelligence" testing.

Not until Heber (1962), functioning as a spokesman for the American Association on Mental Deficiency, proposed that adaptive behavior be included as a second criterion for identifying the mentally retarded was there widespread intellectual interest in conceptualizing and measuring the social aspects of intelligence. This interest was further encouraged with the passage of Public Law 94-142, the *Education of the Handicapped Act* (1975), which mandated that no single procedure could be used in identifying a child as handicapped. Subsequent federal guidelines listed "adaptive behavior" as one of the dimensions that should be measured (*Federal Register*, August 23, 1977).

Definitions of social-behavioral intelligence

Two distinct models have been used to conceptualize social-behavioral intelligence: a decontextualized trait model and a contextualized behavioral model.

Decontextualized trait models

This approach to social behavioral intelligence leans heavily on the conceptual model developed to measure academic intelligence. Borrowing from the medical model, which has dominated the thinking of measurement theorists (Mercer, 1979), this type of model tends to portray social intelligence as a trait or characteristic of the individual applied in many different social situations to deal with the specific demands of those situations. Just as academic intelligence can be used to solve a variety of different mental problems, so social intelligence can be used to guide behavior in a variety of social environments.

Gesell and Amatruda (1941), both medical doctors, conceptualized social development as an orderly maturational process unfolding in a similar fashion in all human beings. Recognizing that some might argue that human reactions are too multitudinous, variegated, and contingent on environment to be measured, these investigators demonstrated that such is not the case. Working almost exclusively with infants and preschool children, they reasoned that the patterning of behavior is fundamentally determined by intrinsic factors:

Development yields to diagnosis because the construction of the action system of infant and child is determined by lawful growth forces. Behavior patterns are not whimsical or accidental by-products. They are authentic end-products of a total developmental process which works with orderly sequence. They take shape in the same manner that the underlying structures take shape. They begin to assume characteristic forms even in the fetal period for the same reasons that the bodily organs themselves assume characteristic forms. . . . All behavior patterns both in prenatal and postnatal life take shape in a comparable manner. . . . Throughout all infancy this same morphogenesis is at work, creating new forms of behavior, new and more advanced patterns. These patterns are symptoms. They are indicators of the maturity of the nervous system. (Gesell & Amatruda, 1941, pp. 5–6)

The procedures for developmental diagnosis developed by Gesell and Amatruda are still widely used in pediatric settings.

Although Doll (1953) placed more emphasis on environmental factors than did Gesell and Amatruda, his concept of social competence was still rather decontextualized. He postulated that a central developmental factor, comparable to Spearman's g, operated to move the individual progressively toward self-direction, ultimately culminating in the direction and protection of others. Doll saw environmental factors as important principally in determining the types of items appropriate for measuring social competence in different societies. The underlying dimension remains as a general factor or trait. The form and scoring of his Vineland Social Maturity Scale (1965) mimicked the Stanford-Binet scales, even including a "social quotient" patterned after the "intelligence quotient" yielded by those scales (Terman &

Merrill, 1937). The Vineland scales have been widely used for several decades. It is noteworthy that the two earliest scales, which were developed from a decontextualized perspective, are designed primarily for infants and young children. The most recent revision of the Vineland Scale (Sparrow, Balla, & Cicchetti, 1984), organizes scores into domains – communication, daily living skills, socialization, and motor skills – and is more contextualized than the original scales. It covers from birth through 18 years, 11 months of age.

When workers in the field use such terms as "social intelligence," "practical intelligence," and "social competence," they are usually operating from a decontextualized mental construct that visualizes the ability to cope with social structure and social interaction as a more or less stable personal characteristic. The ability, or lack thereof, is assumed to generalize across specific social situations and is conceptualized as a relatively enduring trait of the individual. A hypothetical construct, variously called "social intelligence," "practical intelligence," and "social competence," is the focus of measurement. Scores on social competency measures are interpreted as indicators of the "maturity of the nervous system" (Gesell & Amatruda, 1941) or the extent to which the individual has developed a general "social" factor (Doll, 1953).

Contextualized models

The **behavioral** non-*trait* approach to the assessment of social-behavioral intelligence is more recent. These models are grounded in sociological and social-ecological models (Mercer, 1978) and focus on the extent to which behavior meets the normative expectations that others have for persons playing a particular role in a particular group. Those operating from this perspective tend to use terms such as "adaptive behavior" and "social role performance" to describe the phenomenon being measured and do not postulate the existence of a construct or trait that is a general characteristic of the individual, nor do they operate from an implicit medical model (Mercer, 1979). The work reported in this chapter is based on a contextualized behavioral approach that has evolved over a period of years. The terms "adaptive behavior" and "social role performance" are used interchangeably to indicate our contextualized perspective and the terms "practical intelligence," "social intelligence," and "social competence" when discussing decontextualized constructs.

The adaptive behavior scales developed for use in the epidemiological study of mental retardation in Riverside (Mercer, 1973) were a hybrid, consisting of twenty-eight age-graded scales. The scales for infants and children borrowed heavily from the work of Gesell, Amatruda, and Doll. They were decontextualized. However, when scales were being developed for older children, adolescents, and adults it became evident that a more contextualized approach was required. It was simply not possible to conceptualize the adaptive behavior of adults as a general characteristic that can be assessed independent of social status and social role in various social systems. Consequently, the scales for older children and adults inquire about performance in specific social roles in specific social systems.

The Adaptive Behavior Inventory for Children (ABIC) (Mercer, 1979) is explicitly based on a working definition of adaptive behavior that is highly contextualized – the social system model. Adaptive behavior is defined as the child's social role performance in a variety of social systems as evaluated by others in those systems. A child's adaptive topography at any point in time represents that child's level of performance in the major social systems in which the child is participating – the family, the peer group, the community and neighborhood, the school, and the economy.

The social environment is seen as a network of interlocking social systems that form the social structure in which the individual lives. Each social system consists of social statuses that indicate the positions occupied by system members; for example, father, mother, son, and daughter represent statuses within the family. Social roles are the behaviors of persons occupying particular social statuses. Social norms are the group's expectations for role performance. Group expectations are enforced by positive and negative sanctions, the rewards and punishments meted out to those who fulfill or fail to fulfill group norms. Normal behavior is that which conforms to the norms of the group.

Because social systems differ in the statuses, roles, and norms that define their structure, and individuals are constantly moving from one system to another, social adaptation is a continuous process. To negotiate entry to a new social system, the individual must learn the role behaviors required of persons participating in that system and must establish interpersonal ties with other system members. An individual may achieve an adaptive fit in some social systems and not in others. A child whose role performance is quite satisfactory to the family at home may be regarded as a deviant or misfit when participating in the peer group or school.

Superficially, it might appear that such a highly contextualized working definition precludes measurement. Fortunately society is formed of overlapping networks. Certain core expectations and values permeate most of the social systems of a society. Skills learned in one social system are useful in adapting to the expectations of other social systems, creating sufficient coherence in social expectations to permit measurement. Furthermore, as will be demonstrated, there is sufficient consensus, cross-culturally, to generalize our conceptual framework across cultural subgroups in American society and across international borders to Mexican society.

Within each of the major social systems that make up the social world of the child, we have identified those role behaviors and skills that are expected of system participants in addition to the interpersonal skills required for successful functioning in all social systems.

> *Family roles* include interpersonal skills in dealing with other family members; responsibilities around the house, helping and teaching younger siblings; and helping repair and care for family possessions.
>
> *Community roles* include participation in neighborhood groups and community groups; moving independently about the community to visit friends, neighbors and relatives; participation in social, political, religious, and recreational activities; and the use of community facilities, such as the library.
>
> *Peer roles* include interactions with others of the same age group; participation in games and activities; initiating and sustaining interaction; handling disputes; and assuming leadership roles.
>
> *Nonacademic school roles* include those school activities that are not primarily academic, such as holding class offices; participating in sports, musical, and dramatic activities; and working on school projects. Academic performance is explicitly excluded from our definition because measures of academic intelligence focus on the academic dimension.
>
> *Earner/consumer roles* cover various economic activities such as understanding monetary values; being able to make change; earning, borrowing, saving, and spending money; knowing common brand names and products; being able to shop for commodities, order in a restaurant; and so forth.
>
> *Self-maintenance roles* include a wide range of behaviors that are important in adapting to most social systems and the general society, such as the ability to care for one's own physical needs, health, and safety and to recognize dangerous situations; and the ability to prepare food, to dress oneself, to cross busy streets, to schedule time and keep appointments, and to manage one's life.

A complete discussion of our concept of adaptive behavior appears elsewhere (Mercer, 1978, 1979; Mercer & Lewis, 1977).

Criticisms of the concept of social-behavioral intelligence

Although various attempts have been made to measure social competence (Doll, 1965; Cain, Levine, & Freeman, 1963; Gesell & Amatruda, 1941; Lambert et al., 1975; Mercer 1973, 1979; Nihira et al., 1969; Sparrow, Balla, & Cicchetti, 1984), relatively little theoretical work has been done on the construct. Furthermore, compliance with federal guidelines mandating the measurement of adaptive behavior as part of a comprehensive assessment for handicapping conditions has been minimal (Heller, Holtzman, & Messick, 1982; Zigler, Balla, & Hodapp, 1984).

Undoubtedly there are many reasons why there has been so little interest in social-behavioral intelligence. Cleary and associates (1975) expressed two fundamental objections to including social intelligence as a component of their definition of intelligence, which probably reflect the opinions of many in the measurement community.

There are at least two fundamental reasons for rejecting the "adaptation to one's environment" approach to the measurement of intelligence. The first reason is that the definition is so broad as to be virtually meaningless for purposes of criterion development as well as test use. . . . The second reason is that if the environment is too narrowly defined (e.g., the ability to cope with the specific problems of the inner city), the resulting measurement will have too little generalizability. (Cleary, Humphreys, Kenrick, & Wesman, 1975, p. 24)

Zigler, Balla, and Hodapp (1984) propose rescinding the AAMD definition of mental retardation, which includes subnormal adaptive behavior as one of three criteria. These investigators would revert to the IQ test as the single criterion. They argue that "the concept of social adaptation is simply too elusive and ill-defined to be a criterion of mental retardation" (p. 218) and that professionals generally avoid social adaptation indicators because of "limitations of the construct itself." Continuing their attack:

Although the definition of intelligence may remain elusive, workers are light years away from agreeing on the ultimate defining feature of social adaptation; and because social adaptation is so far from basic definition, measures to assess it necessarily lack validity. . . . At the most basic level, exactly what social expectancies must be fulfilled before an individual can be considered socially competent? These change with age and with the fluctuating nature of the social situation. . . . Obviously, social adaptation is not an enduring trait, and it leads to a classification system that allows individuals to flit from category to category. (pp. 226–227)

From their criticisms, we can abstract five theoretical objections to the inclusion of social-behavioral abilities as a component of intelligence:

1. Measures of social adaptation will be unreliable because the criteria for necessary competencies will vary by the "nature of the social situation," which "allows individuals to flit from category to category" (Zigler et al., 1984, p. 226).
2. Measures to assess social adaptation "necessarily lack validity" (Zigler et al., 1984, p. 226). The critics do not specify what types of validity such measures presumably lack.
3. Measures will lack generalizability. A broad definition, such as "adaptation to one's environment," is "virtually meaningless for purposes of criterion development." On the other hand, "if environment is too narrowly defined . . . the resulting measurement will have too little generalizability" (Cleary et al., 1975, p. 24). Rephrasing this objection in terms of the earlier definition, the critics are arguing that a decontextualized concept of social adaptation will be at too high a level of abstraction to permit meaningful measurement, whereas contextualized approaches will be at too low a level of abstraction for generalizability.
4. Measures of social adaptation will be difficult because "social expectancies . . . change with age" (Zigler et al., 1984, p. 226).
5. There is no agreement on the defining features of the construct of social adaptation; such basic agreement is unlikely because "social adaptation is not an enduring trait" but fluctuates with the social situation (Zigler et al., 1984, p. 226).

The critics then contrast the five problems in assessing social-behavioral intelligence with the current status of measurement in the area of academic intelligence. The conclusion? That measures of academic intelligence are adequate in that they are reliable, valid, generalizable, and age appropriate and that there is general agreement on the definition of the construct.

Questions concerning the reliability, validity, generalizability, and age appropriateness of measures of social-behavioral intelligence can also be examined empirically. We shall address these questions by presenting data from the United States and Mexico on a measure of academic intelligence, the Wechsler Intelligence Scale for Children–Revised (WISC–R) (Wechsler, 1974) and a measure of social-behavioral intelligence, the Adaptive Behavior Inventory for Children (ABIC) (Mercer & Lewis, 1977).

The samples

Anglo and Chicano samples

Selected on a random probability basis from the public school population of California, the samples consisted of 700 Chicano and 700 Anglo students aged 5 through 11. The sample design consisted of a three-stage procedure in which school districts were first selected on a random probability basis according to the number of students of that particular group enrolled in the district, as reported in the ethnic survey conducted by the California Department of Education. Schools were then selected within each district on a random probability basis according to the number of students of that particular group enrolled in the school. Finally, individual students were selected randomly from the enrollment files of each school until a cluster of fourteen students of that ethnic group had been selected, one male and one female at each age level, 5 through 11 years. Data from the 5-year-olds is not reported here because there were no 5-year-olds in the Mexican sample. Thirty-six non-Mexican-heritage students were selected for the Chicano sample, representing 5.1% of the total. Of those students with a Mexican heritage, 29.6% had parents who were both born in Mexico, 13.9% had one parent born in Mexico, and 56.5% had both parents born in the United States. Because of the primarily Mexican background of those in the sample, we have designated it as a Chicano sample.

The Mexican sample

Subjects in the Mexican sample consisted of 1,100 public school students enrolled in the schools of the Federal District of Mexico City, fifty boys and fifty girls at each age level, 6 through 16. Fifty primary schools, thirty-nine general secondary schools, and eleven technical secondary schools were selected on a random probability basis according to the number of students enrolled. Students were selected randomly from the enrollment files of each school, one boy and one girl at each age level, 6 through 11 years, in the primary schools and 12 through 16 years in the secondary schools (Gomez-Palacio et al., 1982).

Data-collection procedures

Anglo and Chicano parents were contacted for an interview. One parent, usually the mother, was interviewed for approximately one hour. The interview covered information on the sociocultural background of the family and on the health history of the student and included questions on the student's adaptive behavior, as measured by the ABIC. Both an English and Spanish version of the schedule were developed. Interviews were conducted in either English, Spanish, or a combination of English and Spanish, depending on the preference of the parent. Interviews with Chicano parents were conducted by a team of thirty-eight Chicano women who could speak, read, and write Spanish as well as English. Each interviewer underwent approximately ten hours of training before embarking on fieldwork. During the interview, each parent was asked to give written permission for testing the student. Interviews were completed with 690 Chicano and 699 Anglo parents.

Anglo and Chicano students were tested using the WISC–R, usually in two test sessions, during school hours. Testing of 12% of subjects was conducted by school psychologists who worked for the school district in which the student was enrolled. All other students were tested by psychologists employed by the research project. All psychologists had been given special training in administering the WISC–R to ensure standardized procedures. All scoring was done by the research staff. Tests were completed with 617 Chicano and 669 Anglo students.

The Mexican fieldwork was conducted by a team of psychologists employed by the Dirección General de Educación Especial of the Republic of Mexico. Approximately twenty individuals were involved in some aspect of the fieldwork. Parent interviews were conducted using the Spanish version of the interview schedule, which had been used for the Chicano sample in California. Students were tested by the same team of psychologists who had conducted the parent interviews. All students were tested during school hours.

Operationalizing social-behavioral intelligence and academic intelligence

The Anglo and Chicano students' adaptive behavior was measured using the ABIC, which consists of thirty-five non-age-graded items asked of all students and 207 age-graded items, in order of level of difficulty. When administering the ABIC, the interviewer enters the age-graded sequence at the chronological age of the student and then works backward to establish a floor and forward to establish a ceiling. All questions have multiple-choice responses reflecting three levels of performance on that particular item: mastered, emergent, or latent behavior, scored 2, 1, and 0, respectively. The questions are organized into six scales: family roles, nonacademic school roles, community roles, peer group roles, earner/consumer roles, and self-maintenance roles. In this study, raw scores were calculated for each scale and then converted to standard scores with a mean of 50 and a standard deviation (SD) of 15. The scales were standardized at four-month age intervals. A complete description of the technical aspects of the ABIC may be found in the *SOMPA Technical Manual* (Mercer, 1979).

The academic intelligence of each student was measured using the WISC–R (Wechsler, 1974). All students were tested in English. Examiners were instructed not to test any student who, in their professional judgment, had insufficient command of English for valid testing. Although we developed sociocultural norms for the WISC–R to facilitate more accurate interpretation of the meaning of individual student scores, only data based on the standard norms are presented here.

Adaptive behavior of the Mexican students was measured using the Spanish version of the ABIC. The Spanish version used in the United States was judged completely appropriate for use in Mexico City by the Mexican research psychologists conducting the fieldwork in Mexico City. Only one item was dropped. Because communication by mail is infrequent in Mexican society, the question asking whether the child brings in the mail was eliminated. No substantive changes were made in any of the items. The only issue raised by the Mexican research team related to those questions asking about activities with neighborhood peers. Because families in Mexico frequently live in close proximity to other members of the extended family, it is not unusual for neighborhood peers also to be cousins or other relatives, a situation that seldom occurs in the United States. There was speculation that responses might differ depending on the relationship between the child and neighborhood peers. For this reason, all questions concerning interaction with neighborhood peers were asked in two forms – one asking about activities with relatives and the other about activities with nonrelatives. Subsequent analysis found no important differences in the responses to the two forms of the question. Consequently, the exact item wording used in the original version of the ABIC was retained with very minor exceptions for the final Mexican version. The ABIC was administered only to students aged 6 through 11.

The academic intelligence of the Mexican sample was measured using a modified version of the WISC–R – called the Wechsler Intelligence Scale for Children–Revised Mexicano (WISC–RM). Because there was no Spanish version of the WISC–R, the Mexican research team translated the test into Spanish. The content of some questions was changed to reflect more adequately the Mexican cultural experience. Experimental items were added for the purpose of replacing any items that proved inappropriate when the standardization data were analyzed. Revisions were made in three of the verbal subtests.

Nine items were dropped from the information subtest: "How many ears do you have?" "How many legs does a dog have?" "What must you do to make water boil?" "From what animal do we get bacon?" "What is the main material used to make glass?" "What is the capital of Greece?" "What is a barometer?" "How far is New York from Los Angeles?" "What does turpentine come from?"

Seven new items were added. "What is a baby chicken called?" "Where do we obtain *chicarrón*?" "Who was the president of Mexico who expropriated the oil?" "What is the satellite of the earth?" "How is sound transmitted?" "Who was Hernan Cortez?" "Who was Isaac Newton?"

Other items were modified to make them more appropriate. For example, instead of "How many pennies make a nickel?," the question is, "How many *vientes* make a *peso*?" Instead of "From what country did America become independent in 1776?," the question is, "From what country did Mexico become independent in 1810?" Instead of, "Name two countries that border the United States?," the question is modified to read, "Name the two countries that border Mexico." Rather than asking, "How tall is the average American man?," the question becomes, "How tall is the average Mexican man?" The information subtest consists of twenty-eight questions in the WISC–RM, as compared with thirty in the WISC–R.

Seven words were removed from the vocabulary test: knife, umbrella, clock, hat, thief, hazardous, and imminent. They were replaced by *limosna, gracioso, exportar, improbable, sinfonia,* and *amparo.* The vocabulary subtest has thirty-one items in the WISC–RM compared with thirty-two in the WISC–R.

Five items were dropped from the comprehension subtest: "What is the thing to do when you cut your finger?" "What are you supposed to do if you find someone's wallet or pocketbook in a store?" "What is the thing to do if you lose a ball that belongs to one of your friends?" "Why do we have to put stamps on letters?" "Why is it important for the government to hire people to inspect the meat-packing plants?"

Five items were then added: "Why is it better to drink a glass of milk than a soft drink?" "Why do we register the birth of babies?" "What does this sentence mean: 'El respeto al derecho ajeno es la paz.'" "What value is there in having governors for the states?" "What is the thing to do if you find a book knapsack lying in the schoolyard?"

Table 1. *Comparison of split-half reliability coefficients for subtests of the ABIC[a] for Mexican, Chicano, and Anglo students.[b]*

Subtests	Mexican (n = 600)	Chicano (n = 589)	Anglo (n = 602)
Family	.85	.87	.87
Community	.82	.90	.88
Peer relations	.79	.84	.82
Nonacademic school roles	.79	.88	.87
Earner/consumer roles	.70	.86	.87
Self-maintenance	.78	.81	.83

[a] ABIC, Adaptive Behavior Inventory for Children.
[b] The Mexican reliability coefficients are average coefficients for 6- through 11-year-olds.
Source: Gomez-Palacio et al. (1982, p. 107).

The only change made in the performance subtests was to drop three pictures from picture completion: the comb, fox, and umbrella.

The WISC–RM was administered to students aged 6 through 16 (Gomez-Palacio et al., 1982; Padilla et al., 1982; Gomez-Palacio et al., 1984).

Cross-cultural reliability of the ABIC and WISC–R/WISC–RM

ABIC

Table 1 presents the split-half reliability coefficients for the ABIC corrected for length of test using the Spearman-Brown formula (Guilford, 1954, p. 354). Measurements were made for 600 Mexican students, 589 Chicano students, and 602 Anglo students. The coefficients are slightly lower on all scales for the Mexican sample. Nevertheless, differences are small, ranging from .02 on the family scale to .17 on Earner/Consumer roles. All reliabilities are high, ranging from .70 for the Mexican sample on earner/consumer roles to a high of .90 for Chicanos on the community scale.

WISC–R/WISC–RM

Table 2 presents the reliability coefficients for scaled scores on the WISC–R and WISC–RM. It should be noted that the reliability coefficients for the Mexican sample are based on students aged 6 through 16, whereas those for the Chicano and Anglo samples are based on students aged 6 through 11. Again, there is a tendency for the Mexican reliability coefficients to be slightly lower than those for the Chicanos and Anglos, but the differences

Table 2. *Comparison of the reliability coefficients for scaled scores on the WISC–R[a] for Mexican, Chicano, and Anglo students.[b]*

Subtests	Mexican (n = 1,100)	Chicano (n = 520)	Anglo (n = 604)
Information	.85	.84	.89
Similarities	.75	.84	.85
Vocabulary	.89	.88	.89
Comprehension	.81	.82	.85
Arithmetic	.71	.86	.86
Picture arrangement	.80	.85	.81
Picture completion	.80	.86	.86
Block design	.81	.77	.77
Object assembly	.77	.68	.72
Mazes	.69	.80	.77

[a] WISC–R, Wechsler Intelligence Scale for Children–Revised.
[b] The Mexican sample includes students 6 through 16 years of age.
Source: Data are from Gomez-Palacio et al. (1982, Table 5, p. 86).

are small, ranging from a difference of .01 on vocabulary to .15 on arithmetic. All reliability coefficients are high, ranging from .69 for the Mexican sample on the mazes subtest to a high of .89 for the Mexicans and Anglos on vocabulary and Anglos on information.

Comparing Tables 1 and 2, we conclude that the reliability of the ABIC, a measure of social-behavioral intelligence, and the WISC–R/WISC–RM, a measure of academic intelligence, is stable cross-culturally. Furthermore, the two measures have similar levels of reliability. There is no evidence that academic intelligence can be measured more reliably than adaptive behavior.

Internal validity of the ABIC and WISC–R/WISC–RM cross-culturally

ABIC

One aspect of validity is the extent to which scales are internally consistent. One way to examine internal consistency is to calculate the intercorrelations among the subtest scores. Table 3 presents such intercorrelations for the Anglo, Chicano, and Mexican samples on the ABIC. The intercorrelations are quite high for all three samples, ranging from .84 to .91 for the Mexican sample, from .68 to .82 for the Chicano sample, and from .63 to .83 for the Anglo sample.

Table 3. *Intercorrelations of subtest scaled scores on the ABIC[a] for Mexican, Chicano, and Anglo students.*

	Family roles	Community roles	Peer relations	Nonacademic school roles	Earner/ consumer roles
Mexican (N = 600)					
Community roles	.91	–	–	–	–
Peer relations	.86	.89	–	–	–
Nonacademic					
school	.91	.91	.89	–	–
Earner/consumer	.90	.88	.84	.90	–
Self-maintenance	.94	.88	.88	.91	.90
Chicano (N = 690)					
Community roles	.80	–	–	–	–
Peer relations	.73	.73	–	–	–
Nonacademic					
school	.78	.77	.73	–	–
Earner/consumer	.77	.81	.68	.72	–
Self-maintenance	.82	.74	.73	.77	.76
Anglo (N = 699)					
Community roles	.80	–	–	–	–
Peer relations	.68	.68	–	–	–
Nonacademic					
school	.76	.76	.68	–	–
Earner/consumer	.77	.78	.63	.68	–
Self-maintenance	.83	.74	.68	.75	.75

[a] See Table 1.

WISC–R/WISC–RM

Tables 4, 5, and 6 present the intercorrelations among the subtests of the WISC–R and WISC–RM, for the three samples. They range from a low of .15 to a high of .59 for the Anglo sample, a low of .19 to a high of .65 for the Chicano sample, and a low of .18 to a high of .56 for the Mexican sample. In general, the intercorrelations among verbal tests and among performance tests are higher than intercorrelations across verbal and performance subtests. There is no indication that the correlations are either better or worse for the three cultural groups. They are of about the same magnitude as those reported by Wechsler for the standardization sample (Wechsler, 1974, Table 14).

We conclude that the internal consistency among subtests of the WISC–R and WISC–RM, measures of academic intelligence are comparable across our three cultural groups. Furthermore, we conclude that the internal consistency among subtests of the ABIC, a measure of social-behavioral intelligence, is comparable across the three cultural groups. There is no indication

Table 4. Intercorrelations among subtest scaled scores on the WISC–R[a] for Anglo students (N = 668).

	Infor	Simil	Arith	Vocab	Compre	Digit	PicComp	PicArr	Block	Object	Coding
Similarities	.50	–	–	–	–	–	–	–	–	–	–
Arthmetic	.49	.46	–	–	–	–	–	–	–	–	–
Vocabulary	.59	.56	.47	–	–	–	–	–	–	–	–
Comprehension	.45	.49	.40	.58	–	–	–	–	–	–	–
Digit span	.38	.34	.42	.33	.27	–	–	–	–	–	–
Picture completion	.31	.32	.27	.31	.30	.21	–	–	–	–	–
Picture arrangement	.33	.37	.33	.37	.33	.33	.34	–	–	–	–
Block design	.31	.32	.38	.34	.31	.27	.37	.36	–	–	–
Object assembly	.30	.30	.31	.29	.26	.22	.40	.36	.53	–	–
Coding	.26	.19	.22	.22	.24	.24	.15	.19	.21	.19	–
Mazes	.27	.16	.23	.23	.22	.25	.21	.22	.32	.37	.22

[a] See Table 2.

Table 5. Intercorrelations among subtest scaled scores on the WISC–R[a] for Chicano students ($N = 613$).

	Infor	Simil	Arith	Vocab	Compre	Digit	PicComp	PicArr	Block	Object	Coding
Similarities	.54	—									
Arithmetic	.56	.46	—								
Vocabulary	.65	.64	.45	—							
Comprehension	.53	.50	.34	.65	—						
Digit span	.48	.41	.49	.43	.37	—					
Picture completion	.40	.31	.37	.40	.27	.32	—				
Picture arrangement	.37	.37	.36	.35	.30	.35	.32	—			
Block design	.39	.30	.34	.36	.28	.30	.41	.32	—		
Object assembly	.36	.33	.29	.36	.29	.33	.33	.30	.44	—	
Coding	.28	.20	.33	.28	.19	.22	.23	.28	.30	.20	—
Mazes	.30	.19	.30	.22	.28	.34	.28	.26	.36	.36	.23

[a] See Table 2.

Table 6. *Intercorrelations among subtest scaled scores on the WISC–R[a] for Mexican students ($N = 600$).[b]*

	Infor	Simil	Arith	Vocab	Compre	Digit	PicComp	PicArr	Block	Object	Coding
Similarities	.46	–	–	–	–	–	–	–	–	–	–
Arithmetic	.47	.41	–	–	–	–	–	–	–	–	–
Vocabulary	.56	.51	.39	–	–	–	–	–	–	–	–
Comprehension	.47	.42	.27	.58	–	–	–	–	–	–	–
Digit span	.35	.28	.49	.31	.21	–	–	–	–	–	–
Picture completion	.42	.38	.26	.34	.30	.22	–	–	–	–	–
Picture arrangement	.44	.40	.41	.50	.38	.29	.42	–	–	–	–
Block design	.33	.34	.27	.32	.19	.32	.40	.44	–	–	–
Object assembly	.38	.34	.31	.39	.27	.27	.46	.45	.56	–	–
Coding	.22	.27	.29	.22	.19	.24	.25	.30	.29	.23	–
Mazes	.30	.22	.24	.27	.21	.21	.37	.39	.44	.40	.18

[a] See Table 2.
[b] The above correlations are average correlations for 6- and 11-year-olds.
Source: From Gomez-Palacio et al. (1982, Tables 7, 8, 9, 10, 11, and 12).

Table 7. *Factor analysis of ABIC^a and WISC–R^b subtests for Chicanos and Anglos.*

	Chicano sample				Anglo sample			
Scales	Linear verb	Cor. perf.	Factor 1	Loadings 2	Linear verb	Cor. perf.	Factor 1	Loadings 2
Family	.12	.11	.92	.04	.12	.13	.91	.04
Community	.18	.14	.89	.08	.17	.15	.88	09
Peers	.22	.15	.82	.13	.21	.18	.75	.16
School	.23	.21	.85	.17	.25	.20	.83	.19
Earner/consumer	.18	.14	.85	.09	.11	.11	.85	.03
Self-maintenance	.23	.21	.87	.18	.24	.20	.87	.18
Verbal	–	.59	.12	.79	–	.57	.09	.81
Performance	.59	–	.08	.74	.57	–	.10	.69
% Variance	–	–	81.1%	18.9%	–	–	80.6%	19.4%

^a See Table 1.
^b See table 2.
Source: Varimax Rotated Factors using *Statistical Package for the Social Sciences* (2nd ed.) Norman Nie, Hadlai Hull, Jean Jenkins, Karin Steinbrenner, and Dale Bent. McGraw-Hill Book Company, 1975.

that a measure of adaptive behavior has lower internal consistency, cross-culturally, than a measure of academic intelligence. Quite the contrary, the intercorrelations among the subtests of the ABIC are consistently and significantly higher for all cultural groups than those for the WISC–R and WISC–RM.

Discriminant validity of the ABIC and WISC–R cross-culturally

Another aspect of test validity is the extent to which scales that purport to measure one dimension of performance can be discriminated, statistically, from scales that purport to measure another dimension of performance. A very important question in the study of academic intelligence as compared with practical or social intelligence is the extent to which they comprise two distinct aspects of intelligence and can be differentiated empirically as well as conceptually.

Table 7 presents the linear correlations between the subtests of the WISC–R and the subtests of the ABIC for the Chicano and the Anglo samples and a varimax rotated factor analysis of the subtests. Unfortunately, data were not accessible to do a similar analysis for the Mexican sample.

Correlations between the subtests of the ABIC and WISC–R are relatively low for both samples, ranging from $r = .11$ to $r = .25$. The maximum amount of variance explained is slightly over 6%. In most cases the amount of variance explained is less than 4%. Two factors emerged clearly in the factor analysis: an ABIC factor that accounts for approximately 80% of the variance and a WISC–R factor that accounts for approximately 20% of the variance. Findings are essentially identical for both samples.

It is clear from these analyses that academic intelligence, as measured by the WISC–R and social intelligence, as measured by the ABIC, are distinct dimensions that can be readily identified both empirically and conceptually. Discriminant validity is equally apparent in two different cultural groups.

Cross-cultural age patterning of ABIC and WISC–R/WISC–RM items

Zigler et al. (1984) argue that it is not possible to have a valid measure of social adaptation because "exactly what social expectations must be fulfilled before an individual can be considered socially competent" will "change with age." The fact that performance levels in cognitive development change with age has never been considered an insurmountable obstacle to measuring academic intelligence. In fact, Binet built these developmental changes into the fabric of his test by sequencing items according to the age level at which they are typically passed. The notion of mental age incorporates the age dimension as the fundamental criterion for evaluating the level of an individual performance. A basic method for validating scales that claim to be developmental measures is to correlate raw scores with age. As in the case of measures of cognitive ability, the age patterning of adaptive behavior items provides the rationale for item sequencing, allows for age comparisons, provides a basis for validating the scales, and gives us an excellent opportunity to make cross-cultural comparisons.

ABIC

The ABIC items for the Mexican sample were analyzed following the same procedures as those used for the California samples (Mercer, 1979). A one-way analysis of variance was done on each item by age of the child to determine whether there were significant differences in responses by age. The same thirty-one items that showed no significant difference in response by age in the California samples also showed no significant difference by age in the Mexican sample. Consequently, the non-age-graded items are cross-culturally identical (Gomez-Palacio et al., 1982, p. 110).

The remaining items were assigned to the age category at which the average response to the item was at or near 1.00, the score for "emergent" behavior. Items were then arranged in order within each age category from the easiest (highest average score) to the most difficult (lowest average score). The resulting rank ordering was compared with the rank ordering for the California samples using a rank-order correlation. A correlation of .96 was found between the rank orders in the Mexican population and the California samples. We conclude that the sequence of development and mastery of various social role competencies is essentially identical across the three cultural groups studied.

WISC–R/WISC–RM

The order of difficulty for each of the items in each of the subtests of the WISC–R was compared with the order of difficulty found for the Mexican sample on the WISC–RM. Only those items that appeared in both the WISC–R and the WISC–RM were included in the analysis. The correlations were as follows: information, .87; vocabulary, .85; similarities, .96; comprehension, .96; picture completion, .96; and arithmetic, .99. The order of item difficulty was identical for picture arrangement, digit span, block design, object assembly, coding, and mazes, yielding a correlation of 1.0.

The patterning of items in terms of item difficulty is virtually identical across the three cultural groups studied for both the ABIC and the WISC–R/WISC–RM. Those subtests on the WISC–R in which more cultural impact could reasonably be expected, such as information and vocabulary, yielded slightly lower rank order correlations, but overall we must conclude that measures of adaptive behavior and academic intelligence show very similar patterns of development in the groups studied.

Cross-cultural generalizability of the ABIC and WISC–R/WISC–RM norms

An important aspect of generalizability is the extent to which developmental norms established on the basis of the performance of one cultural group can be generalized to other cultural groups. This question is quite independent of the questions already discussed. It is possible for measures to have similar cross-cultural reliability, internal consistency, and age patterning of items while simultaneously lacking normative generalizability.

Academic intelligence consists of the cognitive processes and structures in the internal world of the individual that are used to manipulate the symbolic systems of the culture to solve the types of intellectual problems which are valued in that culture. Adaptive behavior is the individual's ability to deal with social structures and social interaction and to play a variety of roles considered culturally appropriate. These definitions are based on the assumption that both academic intelligence and social-behavioral intelligence develop with age. Each recognizes that societal expectations for performance in both spheres grow more demanding as the individual matures. The age dimension provides the foundation for operationalizing both definitions and scores are standardized at four-month intervals on both the ABIC and the WISC–R/WISC–RM.

A crucial aspect of generalizability is the extent to which age norms developed on one population can be appropriately applied to other populations. If age standards are universal across all human populations, a single universal normative model can be applied. If age standards differ, generalizability of a single set of norms is limited.

ABIC

Table 8 presents the mean scaled scores on the ABIC for the three cultural groups in our study, based on the United States norms. A one-way analysis of variance indicates that differences in means are all statistically significant at the .001 level of probability. In every case except the family scale, the Anglo mean is highest, the Chicano mean is intermediate, and the Mexican mean is lowest. This is precisely the pattern we would expect based on our knowledge of the cultural differences across the three populations and the fact that the scales were developed in the United States. In general, Chicanos are closer to the Anglos than to the Mexicans, with average means 2 to 3 points lower. Mexican averages are 5 to 16 points below the Anglo averages.

Subsequently, a Scheffé test was performed to identify which pairs of means differ significantly at the .05 level or beyond. All differences between the Mexican sample and Chicano sample and between the Mexican sample and the Anglo sample are significant. Except for means on the family and self-maintenance subtests, all differences between the Chicano and Anglo samples are significant.

Because our large samples make an analysis of variance very sensitive to small differences that may be substantively inconsequential, the last column in Table 8 presents the percentage of the total variance in ABIC scores that lies between cultural groups. The total variance of a test score consists of the variance of the scores of students in each cultural group around the mean of their cultural group (the within-group variance) plus the variance of the group means around the grand mean for all three cultural groups (the between-group variance). We calculated the percentage of the total variance representing between-group variance. This percentage provides a basis for judging the substantive importance of statistically significant differences across the three cultural groups. Between-group differences account for 6% or less of the total variance in ABIC scores on all scales but community. Only the community scale has a substantial percentage of the variance, 18.29%, between cultural groups. We conclude that differences between the cultural groups on the ABIC are relatively trivial, except on the community scale.

Differences in community role performance reflect cultural variance in

Table 8. *Comparison of mean scaled scores on the ABIC[a] for Mexican, Chicano, and Anglo students.[b]*

Subtests	Mexican (N = 600)	Chicano (N = 690)	Anglo (N = 699)	Significance level	Mexican vs. Chicano	Scheffé Mexican vs. Anglo	Anglo vs. Chicano	% Variance explained
Family roles	42.5	49.6	47.7	<.001	<.05	<.05	NS	3.66
Community roles	33.8	46.6	50.2	<.001	<.05	<.05	<.05	18.29
Peer relations	43.0	47.3	51.2	<.001	<.05	<.05	<.05	4.42
Nonacademic school roles	41.3	47.9	50.3	<.001	<.05	<.05	<.05	6.00
Earner/consumer roles	43.2	47.6	50.1	<.001	<.05	<.05	<.05	3.44
Self-maintenance roles	45.2	47.7	49.5	<.001	<.05	<.05	NS	1.36

[a] See Table 1.
[b] Scaled scores are based on the U.S. norms, which are standardized to have a mean of 50 and a SD of 15.

child-rearing practices. In Mexico, young children interact primarily within the extended family, are closely supervised during the younger years, and are less likely to move about the community independently or with peers. Youth organizations, such as scouts, sports leagues, and youth clubs, are much less common in Mexican society than in the United States. Mexican students are older when they begin to attend and participate in community events and to use public transportation.

WISC–R/WISC–RM

Mean scaled scores on the subtests of the WISC–R and WISC–RM are presented in Table 9. Scaled scores are based on U.S. norms (Wechsler, 1974). The Mexican sample includes students aged 6 through 16 (Gomez-Palacio et al., 1982, Tables 3 and 4). A one-way analysis of variance indicates that the mean differences are all statistically significant at the .001 level of probability. A Scheffé test was used to determine whether differences in pairs of means are statistically significant. All differences, except one, were statistically reliable at the .05 level of probability or beyond. Anglos scored higher on all subtests than either the Mexican or Chicano samples. The Chicano sample shows a higher score than the Mexican sample on eight subtests. The Mexican sample scored higher than the Chicano sample on information, vocabulary, and arithmetic, and there was no significant difference between the groups on comprehension. It is important to note that the four subtests on which Mexican student performance is equal to or higher than that of Chicanos are those that were modified by the Mexican researchers to make them more appropriate for the Mexican culture. Apparently, their efforts were partially successful in removing the cultural loading.

Differences in the verbal, performance, and full-scale IQ means were statistically significant except for the verbal IQ, which shows no difference between the Mexican and Chicano samples. The reasons are readily apparent. The Mexican sample scored higher on three of the six verbal subtests, and the Chicano sample scored higher on two verbal subtests, thereby balancing out the total scores on that portion of the Wechsler.

To assess the substantive importance of the findings in Table 9, the right-hand column presents the percentage of the total variance that lies between groups for each of the subtests. Only two of the subtests have less than 5% of the variance between groups – arithmetic and picture arrangement. Five subtests have more than 5% but less than 10% of the variance between cultural groups – vocabulary, comprehension, picture completion, object assembly, and mazes. Five subtests have more than 10% of the variance between groups – information, similarities, digit span, block design, and coding. Verbal IQ has 10.71% of the variance between groups, performance IQ 9.84,, and full-scale IQ 18.95%.

Table 9. *Comparison of mean scaled scores on the subtests of the WISC–R^a for Mexican, Chicano, and Anglo students.*[b]

Subtests	Mexican (N = 1,100)	Chicano (N = 520)	Anglo (N = 604)	Significance level	Mexican vs. Chicano	Scheffé Mexican vs. Anglo	Anglo vs. Chicano	% Variance explained
Information	8.1	7.5	10.5	<.001	<.05	<.05	<.05	10.32
Similarities	6.9	7.6	10.3	<.001	<.05	<.05	<.05	15.79
Arithmetic	9.8	8.7	10.3	<.001	<.05	<.05	<.05	3.26
Vocabulary	9.2	7.9	10.8	<.001	NS	<.05	<.05	9.94
Comprehension	7.9	7.8	10.1	<.001	NS	<.05	<.05	8.62
Digit span	6.4	8.4	10.4	<.001	<.05	<.05	<.05	22.73
Picture completion	8.2	9.8	10.8	<.001	<.05	<.05	<.05	9.25
Picture arrangement	8.6	9.1	10.3	<.001	<.05	<.05	<.05	4.95
Block design	8.2	9.7	10.8	<.001	<.05	<.05	<.05	11.55
Object assembly	8.3	9.7	10.5	<.001	<.05	<.05	<.05	6.35
Coding	7.9	9.7	10.6	<.001	<.05	<.05	<.05	11.76
Mazes	9.2	10.0	11.2	<.001	<.05	<.05	<.05	5.32
Verbal IQ	89.2	87.7	102.0	<.001	NS	<.05	<.05	10.71
Performance IQ	88.0	97.9	103.8	<.001	<.05	<.05	<.05	9.84
Full-scale IQ	87.3	91.9	103.1	<.001	<.05	<.05	<.05	18.95

[a] See Table 2. The WISC–RM (Modified) version of the test was used.
[b] Data include ages 6 through 16.
Source: Mexican data taken from Gomez-Palacio et al. (1982, Tables 3 and 4, pp. 84–85).

Even with the modifications made by the Mexican research team to make the test more appropriate for Mexican society, the WISC–R/WISC–RM is more sensitive to cultural differences and the norms are less cross-culturally generalizable than the ABIC.

Discussion and conclusions

Some members of the psychometric community and workers in the field of child development subscribe to the belief that only academic intelligence can be adequately conceptualized and usefully measured. They hold that attempts to measure "intelligence" should be restricted to assessment of the internal cognitive processes of the individual. Furthermore, they argue that recently developed definitions of mental retardation, which include subnormal adaptive behavior as a second criterion, should be abandoned in favor of a return to a single criterion – subnormal performance on traditional "intelligence" tests, such as the WISC–R. These recommendations are based on the belief that measures of social-behavioral intelligence are unreliable, invalid, ungeneralizable, and unable to deal with changes in role expectations across age. It is also argued that the construct being measured is too elusive and theoretically underdeveloped for effective operationalization. Either the definition is so broad as to be "meaningless" or so narrow as to be ungeneralizable. Despite these criticisms, the most prominent critics (Cleary et al., 1975; Zigler et al., 1984) present no empirical data to support their negative conclusions. For this reason, we must treat their "conclusions" as hypotheses rather than as findings.

Our study was conducted using three samples from culturally distinct populations – Anglos, Chicanos, and Mexicans – to provide a more rigorous test than would be possible using a single cultural group. If findings can be replicated in three such diverse populations, they have greater credibility. These three cultural groups are especially appropriate for study because their cultural characteristics form a natural continuum with Chicanos as the intermediate group sharing some of the cultural characteristics of both the Anglo and the Mexican samples. Because the ABIC and WISC–R were both designed and standardized for use in the United States, we can hypothesize that the direction of any differences found in reliability, validity, age patterning, or generalizability should favor the Anglo group. The scales are least culturally appropriate for the Mexican sample. We would therefore expect their scores to have the lowest reliabilities, internal consistency, and so forth.

Contrary to the expectations of the critics, we found that both academic intelligence and adaptive behavior could be measured with a high degree of reliability in all three cultural groups. There was no evidence that subjects classified by their scores on the ABIC would be any more likely to "flit from category to category" than would those classified by their scores on the WISC–R. High reliabilities are not unique to the ABIC. The lowest split-half reliability for any age level on the revised version of the Vineland adaptive behavior scales is .70. Median reliabilities for the four domains are .89, .90, .86, and .83 (Sparrow, Balla, & Cicchetti, 1984, Table 3.3).

We examined the internal validity of the ABIC and compared it with that of the WISC–R by looking at the intercorrelations among subscales. We found intercorrelations among the subscales of the ABIC to be consistently and significantly higher for all three cultural groups than intercorrelations on the WISC–R/WISC–RM. The lowest intercorrelation on the ABIC (.63) is only slightly lower than the highest intercorrelation (.65) on the WISC–R/WISC–RM.

To ascertain the discriminant validity of the ABIC and WISC–R, we calculated the linear correlations among the subtests of the two measures and did a factor analysis of the subtests. Correlations are all low. Two very distinct factors emerged. Factor 1, which accounted for approximately 80% of the variance in both the Chicano sample and the Anglo sample, consisted of the ABIC subtests, and factor 2 consisted of the WISC–R verbal and performance subtests. It is clear that academic intelligence and practical intelligence can be distinguished empirically, a finding that supports the conceptual distinction between the two types of intelligence.

The issue of changes in social expectations as persons age is not unique to measures of adaptive behavior. All traditional measures of "intelligence" and "achievement" recognize that cognitive abilities increase with age and incorporate that fact into the structure and norming of the test. Age is no more a problem in measuring adaptive behavior than it is in measuring academic intelligence. The study of the correlation between items and age, cross-culturally, provides an additional basis for assessing the cross-cultural validity and generalizability of the notion of adaptive behavior and its measurement.

We found that the same items which were uncorrelated with age in the Anglo and Chicano samples were also uncorrelated with age in the Mexican sample. The list of thirty-five items includes behaviors, such as getting along with parents and siblings, interacting with peers, and emotional responses to various situations. The fact that the same items were not age graded in all three samples provides rather impressive evidence for cross-cultural regularities. Furthermore, the more than 200 items that were correlated with age were rank ordered by difficulty level. The rank-order correlation between the California samples and the Mexican sample was almost unity – $r = .96$. We believe this to be an extremely important finding. It indicates that the developmental sequence for the acquisition and mastery of social roles is essentially identical for the 6- through 11-year-olds in the three cultural groups studied. Childhood socialization patterns are very similar cross-culturally. There is no evidence that changes in social role performance with age create difficulties in measuring adaptive behavior. Rather, the fact that the age sequence is generalizable provides further evidence of the robustness and validity of the dimension being measured. Rank orders of items were also highly correlated across the samples for the WISC–R/WISC–RM, ranging in magnitude from .85 to 1.0.

There is additional evidence of scale generalizability in the fact that virtually no changes were necessary to adapt ABIC items for use in Mexico City. The Spanish version of the ABIC standardized in the United States was directly applicable. On the other hand, a translation and reorganization of several subscales was necessary to adapt the WISC–R for use in Mexico City.

We do not believe the U.S. norms on either the ABIC or WISC–R should be used for Mexican populations. Nevertheless, the ABIC norms are a better fit to the Mexican sample than are the norms for the WISC–R. Overall, significantly less of the total variance in scores on the ABIC lies between cultural groups than on the WISC–R/WISC–RM. Ten of the twelve scales on the WISC–R/WISC–RM (83%) had more than 5% of the total variance lying between groups, whereas the ABIC had only two of six scales (33%), with more than 5% between groups variance.

The final issue relates to the belief that the concept of social adaptation is much more elusive than that of "intelligence" and that "workers are light years away from agreeing on the ultimate defining features of social adaptation" (Zigler et al., 1984). Cleary et al. (1975) also argue that problems of definition are too formidable for measurement. Why do psychometricians perceive the definitional problems as insurmountable in the case of social adaptation? We believe that the difficulty arises at least partially from the decontextualized perspective they are adopting and a failure to recognize the existence of contextual behavioral paradigms.

As we discussed at the outset, early workers in the area of social competence, including Doll, Gesell, and Amatruda, modeled their theories of social development after the paradigm used in "intelligence" testing. They visualized social competence as the manifestation of a central factor, a characteristic of the individual. The view that social adaptation is a trait of the individual, a hypothetical "something" that permeates all social interactions and can be abstracted and measured, leads to the same sort of theoretical elusiveness that has plagued the field of "intelligence" testing since its inception. Trait thinking is fraught with ambiguities. Different researchers define the trait construct differently, thereby creating a variety of mental abstractions bearing the same label. Even when there is agreement on the definition of the construct, there is no definitive mechanism for verifying that a particular instrument is adequately measuring the hypothetical entity being defined. Reification of constructs is a perennial problem. No satisfactory solution to these dilemmas has been found by scholars using trait models to explain behavior. It is clear that Zigler et al. (1984) are conceptualizing the problem from a decontextualized trait perspective when they conclude that no agreement on the definition of social adaptations is possible because "obviously, social adaptation is not an enduring trait."

"Traits" are simply mental constructs created by theorists as a device for categorizing and naming certain regularities in behavior that have been observed in the real world. Because they are abstractions, ways of classifying real-world observations, "traits" exist only in the mind of the beholder. They are part of the cognitive map an individual uses to make sense of the experiential world. They have whatever attributes the definer chooses to ascribe to them. They do not exist in an existential sense. Whether social adaptation is viewed as an enduring or transitory trait is a definitional, not an empirical, question.

The findings presented in this chapter can be interpreted from either a decontextualized or a contextualized perspective. The fact that the ABIC subtests are highly intercorrelated, even though the items cover behaviors in different social systems, can be explained, theoretically, as a result of social adaptivity applied in different social situations. Similarly, the cross-cultural reliability of the ABIC can be interpreted as evidence of the stability of an underlying social trait, variously called "practical intelligence" or "social intelligence." The near-identical patterning of the difficulty levels of items, cross-culturally, can be ascribed to an intrinsic social maturational process that emerges in children being socialized in different cultural settings. The marked differentiation between adaptive behavior and academic intelligence can be viewed as evidence for distinct psychological dimensions within the individual.

On the other hand, the same findings can be interpreted from a contextualized behavioral model. Such a model would explain the high intercorrelations among ABIC subtests as the result of shared values, norms, and expectations across social groups in the same society. Children who perform successfully in one social group, such as the peer group, are also likely to perform successfully in other social systems, such as the school, because the social skills learned in one subsystem are useful in other subsystems with similar norms and expectations.

Society is made up of interlocking social groups, not discrete and isolated units. The high reliability of the ABIC is based on systemic as well as individual regularities. The similar developmental sequencing of the social role performance of children in the three cultural groups can be attributed to increasing societal demands for performance placed on maturing children by the various groups in which they participate. The fact that these demands follow a similar sequence in the United States and Mexico is sociologically informative, the result of important uniformities in childhood socialization in the two societies. Fortunately for the individuals trying to negotiate their way through a complex society and for social scientists trying to measure their success in doing so, there is sufficient coherence in expectations to allow for transfer of learning and for reliable measurement.

The differentiation between adaptive behavior and academic intelligence found in the factor analysis can be interpreted as evidence that the social norms for cognitive and academic performance are very different from the social norms for interacting in social groups. Because the behaviors involved are so different and are judged by such different criteria, a person who is successful in one area might not be successful in the other. There is no reason to expect that persons who can solve math problems or who have large vocabularies will be either more successful or less successful in their interpersonal relations than those who do not. The perspective adopted by an investigator when interpreting findings is frequently a matter of disciplinary emphasis.

Although distinctions between contextualized and decontextualized models have been maintained throughout this chapter, the differences are a matter of perspective and should not be exaggerated. Decontextualized models focus on the internal psychological organization of the individual's social experience using trait constructs. These models visualize the patterning of the individual's social learning as a coherent measurable structure acquired through social learning. The existence of the social world is taken for granted. On the other hand, contextualized models focus on behavior in the external social world. These models visualize the demands of various social systems as forming a relatively coherent pattern of external social expectations. Whereas requirements for social role performance do vary from subsystem to subsystem, many of the skills necessary to succeed in one subsystem can be applied to others. Emphasis is on the external world, producing consistency in behavior that can be measured reliably. The fact that this consistency will be reflected in the organization of the internal psychological world of the individual is taken for granted. The two perspectives are but opposite sides of the same coin and complement rather than compete with each other.

We conclude that definitional questions are not insurmountable. For those who prefer decontextualized trait models, the data supporting the concept of practical intelligence are similar to those supporting the concept of academic intelligence. For those who prefer contextualized models, there is no need to hypothesize underlying traits. Behavior in a variety of social and cultural groups can be measured reliably and evaluated relative to the norms for those groups.

References

Binet, A., & Simon, T. (1905). Sur la necessité d'etablir un diagnostic scientifique des etats inferieurs de l'intelligence. *Année Psychologique, 11,* 1–28.

Cain, L. F., Levine, S., & Freeman, F. E. (1963). *The Cain-Levine social competency scale.* Palo Alto, CA: Consulting Psychologists Press.

Cleary, T. A., Humphreys, L. G., Kenrick, S. A., & Wesman, A. (1975). Educational uses of tests with disadvantaged students. *American Psychologist, 30,* 15–41.

Coulter, W. A., & Morrow, H. W. (1978). Theoretical aspects of adaptive behavior. In W. A. Coulter, & W. Henry (Eds.), *Adaptive behavior: Concepts and measurements.* New York: Grune & Stratton.

Doll, E. A. (1953). *Measurement of social competence: A manual for the Vineland Social Maturity Scale.* Minneapolis: American Guidance Service.

Doll, E. A. (1965). *Vineland Social Maturity Scale: Manual of Direction* (condensed rev. ed.). Minneapolis: American Guidance Service.

Federal Register, Tuesday, August 23, 1977: Part II, Department of Health, Education and Welfare: Office of Education, Education of Handicapped Children: Implementation of Part B of the Education of the Handicapped Act. Vol. 42, 163, 42474–42518.

Gesell, A. L., & Amatruda, C. S. (1941). *Developmental diagnosis: Normal and abnormal child development.* New York: Hoeber.

Gómez-Palacio, M., Hinojosa, E. R., & Padilla, E. (1982). *Estandarización de la Batería de Pruebas SOMPA en México D. F.: Informe sobre teoria y resultados.* Mexico, DF: Dirección General de Educacion Especial.

Goméz-Palacio, M., Padilla, E. R., & Roll, S. (1984). *WISC–RM.* Mexico City: El Manual Moderno, S. A. (Distributed in the United States by Southwestern Psychological Services, P. O. Box 10263, Alameda, NM 87184.)

Grossman, H. J. (Ed.). (1983). *Classification in mental retardation.* Washington, DC: American Association on Mental Deficiency.

Guilford, J. P. (1954). *Psychometric methods* (2nd ed.), New York: McGraw-Hill.

Heber, R. A. (1962). *A manual on terminology and classification in mental retardation* (2nd edition). *American Journal of Mental Deficiency.* (Monograph Supplement 64.)

Heller, K. A., Holtzman, W. H., & Messick, S. (1982). *Placing children in special education: A strategy for equity.* Washington, DC: National Academy Press.

Lambert, N. M., Windmiller, M., Cole, L., & Figueroa, R. (1975). *AAMD adaptive behavior scale: Public school version* (1974 rev.), Washington, DC: American Association on Mental Deficiency.

Leland, H., Nihara, K., Foster, R., Shellhaas, M., & Kagin, E. (Eds.) (1966). 1966 Conference on measurement of adaptive behavior: II. Parsons, KS: Parsons State Hospital and Training Center.

Leland, H., Nihara, K., Foster, R., & Shellhaas, M. (1967). The demonstration and measurement of adaptive behavior (Adaptive behavior project). Parsons, KS: Parsons State Hospital and Training Center.

Mercer, J. R. (1965). Social system perspective and clinical perspective: Frames of reference for understanding career patterns of persons labeled as mentally retarded. *Social Problems, 13*(1).

Mercer, J. R. (1970). Sociological perspectives on mild mental retardation. In H. C. Haywood (Ed.), *Social/cultural aspects of mental retardation: Proceedings of the Peabody NIMH conference.* New York: Appleton-Century-Crofts.

Mercer, J. R. (1973). *Labeling the mentally retarded: Clinical and social system perspectives on mental retardation.* Berkeley: University of California Press.

Mercer, J. R. (1978). Theoretical constructs of adaptive behavior: Movement from a medical to a social-ecological perspective. In W. A. Coulter and H. W. Morrow (Eds.), *Adaptive behavior: Concepts and measurements.* New York: Grune & Stratton.

Mercer, J. R. (1979). *System of multicultural pluralistic assessment: Technical manual.* New York: The Psychological Corporation.

Mercer, J. R. (1984). What is a racially and culturally nondiscriminatory test? A sociological and pluralistic perspective. In C. R. Reynolds and R. T. Brown (Eds.), *Perspectives on bias in mental testing.* New York: Plenum.

Mercer, J. R., & Lewis, J. F. (1977). *SOMPA: Parent interview manual*. New York: The Psychological Corporation.

Mercer, J. R. (1978). *SOMPA: The student assessment manual*. New York: The Psychological Corporation.

Nihara, K., Foster, R., Shellhaas, M., & Leland, H. (1969). *Adaptive behavior scale*. Washington, DC: American Association on Mental Deficiency.

Padilla, E. R., Roll, S., & Gomez-Palacio, M. (1982). The performance of Mexican children and adolescents on the WISC-R. *Interamerican Journal of Psychology, 16*(2), 122–128.

Public Law 94-142. Amendment to the Education of the Handicapped Act. 94th Congress. S. 6. November 29, 1975. 20 usc 1401.

Robbins, R. C., Mercer, J. R., & Meyers, C. E. 1967. The school as a selecting–labeling system. *Journal of School Psychology, 5*, 270–279.

Sparrow, S. S., Balla, D. A., & Cicchetti, D. V. (1984). *Vineland Adaptive Behavior Scales: Survey form manual*. Circle Pines, MN: American Guidance Service.

Sternberg, R. J. (1981). Testing and cognitive psychology. *American Psychologist, 36*, 1181–1189.

Sternberg, R. J. (1982). Thinking and learning skills: A view of intelligence. *Education Digest, 27*, 20–22.

Terman, L., & Merrill, M. A. (1937). *Measuring intelligence: A guide to the administration of the new revised Stanford-Binet tests of intelligence*. Cambridge, MA: Houghton Mifflin.

Wechsler, D. (1974). *Manual for the Wechsler Intelligence Scale for Children–Revised*. New York: The Psychological Corporation.

Zigler, E., Balla, D., & Hodapp, R. (1984). On the definition and classification of mental retardation. *American Journal of Mental Deficiency, 89*,(3), 215–230.

14 Intelligence and literacy: the relationships between intelligence and the technologies of representation and communication

David R. Olson

One day we shall have to revolutionize psychology by looking at the human mind as an organ for interacting with objects of the third world [the world of man-made artifacts and symbols]; for understanding them, contributing to them, participating in them; for bringing them to bear on the first world [the natural world]. (Sir Karl Popper, 1972, p. 156)

This chapter addresses an aspect of the task mentioned by Popper, namely, that of examining intelligence not so much as a general adaptive quality of mind but as the forms of competence involved in dealing with cultural artifacts or technologies. This line of argument has been developed by such investigators as Vygotsky (1962), Luria (1976), and Cole and colleagues (LCHC, 1982), who stress the role of culture in cognition. My emphasis will be on one particular aspect of culture, namely, that having to do with the technologies of communication, in particular those of writing and computing. Skills with these media make up important forms of practical intelligence in a literate bureaucratic society, forms of competence that are so widely applicable that they have succeeded in essentially preempting the entire concept of intelligence for themselves. My concern is with the structure of literate competence, with showing how what we frequently call "intelligence" is little more than this form of literate competence, with examining the contexts in which such competence is useful, in examining the relations between literate and computational competencies and in advancing some general reflections on the concept of intelligence as an explanatory as opposed to a descriptive concept.[1]

Intelligence as a descriptive concept: the testing movement

The concept of intelligence is likely to be with us for some time. Intelligence, along with charm, poise, open-mindedness, and left-leaning, are ways in which we characterize our friends; these characterizations in part contribute to our decisions as to whom we would care to have a conversation with, marry, avoid, or employ.

Moreover, such categorical descriptions can be quantified. In the hands

338

of Binet and the testing movement, intelligence tests were shown to be reliable and predictive: One could account for general learning capabilities by sampling performance on a range of high-level intellectual tasks. The success of the enterprise invited the inference that such tests were not merely descriptive but explanatory. That is, they were taken not as a sample of performance in a particular domain but as an explanation of why there was a high level of performance in that domain. They explained performance on the basis of a general quality of mind, roughly describable as intellectual potential, which was tapped by those tests. Tests were not seen as merely descriptions or samples of competence, but rather as underlying that competence. A favorite metaphor was that intelligence specifies the limits of what a person could achieve, whereas language, culture, and education determine the extent to which one achieves that potential.

Furthermore, because intelligence was seen as potential for learning, it was seen as being the part of mind that is essentially independent of knowledge, beliefs, desires, goals, or conventions. It could be seen as a universal, essentially biological property or quality of mind. Indeed, it claimed its explanatory power on precisely these grounds. Intelligence could explain performances on various tasks because it was seen as underlying those performances. Again, it was not the beliefs, goals, or strategies of a person but the quality of mind that made those beliefs, goals, and strategies possible. It was a more basic quality of the mind/brain. As we shall see, that is still a common view, and much research has gone into an attempt to find that elusive quality of the mind/brain.

But, do tests of intelligence measure some underlying quality of mind and thereby explain intelligent performance? Or do they simply, as I prefer to say, sample a domain of competence, thereby providing a *description* of a range of cognitive competence but not an *explanation* of how or why such competence would arise? To focus this question more sharply, do tests of intelligence give access to some underlying quality of mind that would explain a person's performance on cognitive tasks, or do they merely sample that competence in such a way as to give an indication of level of performance in a domain, but in no way explain that level of competence?

There is no doubt that some people reliably perform at a high level on IQ tests and that performance on these tests correlates with, "predicts," if you like, performance on other tasks. In the simplest case, IQ predicts reading comprehension. But why? What are these tests measuring? A basic quality of the mind that makes learning to read easy? Or a sample of a specialized use of language common to both tests of intelligence and tests of reading. If it is the first, the IQ test would explain the good or poor reading competence; if the latter, it is simply a sample of the good or poor reading competence itself. In that case, it would provide a description of the poor reading but not an explanation for that level of reading competence. An explanation of why someone was a good reader would have to be sought elsewhere — in the knowledge, strategies, and goals of the reader, for example.

This is the construct validity problem: What do tests of intelligence measure? Do they sample and thereby describe, or do they explain? One way to answer that question is to look more closely at the questions that are central to IQ tests and attempt to reconstruct the processes that go on in their solution. Instead of adding to the earlier views of intelligence, this strategy yields a completely new conception of intelligence, a view of intelligence that is represented in the work of Piaget (1950) and in the recent work in cognitive science.

Before we consider an alternative to the "quality of mind" view, let us briefly examine two of the kinds of questions that can be used to measure intelligence.

Consider the question, "I have two coins. Together they make 55 cents. One of them is not a nickel. What are they?" You may have failed such an item. Failure, I hesitate to mention, indicates lower IQ, lower creativity, lower open-mindedness. (This test item, as I recall, was used by Milton Rokeach to measure closed-mindedness but it measures everything else as well.) But you should not be too alarmed. Failing it does not prove, or even provide evidence, that you have a propensity toward being dull, rigid, or banal. However, failure may indicate that you are not highly sensitive to the function of the pronoun "one" in the above question. If you read (understood) the second sentence as, "Neither of them is a nickel," you will get the question wrong. If you read "one of them" strictly, you will realize that whereas one of them is not a nickel, the other one could be a nickel, and the problem is solved. Most people are neither knowledgeable about, nor interested in, such subtle linguistic distinctions. People vary greatly in vocabulary and in sensitivity to linguistic nuance and implicature – those features, as I shall argue, that tests of intelligence are particularly attuned to.

For another example, consider one of the test items made famous by Luria (1976). He asked unschooled subjects in a traditional society "test" questions of the following sort: "In the Far North, where there is snow, all bears are white. Novava Zemlya is in the Far North and there is always snow there. What color are the bears there?" Like young schoolchildren in our society, these subjects frequently replied to the effect, "I don't know. There are many sorts of bears." When pressed to pay particular attention to the wording of the question, one subject replied: "Your words can be answered only by someone who was there, and if a person wasn't there he can't say anything on the basis of your words" (pp. 108–109). Such answers are perfectly reasonable, but they violate one of the canons of literacy, namely, that there is a strict relationship between a "text" and the interpretation that one is to assign to it. The subject in this case failed to treat the story as an autonomous text, to see, we may say, that language is an object about which one can be asked questions. Again, it involves a particular orientation to language and texts.

Just because such test questions reflect orientation to and sensitivity to particular aspects of language, some writers have concluded that performance on these verbal questions is at best of minor significance. Admittedly, they do not reflect an absence of rationality or an inability to draw inferences or an inability to comprehend texts as some theories of "primitive thought" have argued. Yet, the distinctions on which such questions are based are extremely important to many forms of intellectual activity in a literate society.

It is easy to show that sensitivity to the subtleties of language are crucial to some undertakings. A person who does not clearly see the difference between an expression of intention and a promise or between a mistake and an accident, or between a falsehood and a lie, should avoid a legal career or, for that matter, a theological one. A person who does not see the oddity of: "I *know* you'll change your mind," should, perhaps, avoid a career in logic or linguistics. A person who does not clearly see the difference between an explanation and a description should avoid a career in science. That is to say, tests that measure sensitivity to nuance of meaning, at least to nuance of meaning in important conceptual domains, have predictive power. Their measurement has practical significance to a domain of activity.

But this fact does not help us with the construct validity problem. Tests may have predictive power either by sampling the domain or by detecting some underlying quality that explains that level of performance. Traditionally, intelligence is not taken simply as a description of what one does well; it is taken as an explanation of *why* one does well. Why did you fail the item about the coins mentioned above? Because, the story goes, you are less intelligent than someone who passed it. It is at this point that the concept of intelligence has become seriously misleading.

Because measures of "intelligence" have been shown to be highly related to certain competencies valued by the society, test performance is used as the basis for judgments as to the educability of children and the employability and promotability of adults. When the concept of intelligence carries the extra, and in my judgment, unwarranted, implication of indicating an underlying quality of mind, it may be overvalued relative to the actual levels of competence achieved at work or at school and in this case may be individually and socially harmful. That is, it may be used to exclude people from an education or from jobs rather than as an indication of what education and training is required. And as a by-product, the tests lose their predictive value; a sample of performance will be a better predictor than a general IQ test score.

To summarize this point, as a *description* of the performances of people on a wide variety of these somewhat special tasks, the concept of intelligence is perfectly appropriate, indeed useful. As an *explanation* of that variability, it is vacuous. It is as vacuous as an explanation as was Molière's famous explanation of the effects of sleeping potion; that is, sleeping potion makes people sleep because of its dormative properties. People perform well on IQ questions, it is said, because they have high intelligence. One can break this circularity only by finding some quality of mind/brain that lies outside the sampled performance, an enterprise that has been conspicuously unsuccessful, or by changing or at least redirecting the concept of intelligence significantly. As we shall see, "intelligence" in the hands of both Piaget and artificial intelligence theorists has gone for the latter, and thereby provides quite a different form of explanation of complex cognitive activity.

Before we consider that alternative, let us consider two current theories of intelligence, one of which is an extreme form of the traditional view of intelligence, that of Jensen (1984), and the other of which appears to stand halfway between the traditional and the Piagetian/cognitive science view, that of Sternberg (1984). Jensen argues that variability in test performance is to be explained by appeal to variability in the basic mental mechanisms (assumed to be reliably measured by simple reaction times). Indeed, he goes one step further: "speed of elemental information processing may not be the most basic source of individual differences in intelligence but may be only a secondary phenomenon, derived from a still more basic source of individual differences – a hypothetical construct I have termed "neural oscillation" (p. 296). By this putative explanation, people with more rapid neural oscillations, a purely biochemical property of the nervous system, benefit more from experience. IQ is taken to be an underlying quality of the mind/brain.

Lost to such a theorist is the possibility that a subject's speed or skill on elementary tasks, such as letter recognition, or search through a memory set for a specified letter, may itself simply be further samples of the performances that the tasks were designed to explain. That is, people who are fast, or competent, in interpreting texts, may be fast, or competent, on any constituent task that makes up that competence: recognizing a word, identifying a letter, comparing a letter or word or phrase against a set stored in memory, and the like. One may measure reading speed by determining how long it takes an individual to read a whole book, a page, a sentence, a word, or a letter. Rather than get outside the domain and thereby explain skill in that domain, such tests, I suggest, merely take smaller and smaller samples of that domain. Again, that is not to say that it is unimportant to find out what activities are constituents of complex activities and thereby may serve as samples of those complex activities; it is only to say that such tasks never get outside that domain to tap some underlying "quality of mind" that would explain those performances.

Lost, too, in such a theory is the possibility that biologically based in-dividual differences, if and when they are isolated, may consist of predis-positions to certain ideas, beliefs, strategies or procedures, rather than to simple quality of mind differences. As more explicit theories of intelligence develop, primarily under the impact of artificial intelligence, it seems more and more difficult to think of these differences in any other terms. As C. S. Pierce once noted, people seem predisposed to have ideas that are true. Perhaps some people are more so predisposed than others. This is quite a different assumption than the general quality-of-mind assumption.

Even theories that are dramatically more sensitive to the uses of the mind in various cultural contexts, such as the recent elaborate theory proposed by Sternberg (1984), never quite abandon the notion that intelligence is at bottom an underlying quality of mind that explains performance in a variety of tasks. Although the major focus of Sternberg's work is on the structure of intellectual tasks, particularly that of analogies, and so falls into what I shall describe presently as an explanatory theory, he assumes that these structures must come from somewhere and that people must vary in their ability to make up and manipulate structures. Thus Sternberg assumes, like Jensen, that "intelligence" is a personal quality of mind, a trait, which differs importantly from individual to individual, which is prior to and independent of experience, learning, and achievement, and which thereby causes and explains variation in human competence. It consists, he says, of "the *ability* to deal with novel . . . demands" and "the *ability* to automatize information processing" (p. 279, emphasis added). Thus, although the vehicles by means of which one measures these "abilities" will need to differ across social groups, he argues that the underlying mechanisms to be measured are com-mon to all groups. A theory of intelligence, Sternberg says, is concerned with how individuals vary, not in their mechanisms and functions, for these are universal, but in their *abilities* with these mechanisms and functions. These *abilities* ultimately explain differences in intelligence. Leaving aside the latent circularity of explaining abilities by appealing to still other abilities, Sternberg's fundamental assumption is clear and identical to that of Jensen: Intelligence is a quality of mind, the quantity of which differs from individual to individual, which explains intelligent actions.

But even if this assumption is shared by laypersons and intelligence theor-ists, it suffers from three weaknesses. First, there is no good reason to believe that it is true. LCHC (1982) expresses doubts about the possibility of even understanding intelligence, let alone measuring it, without a deep analysis of the cultural practices in which people participate. Second, it leads researchers to confuse descriptions with explanations so as to treat samples of intellectual performance as explanations of that performance. Third, the search for that particular underlying (explanatory) quality has diverted attention from the structure and development of the full range of intellectual competencies that are personally fulfilling, which are socially useful, which may be acquired through education and practice, and which may be refined to high levels of expertise.

Intelligence as an explanatory concept: Piaget and cognitive science

The attempt to formulate a genuinely explanatory theory of intelligence has not been completely neglected. Piaget simply abandoned the search for intelligence, construed as an underlying quality of mind. He viewed intelligence as the system of schemes or structures of mind deployed in thought and action. Although intelligence presupposes biological structures and an environment in which to operate, it was for Piaget basically interactive. No basic quality of mind was postulated to explain the degree to which one benefits from experience or even the level of competence one could achieve. Intelligence is simply the assembly of mental structures used in coping with the physical and social world, and intelligence develops through a series of quite fundamental reorganizations of cognitive structure. Intelligence is the set of structures for doing things; it is not something that underlies or makes possible the acquisition of those structures. Again, intelligence is not the ability to reorganize cognitive structures – it is those reorganized cognitive structures. Intelligence is not the *ability* to assimilate and accommodate – it is that assimilation and accommodation. Intelligence is not the ability to automatize (restructure) procedures – it is those automatized procedures.

As in Piagetian theory, recent work in cognitive science and artificial intelligence attempts to explain a range of intelligent performances by specifying the rules and representations underlying those performances. Thus, the more recent analyses of cognitive tasks into the structures and procedures that subjects use in solving those tasks, whether in the work of Piaget (1950), Case (1985), or Sternberg (1984), provide explanations of those performances. So too, Ellen Bialystok and I attempted to explain children's and adults' performances on a large variety of spatial tasks by finding the set of mental representations and operations that could most economically account for their spatial perceptions and spatial judgments (Olson & Bialystok, 1983).

A theory of intelligence explains mental activities if it specifies the representations (roughly, beliefs) and the rules for operating on those representations that subjects use in answering questions, making judgments, solving problems, and so on. One also explains individual differences in such a theory by noting the presence or absence of a particular representation, a special set of relationships among those representations, or a different set of rules for operating on those representations. But, one does not add to the theory an additional *ability* to make up representations. The theory has to stand on its own feet, so to speak. Recall that it was precisely on this point that I criticized Sternberg for adding "intelligence" as an explanation of where these representations come from – he claiming that intelligence lies behind these structures, me claiming that intelligence is those structures.

This same point is made in theories of artificial intelligence. There the question is framed: What makes a system intelligent? McCarthy (1979), for example, argues that a computer is intelligent when it operates on the basis of beliefs and goals, when it alters means in the course of seeking those goals, when it alters beliefs in the light of new information, and when it subordinates beliefs to one another. Intelligence is a way of characterizing a system in which actions and decisions are based on beliefs, plans, and goals. The more beliefs, the better organized, efficiently used and so on, the more intelligent the system. Intelligence, then, is the structure of the beliefs, and so forth, and not something that putatively lies behind those beliefs. Again, intelligence is explained by finding the sets of beliefs and goals of the machine, the structure of knowledge, and the operations applied to that knowledge.

Gardner (1983) too has argued against the view that there is a single quality of mind called intelligence and has offered in its place the view that there are a number of distinctive ways in which one can be highly skilled. These forms of competence, or "intelligences," reflect the degree of mastery of the distinctive forms of symbolic systems evolved and exploited by a culture as means for representing and acting on the world. The task for a theory of intelligence, in this view, is to characterize the structure, development, and education of those forms of competence.

What are those major forms of competence? I shall try to characterize two such general and practical forms of intelligence.

Literacy, language, and thought

If IQ tests sample a domain, as I have argued, just what domain is it that they sample? And why is that sample representative of a sufficiently large and important set of cognitive activities to warrant their use in such a broad range of contexts? In what follows, I shall develop the argument that intelligence tests sample precisely those aspects of linguistic competence that are associated with literacy. Writing is one of the technologies that help make up Popper's "World Three," and literate competence is one of the ways in which the mind is specialized to deal with that technology. The question is whether we can trace some of the properties we usually associate with ability in general and verbal ability in particular to the characteristics of written language.

During the past two decades, an enormous amount of progress has been made in understanding the differences between speech and writing, on one hand, and the cultural institutions that have grown up with each of them. I shall review the high points of this increased understanding and then consider some of the ways that the specialized uses of language associated with literacy are the very competencies we take as marks of intelligence.

The first of these differences has come from detailed study of the structure and uses of language in an oral society, a society that relies primarily on human memory for the storage and retrieval of knowledge, as opposed to a literate society that relies on written records for those purposes. Obviously, in the latter, increased emphasis falls on such cognitive activities as reading and writing, study, translation, and interpretation, as well as on explicit forms of organization of knowledge through lists, indexes, encyclopedias, and dictionaries.

So which cognitive processes are encouraged by the uses of oral language in an oral society and which by written language in a literate society? Although this work is the product of many scholars, including Parry (1971), Lord (1960), McLuhan (1962), Goody and Watt (1963) and others, the cognitive implications of these developments have been described most clearly by Havelock (1963, 1973). Speech which has been shaped by the requirements of auditory memory, Havelock calls *poetized* speech. But these requirements put a bias on the sorts of things that can be said and remembered. The syntax of memorized rhythmic speech permits some kinds of statements and discourages others. Definitions, logical principles, and statements of causes are not easily generated in oral contexts nor readily remembered; even now, children who are required to memorize such things have to develop alphabetic mnemonics to handle them. Rather, oral tradition is compatible with the types of statements we call "sayings." Havelock says:

Neither principles nor laws nor formulas are amenable to a syntax which is orally memorizable. But persons and events that act or happen are amenable. . . . Orally memorized verse [such as the Homeric epic poems] is couched in the contingent: it deals in a panorama of happenings, not a program of principles. (1973, p. 51)

In this way, Havelock is able to account for at least part of the characteristics of the Homeric epic tradition and for the abrupt change in the patterns of language and thought that replaced the Homeric tradition at the time of the literate, classical Greeks. The invention and wide deployment of writing, Havelock argued, gave classical Greek culture the qualities it retains to this day:

For the first time the governing word ceases to be a vibration heard by the ear and nourished in the memory. It becomes a visible artifact. . . . The documented statement, persisting through time unchanged, is to release the human brain from certain formidable burdens of memorization while releasing the energies available for conceptual thought. The results as they are to be observed in the intellectual history of Greece and of Europe were profound. (p. 60)

Literacy, then, inaugurated a series of changes in the orientation to and uses of language. The formulation of documented statements, the organization of such statements into prose text, the elaboration of literary genres including those of science, philosophy, and theology were all tied to the development of literacy. With specialized forms of language came specialized attitudes to language, truth, rationality, and logic. Havelock argues that Plato's *Republic* was in part an attack upon the oral poetic tradition. The literate Greeks came to prefer the sorts of statements we call rational or logical to poetic ones. Such statements substituted general principles for dramatic happenings.

With a change in language from poetic to prosaic comes a change in the uses of intellect. The primary intellectual activity is no longer memory for the information embodied in oral, poetic forms, but rather the study, analysis, and interpretation of both texts and nature. And rather than inviting participation in an oral form, it invites reflection and analysis of an objective written form.

The classical literate tradition was essentially lost with the fall of the Roman Empire and had to be rediscovered and recovered in the later Middle Ages and the Renaissance. In his careful study of the growth of literate practices in the later Middle Ages, Stock (1983) points out that the techniques of analysis developed for the interpretation of Scripture were directly applicable to the interpretation of the natural world. Categories like the real and the apparent, the form and its meaning, the text and its interpretation, were used equally for understanding the sacraments and for understanding the natural world: "The interest in empirical reality already evident in discussions of the sacrament was consequently supported by a genuine appreciation of science" (Stock, 1983, p. 318).

But the techniques and the conceptual categories for the interpretation of written texts are not identical to those implicated in oral memory. The model of conceptual analysis that evolved in the later Middle Ages and continues to this day, is written language: "Analogies from written, i.e., learned, language occur [frequently]. Elements . . . are like letters, that is, the indivisible parts of syllables" (p. 319). "Reason," one such early writer said, "is to be sought in all things." Yet, as Stock comments, his reason "is inseparable from the logical, linguistic and meaningful relations of texts." (p. 320).

It is not only the studies of cultural change by the classicists that have contributed to our understanding of the ways that literacy altered both language and patterns of thought but also the parallel studies conducted by philosophers, linguists, and psychologists.

In hermeneutics, the systematic study or theory of the interpretation of written texts, Ricoeur (1981) has presented arguments that the interpretation of written texts is fundamentally different from the comprehension of speech in two ways. The world referred to in speech, the immediate contextual world, becomes, in written texts, the world of texts, of literature. Second, the relationship between speaker and utterance is altered in writing, for in writing, the author is separated from the text and, in a sense, is merely the first reader. As a result, in dealing with written texts, Ricoeur argues, one acquires both an altered conception of the world and an altered conception of language. For example, the interpretation of a text involves more than simply the recovery of the intention of the writer, whereas in speech such recovery would be perfectly adequate.

Recall Luria's anecdote about the white bears. The question is really a literate one. It treats the question and answer as part of a text – the answer must be formulated by appealing to the text. The "naive" answer comes from treating the question as if it were simply a conversational, oral, one. With writing, the text comes to be treated as an autonomous representation of meaning: "A text is really a text only when it is not restricted to transcribing an anterior speech, when instead it inscribes directly in written letters what the discourse means" (Ricoeur, 1981, p. 146).

In linguistic studies of literacy, Chafe (1985) has shown that the linguistic structure of written statements generated by contemporary speakers of English tends to be grammatically complex and informationally dense relative to the oral utterances of the same speakers. In my own cognitive psychological research, I have provided some evidence that the important conceptual distinctions between what is said and what is meant by it, between what is given and what is interpreted, and between what one knows and what is "known" are either directly or indirectly related to literate as opposed to oral conversational competence (Olson, 1977; Olson & Torrance, 1983; Olson & Astington, 1986; Olson, in preparation).

The point of such analyses is to make clear that verbal competence as reflected in oral conversational language and in oral poetic tradition is quite different from verbal competence in the comprehension and analysis of written texts. The primary qualities of mind required for the latter are an enormously extended vocabulary, commonly known as a reading vocabulary, mastery of a set of complex grammatical forms involving devices for subordination of clauses, and organization of sentences into higher-order structures such as paragraphs, essays, and the like, and the systematic application of such argument categories as claims versus evidence, facts versus theories, observations versus inferences, and statements versus interpretations. These devices characterize the production and comprehension of written texts, but they are also more general tools of thought.

Third, the use of writing to formulate statements and to revise them in the light of further discoveries makes written texts instruments for the progressive accumulation of knowledge (Eisenstein, 1979). It is these accumulated bodies of organized knowledge that contrast so conspicuously with the lack of generalizability of problem solutions in traditional societies (Goodnow, 1976; Greenfield, 1972; Scribner & Cole, 1973). Knowledge can accumulate in a unique way in a literate society; so while knowledge evolves, the human organism remains much the same. Not only does knowledge evolve, but instruments for the construction, storage, and retrieval of that knowledge change. To be intelligent is to have access to both the technologies and to these accumulated bodies of knowledge.

Admittedly, once developed for the drafting and analysis of written texts, and marked in the vocabulary and grammar of the language, literate concepts may occur in both writing and in speaking. One mark of a "literate" person is that the concepts of significance for the analysis of texts are applied to everyday experience – to interpret social interactions (Schroter, 1985), for example. And children from literate families will be more likely to pick up and apply such distinctions and the corresponding linguistic forms. Finally, it is competence with just those specialized linguistic forms that is taken as an indication of intelligence.

Literacy and tests of intelligence

I have discussed the application of one technology, alphabetic writing systems, to the invention of categories for interpreting language and for interpreting nature, and I have tried to indicate how this specialized form of written language contributed to the cognitive characteristics of abstraction and rationality that we take to be indicative of intelligence.

Intelligence tests differ from achievement tests in that the latter assess people's knowledge of that accumulated literate tradition. What, then, do intelligence tests measure? Not the knowledge itself, but the categories or concepts used for constructing and operating on those systematic bodies of knowledge – definitions of terms, semantic relationships between synonymous and antonymous terms, inference and interpretation. Far from being ordinary language processes, these are the catgories and relationships required for dealing with written, archival texts. The ability to cope with them indicates the degree of familiarity with that literate tradition.

One indication of the relationship between tests of intelligence and literacy is the well-known correlation mentioned earlier between IQ and reading scores. IQ tests are subtle tests of literacy. There is a similar radical cultural bias to all intelligence tests. The literate bias, that is, the reliance on competence with the specialized language of literacy, is seen most clearly in the most universal form of tests of intelligence, namely, the vocabulary test.

Vocabulary tests make a series of literate assumptions (see Watson & Olson, in press). First, those tests assume the existence of a metalinguistic notion of a word. Some time ago, Goody and Watt (1963) showed that in a traditional society there is no concept of a word as a linguistic unit. But the question "What does the word, *jump* mean?" presupposes the concept of a word. Furthermore, the question presupposes a concept of meaning: "What does it mean?" Meaning is also a metalinguistic concept. Second, *mean* is a verb that takes a word for its subject rather than a speaker for its subject in these definition questions. In other words, it asks the question, "What does *it* mean?," not "What do *you* mean?" Again, it involves a highly metalinguistic form of analysis. Third, the form of the definition is not conversational, as would be the case if one were merely soliciting information. Rather, it requires a particular linguistic frame, an equative verb of being, *is*, and a syntactic formula, *NP* is *NP*. That this is not a natural linguistic form is suggested by the following exchange reported by Watson (1982):

Teacher: What's a lullaby?
Child 1: It puts you to sleep.
Teacher: But what *is* it?
Child 2: It's a song.
Teacher: Right.

Such dialogues suggest that vocabulary test performance is a rather direct reflection of a literate attitude to language, an attitude expressed by such metalinguistic terms as say, mean, and the like, a form of competence carefully taught by teachers and by literate parents.

Faced with such arguments, test makers and intelligence theorists have for years attempted to circumvent cultural bias to find some more direct indication of "intelligence." But even such nonlinguistic tests as the Raven's Matrices are hopelessly culturally biased and highly related to tests of literacy. Why? One possibility is that the Raven's requires the same analytical rules, rules for analysis, coding, and transforming relationships required by the analysis of texts.

The notion of a culture-free measure of intelligence, we may note, is based on the presupposition we considered at the beginning of this paper, namely, that intelligence is a quality of mind that lies behind any skilled performance. I argued then that rather than lying behind competence, such tests simply sampled competence. Now, we can add, by and large, they sample literate competence.

Brain, technology, and intellect

What is the contribution of the brain to literate competence? Intellectual competencies are achieved by coupling impressive but limited biological resources with technologies which have been invented to circumvent those limitations. An ability is the product of resource plus artifact. Indeed, it is almost impossible to separate the two. What mathematics could a brain do without a number system? Mathematical ability is the ability to use the number system for a broad range of purposes. Verbal ability involves the use of language, primarily the language as specialized under the impact of writing, for a broad range of purposes. Changes in the technologies have the effect of making some of the possible uses of the mind irrelevant or obsolete. Oral memory based on assonance, rhyme, rhythm, a form of memory so important in an oral tradition, became largely irrelevant with the invention and exploitation of a written tradition. But written language placed a new set of possibilities and a new set of demands on the individual users, demands we may express with concepts such as interpretation, meaning, intention as well as a large set of speech act and mental state concepts.

We may state these relationships in a somewhat more radical way. Technologies of the intellect, as Goody (1977) calls them, are not simply external devices that may be exploited for cognitive purposes. Rather, the technologies are invented and elaborated to suit the biological structures of the mind. Even the most recent cultural inventions are inventions that must respect the cognitive structures of their users. Otherwise, they could not be learned and used. From this perspective, one may view the structures of cultural artifacts as explications of mind, as "the extensions of man" (McLuhan, 1962).

When symbol systems and technologies are viewed in this way, it becomes clear why intelligence tests do not measure an underlying ability but rather sample competence with these systems. The technologies already correspond to the basic psychological processes and categories that are available to the human nervous system. The only question is the degree to which any individual or group has learned to cope with the explicit representations of these forms of activity. They are learnable only because they correspond in some way to the basic structures of the mind. But the degree of competence an individual acquires with a technology depends upon such things as exposure, practice, and relevance as well as predisposition to that technology.

The task for psychologists and educators is to isolate the primary forms of competence that combine the resources of the mind with the most powerful technologies – literacy is the one of greatest generality in a literate society – to analyze the structure of that competence in terms of basic representations and operations, and to provide suggestions for how these competencies could be enhanced through education. The second task is to design, invent, and refine newer technologies that will bring a set of worthwhile goals within the reach of every member of the society.

Computers as tools of the intellect[2]

I have argued that intelligence is not simply a basic quality of mind but must be seen as a product of the relationship between the structures of mind and the properties of the "technologies of intellect." These technologies include the means for representing quantities by number systems, for representing spatial relationships by means of maps and diagrams, and representing language by means of writing and printing. In general, these symbol systems constitute the media of expression and communication (Eisner, 1982).

But if we are coming to see intelligence as a form of competence for dealing with literate artifacts, we may raise the question as to the forms of competence that are presupposed and that will be developed by our growing reliance on computer technologies. We may begin to answer this question by applying the principles we have used for examining the relationships between literacy and cognition to the problem of the relationships between computing and cognition.

We may differentiate two possible ways in which computers could alter the functions of the mind – first, through altering the knowledge base of the thinker, and second, through altering the operations that one could apply to that knowledge base. As we shall see, the problem does not come apart as simply as that, and yet these categories provide some access to the consequences of computing.

Alterations in the knowledge base

Literacy changed language from an ephemeral means of communication to a permanent, visible object, the written word. Once the written word is seen as an object, the spoken word can also be treated as an object. What are the properties of this object? Writing preserves the wording, what is "said," but it does not preserve the "meaning"; the meanings and intentions of the speaker or writer are left behind, so to speak. Preserving language as an object raises what we may call the problem of interpretation – problems of unresolvable ambiguity, of intended meaning, alternative interpretations, the question of whether one means what one says. Attempts to solve these problems call for strict attention to the very words and their "literal meanings" and for the elaboration of concepts and terms to distinguish these meanings. Mental state concepts such as *intend, interpret*, and *infer* come to be distinguished, as do speech act concepts such as *assert, claim, state*, and *declare*.

The evolution of a literate tradition involved the invention of these concepts, and the preservation of a literate society requires competence in the application of these conceptual distinctions to the problems of interpreting both oral and written language. Not only must people be able to distinguish what was said from its possible interpretations, they must recognize the residual ambiguity of most language, exploiting it in some forms of talk and writing such as poetry and minimizing it in others, such as scientific prose.

The difficulty children have in differentiating what is said from the interpretations one may make of it is clearly illustrated in the sorts of communication games studied by Robinson and Robinson (1982) and by Robinson, Goelman, and Olson (1983). Children appear not to recognize that the interpretation they assign to a sentence may be different from what another person assigns to it. Children tend to assume that others will assign the same interpretations and make the same inferences that they themselves make when they hear or see something.

The recognition of the ambiguity of language – its openness to interpretation – is not something that is recognized by preliterate children nor is it recognized, apparently, in at least some nonliterate societies. In his remarkable work on witchcraft and oracles of the Azande, Evans-Pritchard (1937) commented on these problems of interpretation: "Anything that a suspected witch may say is interpreted in a different sense from the one he intended to give to his words" (p. 133). Evans-Pritchard was surprised that these "interpretations" were attributed directly to the speaker and used to prove his guilt. Clearly, these were not interpretations in a literate sense – they were not thought of as having been made up by the hearer as we would think of them. Rather, any interpretation invented by the listener was ascribed to the speaker. The Azande interpret language just as any language user does, but they do not differentiate their interpretations from what the speaker actually said or intended.

This is just the problem that children in our society have with the ambiguity of language. They assume that the intention or interpretation is exactly what the speaker said. When they arrive at an interpretation, they are convinced that the sentence could not be interpreted any other way (Beal & Flavell, 1984).

These conceptual distinctions are not only useful for interpreting texts; they are extremely important in understanding a speaker's or agent's intentions relative to their utterances or actions and they are extremely important to adopting what may be called a theoretical stance toward nature. Yet, the distinction itself is rooted in literacy, as I have recently attempted to show (Olson, in preparation).

What about computers and knowledge? Computing appears not to displace these conceptual distinctions but rather to impose them more severely. In writing, it is extremely important to recognize that what a sentence means may be different from what a writer means by it and then to shape up what is said so that it is an accurate and explicit representation of meaning or intent. If explicitness of meaning is important to writing, it is absolutely central to computing. Computers can only "decode" the meaning already explicit in the text; they cannot "interpret" that text. All the required interpretations must be explicitly marked in the program. Ambiguous statements are not computable.

Can this requirement of explicitness have an effect on cognition? It is reasonable to expect that it will help provide a clearer line between what is represented in the language and what is added by the reader or listener in creating an interpretation of that representation. A clear understanding of that distinction would permit programmers, writers, and speakers to tailor their utterances so that they are less open to interpretation. It would promote a high degree of explicitness of expressions. This is a possibility that could be examined empirically.

Computers impose the distinction between what a text says and the interpretations one assigns to it with a vengeance. A good deal of work in computer science has gone into designing computers that can cope with these problems of interpretation by providing a rich context for the sentences encountered. Theories of "scripts" and "frames" are such attempts. But a computer cannot come up with personal, subjective, and private interpretations – only wrong ones. A computer deals only with formal, explicit representations and operations on those representations even if the context for interpretation is extremely elaborate.

Computers provide an interesting and promising way of helping children to deal with the problem of ambiguity in language. Adults know that computers do not interpret, they only decode; computers do not make the unwarranted inferences and extrapolations ordinarily made by humans. One solution, the one pursued in artificial intelligence, is to make the computers more "intelligent" by building in a richer knowledge base to guide interpretation. The other solution is to equip people, including children, to make their meanings more explicit and less open to interpretation or misinterpretation. Computers provide immediate feedback as to how an instruction is interpreted. Hence, computers set a new standard of explicitness that anyone dealing with a computer soon discovers. This is not an impossible standard. Recall that literacy has already taken us halfway toward the goal of making meanings fully explicit.

Can children be taught to recognize the distinction between what is actually said and the interpretation they tend to assign more readily in dealing with a computer than they would in dealing with a human being? Although children readily assume that others see, hear, infer, and interpret in the same way that they do and have difficulty seeing that others could come up with a different interpretation, will they make that assumption about computers? It seems reasonable to suppose that computers do not invite the assumption of equivalence with other minds that human interlocutors do. But that hypothesis could be investigated. My hunch is that children will not, at least not as readily, assume that computers will make the same inferences and interpretations that they themselves do and that they usually ascribe to other people. As a result, they will be thrown back upon what exactly was said, that is, what is explicitly represented in the language. Specifically, children may more readily blame the message in cases of communication failure when working with a computer than when working with another human. They will recognize that computers only decode what is there, not "read between the lines." Furthermore, the children's recognition that some messages are ambiguous when directed to the computer may transfer back in the recognition of ambiguity in their own speech and writing. Learning to use a computer, then, could contribute to a child's competence with an important conceptual distinction.

If the results from such an experiment are as predicted, we will know something both about computers and about children's understanding of language. In dealing with computers, as in dealing with literate language, children must learn to distinguish what is intended from what is actually expressed in the message and they must attempt to make what is intended fully expressed in the message or text. That is, computing is dependent on explicit language to an even greater degree than is writing. Second, we will know that children can be led to make this distinction more readily with computers. We may infer that they succeed more readily because they are not so prone to ascribe the same thoughts to computers that they do to themselves and others. Indeed, it may be the case that the immediacy and directness of feedback and the inability of the computer to "read" their intentions discourages children from ascribing any thoughts to computers whatsoever.

This suggestion bears on that advanced by Turkle (1984) in her popular book on computers and children, in which she suggests that working with computers leads children to ascribe mental states both to computers and to themselves. My suggestion is that children will quickly realize that computers cannot "interpret" or read between the lines or entertain any other subjective mental states. Far from enhancing notions of subjectivity, computers may eradicate them altogether. Alternatively, the absence of such states in computers may lead children to an awareness of their own in their attempts to make expressions unambiguous.

Alterations in cognitive operations

As to the mental operations that computers may enhance, it is important to notice that computers are not "tools of the intellect" in the same sense as writing was and is. Computers are "intelligent" in their own right. The potential impact of computers on cognition lies, in fact, on coupling the resources of the mind with the resources of the computer.

Which aspects of intellectual competence can be assigned to the computer? We can get some indications by reconsidering the impact of literacy on cognition.

With literacy, the function of memory has been altered from an exclusive concern with preservation of content to a concern with organization and retrievability. One has simply to recall how the development of libraries and indices for collecting and locating information changed this primary cognitive function. Of course, memory is involved in both an oral and a literate society. But in a literate society, the emphasis falls on knowledge of the logical structure of information as that is crucial to locating information; hierarchically related categories become more important than the episodic, narrative memory for events. Secondly, the archival resources of a library are much greater than those of a traditional wise man; what is known is vastly greater than what any individual knows.

It appears that just as literacy reorganized and extended memory, so computers extend the organization of planned action far beyond what any mind could do. Our society has succeeded in putting an enormous amount of information and much of the organization of planned action into the environment, some of it in the form of computer programs. In doing so, our culture and technology permit us to put a man on the moon and run complex social and economic programs.

Almost any form of human competence is a joint product of the resources of the mind and the potentials of those technologies. Almost any form of human cognition requires one to deal productively and imaginatively with some technology. To attempt to characterize intelligence independently of those technologies seems to be a fundamental error. To use a technology to achieve any particular goal, you may either elaborate the competencies of the user or elaborate the technology so that it is employable with limited human competencies. To refer to our earlier example, if the computer requires it, one can learn to program, write, and speak more explicitly. Alternatively, if the demands are too formidable, one can alter the technology to compensate for the limited resources of the user. But neither the properties of the computer nor the properties of the mind are fixed entities; they are interdependent. Technological invention is a major way of finding out the, as yet undetermined, properties of the mind.

As to our more limited concerns with children's cognition and its relationship to the growing use of computers in the schools and in society at large, even "user-friendly" computers require a degree of explicitness in language that is vastly greater than that involved in ordinary conversational language. Computers never understand ambiguous utterances and they never read between the lines, whereas humans are extremely able to (or do) just that. In learning to deal with computers, children will learn to make their meanings fully explicit. This is a goal that is already pursued to a lesser extent in literate language. Computing, then, may require both a conception of ambiguity of messages and texts and a clear criterion for determining when the goal of explicitness of meaning has been achieved.

Seen from this perspective, computers simply raise, by an order of magnitude, the requirement of making meanings explicit that was begun by giving communication systems a semantics and by then making that semantics more explicit and elaborate through literacy. Far from being obsolete, literate competencies are basic to computational ones. To be intelligent in the society of computer users is to be skilled in making one's meanings explicit.

A summing up

If we are to forgo the simple assumption I have attacked above, namely, that intelligence is an underlying quality of mind that explains why some people are better at some tasks than are others, what role is left for a theory of intelligence? One is the theoretically modest but practically useful descriptive role I have discussed above. Types and levels of intelligence are purely descriptive notions that provide a general characterization of the performance one may expect in a broad range of tasks on the basis of sampling of one or two tasks in that domain. Criterion-referenced tests, in fact, do just this, but because they sample particular domains of knowledge rather than more general uses of literate language, they are useful for very restricted purposes. Intelligence tests measure a form of competence which is more general than that measured by any particular content-based test. What they measure, I have argued, is not a general quality of mind but competence with the specialized language tied to literacy – competence in carefully analyzing linguistic form, in recognizing nuance of word meaning, in making careful distinctions between what a text actually says and the interpretations assigned to it, and in generally treating language as autonomous representation of meaning.

These are not universal operations of the mind. They are operations required for dealing with a human-made artifact – written language. But just because they are not universal does not imply that their measurement is not valid or useful. They are valid measures of level or degree of competence with a particular cultural form, namely written language. And they are useful indicators of competence with the primary technology of a literate bureaucratic society. The best indication of how well someone will do in learning from, criticizing, and applying such information in a literate society is how well they are currently able to handle that information. Good tests accurately sample that current level of competence. Intelligence tests are misused only when test scores are overinterpreted to mean "quality of mind" and then valued above more direct measures of the more limited domain for which actual competence is required. Thus, IQ has been used to exclude people from educational opportunities from which they would benefit and from certain jobs that they are entirely capable of handling.

Because the tests do not assess "underlying ability," there is no value in trying to invent a test that is universally applicable or one that is "culture fair." The whole concept rests on a fundamental error. Intelligence is always directly tied to cultural technologies, in our case, to literacy. It is, therefore, impossible to test intelligence in other cultures unless we know more about their technologies. But once we recognize that quite different forms of competence are involved in dealing with radically different technologies, it becomes clear that we are unlikely to find anything in common across those competencies. To illustrate, if a test is designed to provide a good description of competence in an oral society, it is unlikely to have anything in common with a test designed to provide a good description of competence in a literate society. They are not, I have argued, both measures of an underlying, and common, intelligence.

What about biological predispositions to forms of literate competence? Admittedly, in our society, children's competence with these somewhat specialized linguistic skills may reflect an underlying predisposition to handle such language. But such predispositions, if they exist, are impossible to distinguish from the effects of varying degrees of exposure to and use of these somewhat specialized linguistic forms. For people from traditional societies, intelligence tests do not at all reflect those speaking and thinking practices; for children from less literate households, tests poorly represent those linguistic practices. Hence, intelligence tests do not apply across cultural groups, they correlate highly with social class, and performance is dramatically affected by schooling (Olson, 1970; Scribner & Cole, 1981). Yet some may think it possible and interesting to attempt to devise means to detect underlying predispositions. That is not outside the realm of possibility. But, as I have emphasized, it is incorrect to assume that existing measures of intelligence assess these underlying abilities.

There is an alternative to the "underlying quality of mind" view of intelligence. I have argued that an appropriately formulated theory of intelligence could indeed explain high-level cognitive processes. It would do so by following on the leads of Piaget and recent work in the cognitive sciences. Explanations come from specifying the structures of beliefs and knowledge and the procedures used for operating on those structures which are held by "intelligent systems," whether human, animal, or mechanical.

Theories of intelligence have in the past discredited themselves by claiming too much. If they are seen as sampling particular domains of competence, much as any achievement test does, they can usefully describe levels of competence valued by a society. Our understanding of the full range of such competencies depends, not on finding a common general factor, but on characterizing the structure of complex cognitive activities involved in exploiting the possibilities of the symbols and technologies evolved and used in different cultures and social groups.

Notes

1. Preparation of this chapter was supported by grants from The Spencer Foundation and from the Social Sciences and Humanities Research Council of Canada.
2. An early vision of this section has been published separately under this title in *Educational Researcher*, May 1985.

References

Beal, C., & Flavell, J. (1984). Development of the ability to distinguish communicative intention and literal message meaning. *Child Development, 55*, 920–928.

Case, R. (1985). *Intellectual development: Birth to adulthood*. New York: Academic.

Chafe, W. (1985). Linguistic differences produced by differences between speaking and writing. In D. Olson, N. Torrance, A. Hildyard (Eds.), *Literacy, language and learning: the nature and consequences of reading and writing* (pp. 105–123). New York: Cambridge University Press.

Evans-Pritchard, E. (1937). *Witchcraft, oracles and magic among the Azande*. Oxford: Oxford University Press.

Eisenstein, E. (1979). *The printing press as an agent of change: Communications and cultural transformations in early-modern Europe*. New York: Cambridge University Press.

Eisner, E. (1982). *Cognition and curriculum*. New York: Longman.

Gardner, H. (1983). *Frames of mind: The theory of multiple intelligences*. London: Basic.

Goodnow, J. (1976). The nature of intelligent behavior: Questions raised by cross-cultural studies. In L. Resnik (Ed.), *The nature of intelligence* (pp. 169–188). Hillsdale, NJ: Erlbaum.

Goody, J. (1977). *The domestication of the savage mind*. Cambridge, England: Cambridge University Press.

Goody, J., & Watt, I. (1963). The consequences of literacy. *Comparative Studies in Society and History, 5*, 304–345.

Greenfield, P. (1972). Oral and written language: The consequences for cognitive development in Africa, the United States and England. *Language and Speech, 15*, 169–178.

Havelock, E. (1963). *Preface to Plato*. Cambridge, MA: Harvard University Press.

Havelock, E. (1973) Prologue to Greek literacy. In C. Boulter (Ed.), *Lectures in memory of Louise Taft Semple, second series, 1966–1971* (pp. 329–391). Cincinnati: University of Oklahoma Press for the University of Cincinnati.

Jensen, A. (1984). Mental speed and levels of analysis. *The Behavioral and Brain Sciences, 7*, 295–296.

Laboratory of Comparative Human Cognition. (1982). Culture and intelligence. In R. Sternberg (Ed.), *Handbook of human intelligence* (pp. 642–719). Cambridge: Cambridge University Press.

Lord, A. (1960). *The singer of tales*. (Harvard Studies in Comparative Literature, 14.) Cambridge, MA: Harvard University Press.

Luria, A. (1976). *Cognitive development: Its cultural and social foundations*. Cambridge, MA: Harvard University Press.

McCarthy, J. (1979). Ascribing mental qualities to machines. In M. Ringle (Ed.), *Philosophical perspectives in artificial intelligence* (pp. 161–195). Atlantic Highlands, NJ: Humanities Press.

McLuhan, M. (1962). *The Gutenberg galaxy*. Toronto: University of Toronto Press.

Olson, D. (1970). *Cognitive development: The child's acquisition of diagonality*. New York: Academic.

Olson, D. (1977). From utterance to text: The bias of language in speech and writing. *Harvard Educational Review, 47*, 237–281.

Olson, D. (In preparation). *The world on paper*.

Olson, D., & Astington, J. (1986). Children's acquisition of metalinguistic and metacognitive verbs. In W. Demopoulos & A. Marras (Eds.), *Language learnability and concept acquisition* (pp. 184–199). Norwood, NJ: Ablex.

Olson, D., & Bialystok, E. (1983). *Spatial cognition: The structure and development of mental representations of spatial relations*. Hillsdale, NJ: Erlbaum.

Olson, D., & Torrance N. (1983). Literacy and cognitive development: A conceptual transformation in the early school years. In S. Meadows (Ed.), *Issues in childhood cognitive development* (pp. 142–160). London: Methuen.

Parry, A. (1971). *The making of Homeric verse*. A. Parry (Ed.), *The collected papers of Milman Parry*, Oxford: Oxford University Press.

Piaget, J. (1950). *The psychology of intelligence*. New York: Harcourt, Brace.

Popper, K. (1972). *Objective knowledge: An evolutionary approach*. Oxford: Oxford University Press.

Ricoeur, P. (1981). *Hermeneutics and the human sciences: Essays on language, action and interpretation*. New York: Cambridge University Press.

Robinson, E., & Robinson, W. (1982). Knowing when you don't know enough: Children's judgments about ambiguous information. *Cognition, 12*, 267–280.

Robinson, E., Goelman, H., & Olson, D. (1983). Children's understanding of the relation between expressions (what was said) and intentions (what was meant). *British Journal of Developmental Psychology, 1*, 75–86.

Schroter, C. (1985). *Differentiation of perception and inference: A sociocognitive competency*. Unpublished doctoral thesis, University of Toronto.

Scribner, S., & Cole, M. (1973). Cognitive consequences of formal and informal education. *Science, 182*, 553–559.

Scribner, S., & Cole, M. (1981). *The psychology of literacy*. Cambridge, MA: Harvard University Press.

Sternberg, R. (1984). Toward a triarchic theory of human intelligence. *The Behavioral and Brain Sciences, 7*(2), 269–287.

Stock, B. (1983). *The implications of literacy*. Princeton, NJ: Princeton University Press.

Turkle, S. The second self: Computers and the human spirit. New York: Simon and Schuster.

Vygotsky, L. S. (1962). *Thought and language*. Cambridge, MA: MIT Press.

Watson, R. (1982). *From meaning to definition: The development of word meaning in the school-aged child*. Unpublished doctoral thesis, University of Toronto.

Watson, R., & Olson, D. (in press). From meaning to definition: A literate bias on the structure of word meaning. In R. Horowitz & J. Samuels (Eds.), *Comprehending oral and written language*. New York: Academic.

15   The search for intraterrestrial intelligence

Richard K. Wagner

Accounts of the search for extraterrestrial intelligence (SETI) are prominent in the news. Professional and amateur scientists are observed to be speculating with excitement about important new questions. What is the probability that intelligent life exists elsewhere in our galaxy? In what direction should antennas be directed to maximize the probability of detecting radio waves from another planet? What frequencies should be monitored, and at what bandwidths? How will we recognize intelligent life?

Although not yet as newsworthy, the accounts presented in this volume of the search for "intraterrestrial intelligence" – the intellectual competencies required for handling worldly affairs – reveal a search that is in every way as challenging, exciting, and pioneering as that for intelligence in the Crab nebula. The challenge for researchers in practical intelligence is to understand and describe some of the complexities of intelligent performance in natural settings in a way that transcends a simple assemblage of vignettes of practically intelligent behavior, collected to be shared with one's colleagues as one might show a butterfly collection to a visitor. If our understanding of practical intelligence remains specific to an individual, a setting, and a moment in time, there is no hope of informing a theory of human intellectual competence.

The original search for intelligence began to pay off in a dramatic way with Binet's test for determining who was fit, intellectually, for a public school education. The close resemblance of the current crop of IQ tests to early revisions of Binet's test can be viewed as a tribute to the remarkable foresight of Alfred Binet, or as a disconcerting reminder of how little progress has been made subsequently in understanding and measuring intelligence. A point of view shared by contributors to this volume is that IQ tests measure, at best, only a subset of the intellectual competencies that laypersons and experts alike include in their conceptions of intelligence (Sternberg, Conway, Ketron, & Bernstein, 1981). This schism between what is meant by intelligence and what is measured by IQ tests is not new: Binet, the father of the IQ test, regarded intelligence as the collective faculties of practical sense, judgment, initiative, and the ability to adapt to one's circumstances (Binet & Simon, 1905, Chapter 8).

Each of the contributors to this volume has responded in a unique and informative way to the challenge of getting beyond IQ to an understanding of intelligent performance in natural settings that is sufficiently general to be able to contribute to our understanding of human cognitive functioning. The methods employed have at times been ingenious. Their conclusions about the nature of practical intelligence show a surprising amount of agreement and, to be sure, a fair amount of disagreement.

The purpose of this chapter is to identify some important questions for a psychology of practical intelligence and to illustrate alternative positions on the questions with one or two representative examples drawn from the chapters. This chapter is organized into four parts, each of which addresses in turn the following related questions. First, what is meant by the term practical intelligence? Second, what are viable approaches for understanding practical intelligence? Third, how can practical intelligence be measured? Fourth, what are some important questions for the future?

What is practical intelligence?

Outright attempts to define intelligence have never been particularly helpful, beginning with the time, in 1921, that the *Journal of Educational Psychology* asked seventeen leading researchers to define intelligence and got fourteen different answers and three nonreplies. On the other hand, working definitions often have heuristic value, and they can be informative about presuppositions associated with alternative research approaches. For these reasons, working definitions of practical intelligence will briefly be considered, before turning to a consideration of alternative views of the relations between practical and other kinds of intelligence.

Working definitions of practical intelligence

Definition by exclusion. One way to define practical intelligence is by exclusion, that is, by what it is not. Thus, practical intelligence is defined as intelligence that is not of the "academic" sort. A clear-cut example of an exclusionary definition of practical intelligence is provided by Frederiksen, who considers practical intelligence to be reflected in one's cognitive responses to almost everything that happens outside the school. Problems formally presented in school settings are characterized by being (1) well defined; (2) linear, in the sense of having but one correct solution and one method of obtaining it, (3) disembedded from an individual's ordinary experience and of little intrinsic interest; and (4) complete, in that all needed information is available from the start (Neisser, 1976; Wagner & Sternberg, 1985). Thus, a practically intelligent individual is one who is able to solve the ill-defined problems that arise naturally in daily life, for which there may be multiple solutions and multiple ways of obtaining them.

An advantage of the exclusionary approach is that with such a wide bandwidth, it is unlikely that an important aspect of practical intelligence will be excluded from consideration a priori. However, a working definition that defines by exclusion is rarely much help in deciding just what it is that one should study, and how to go about studying it. Frederiksen's pioneering work with the in-basket technique shows that such limitations need not be fatal. He presented various kinds of managers with a simulated situation chock-full of the kinds of ill-defined problems found on the job. Records of how a sample of the managers responded were analyzed qualitatively to determine categories of responses (e.g., asks for more information, delegates, asks supervisor for advice) to be used in scoring the responses of all the managers. The upshot of large-scale studies carried out with Air Force officers, government administrators, school principals, and medical students was that the performance of managers in situations that simulated the kinds of problems they faced on the job depended primarily upon two elements: knowledge of the problem domain, and ideational fluency, or the ability to make broad searches of long-term memory in order to retrieve relevant ideas and information.

If defining something by what it is not leaves one uneasy, how might practical intelligence be characterized further? Three representative attempts to get beyond exclusionary definitions will be considered.

Practical know-how. Berry and Irvine base their cross-cultural analysis on the concept of the *bricoleur* – a worker who accomplishes odd jobs through devious use and adaptation of whatever resources are at hand, in contrast to the more formal approach of the skilled craftsman and repairman who relies on technical manuals and tools. Their point is that practical knowhow can be found throughout the peoples of the world, including peoples who have been viewed by Western cultures as savages. Their review provides a useful compilation of examples of complex everyday intellectual behavior among diverse peoples, such as the discovery in the Biaka Pygmy people of a highly structured and systematic conceptual organization for their more than 300 medicinal uses of plants. Berry and Irvine argue that not only are such examples of practical know-how widespread, but that the abilities they represent meet the highest possible standard, that of the continuing adaptation and survival of the group. They view their task as documenting cross-cultural examples of practical know-how, and eventually, determining implications of the examples of practical know-how for the psychology of cognition more generally.

Wagner and Sternberg's analysis of *tacit knowledge* used by academic psychologists and business managers in their work-related judgment and decision-making is another example of viewing practical intelligence in terms of its manifestation as practical know-how. On their view, an important determinant of professional competence is acquiring tacit knowledge – knowledge that is not openly expressed or stated. Such knowledge serves in effectively managing oneself, one's tasks, and others. In a series of five experiments, level of tacit knowledge was found to vary across groups as a function of level of professional advancement. Furthermore, within-group differences in tacit knowledge were related to criterion measures of career competence for academic psychologists, business managers, and for graduate students in each domain.

An important task for those who study practical knowledge is to provide an explicit account of the relation between practical *know-how* and practical *intelligence*. Consider the case of IQ tests. Traditional IQ tests largely are tests of achievement for knowledge acquired over the past several years. By making certain assumptions about equal opportunity to learn, and equal familiarity with the test materials, individual differences in underlying abilities are *inferred* from individual differences in current levels of knowledge. Should differences in practical know-how, determined either on the basis of performance on Wagner and Sternberg's tacit-knowledge questions or from cross-cultural observations, be regarded as manifestations of underlying differences in relatively stable practical abilities, or do they have some other origin? Studies of the development of practical know-how are a first step toward answering this question.

Social judgment. Working definitions of practical intelligence differ from conceptualizations of academic intelligence in their emphasis on competence in dealing with others. In fact, for Mercer, Gomez-Palacio, and Padilla, practical intelligence is synonymous with social competence. They define social competence as the extent to which individuals meet the normative expectations that others have for persons playing their particular role in their particular group. Six kinds of social roles are described: family roles, community roles, peer roles, nonacademic school roles, earner/consumer roles, and self-maintenance roles. A wide variety of behaviors are included in a given social role. For example, family roles includes interpersonal skills in dealing with family members, on the one hand, and helping to repair family possessions, on the other. Mercer has developed a psychometric instrument for assessing the social-role performance of children called the Adaptive Behavior Inventory for Children (ABIC) (Mercer, 1979). The ABIC consists of a structured set of questions about a child's social role performance that are answered by the child's caretaker. That the ABIC is sampling something other than academic intelligence was demonstrated in Mercer, Gomez-Palacio, and Padilla's ambitious cross-cultural study involving nearly 2,000

Anglo, Chicano, and Mexican children, in which virtually no relationships were found between ABIC and scores on an IQ test (WISC–R).

Another striking characteristic of this massive set of data is that the intercorrelations among ABIC subtests suggest that social competence as measured by the ABIC is general to a wide variety of social roles. ABIC subtest intercorrelations ranged from .84 to .91, with a median of .89 for the Mexican sample ($N = 600$); .68 to .82, with a median of .76 for the Chicano sample ($N = 690$); and .63 to .80, with a median of .75 for the Anglo sample ($N = 699$). The absolute magnitude of these intercorrelations is probably inflated to some degree because they are based on samples ranging in age from 6 to 16 for the Mexican sample and 6 to 11 for the Chicano and Anglo samples, a fact reflected in the higher intercorrelations for the Mexican sample compared to the Chicano and Anglo samples. But the important point is that these intercorrelations are higher than those of the WISC–R subtests for the same samples, which suggests that variance in social role performance is largely accounted for by a single factor. Mercer, Gomez-Palacio, and Padilla point out that these data could be interpreted as support either for viewing social competence as a general underlying ability or for viewing social expectations as general across the social roles assessed.

Ford's view of practical intelligence also emphasizes social competence, although perhaps to a lesser degree than the view of Mercer, Gomez-Palacio, and Padilla. Ford considers practical intelligence to be embodied in the attainment of important transactional goals – goals dealing with effects outside the person. On the basis of the results of several studies employing methods such as asking students to describe the most socially competent child they knew and how important it was to obtain various goals by age 18, Ford suggests that practical intelligence involves skill at (1) establishing and maintaining social relationships, and (2) completing tasks, both of which rest on a foundation of personal well-being.

Prototypes of practical intelligence. Neisser (1979) has rejected the notion that it is possible to define practical intelligence as any one thing. Instead, he views the concept of intelligence in terms of Rosch's theory of concepts (Rosch, 1978; Rosch & Mervis, 1975; Rosch, Mervis, Gray, Johnson, & Boyes-Braem, 1976). On this view, one's practical intelligence is the extent to which one resembles the prototypically intelligent person. Two examples of the prototype approach will be described because their results are relevant to a working definition of practical intelligence.

Sternberg, Conway, Ketron, and Bernstein (1981) set out to determine people's implicit conceptions of intelligence. Laypersons and experts were asked to rate how characteristic 250 descriptors were of an "ideally" (1) intelligent person, (2) academically intelligent person, and (3) everyday intelligent person. Factor analysis of the laypersons' ratings of everyday intelligence for a subset of the descriptors yielded four interpretable factors: practical problem-solving ability, social competence, character, and interest in learning and culture. A factor analysis of the experts' ratings of everyday intelligence for a slightly different pool of items yielded three interpretable factors, two of which were identical to factors identified for the laypersons' ratings: practical problem-solving ability, practical adaptive behavior, and social competence. The similarity between the laypersons' and experts' conceptions of everyday intelligence was reflected in the correlation of .81 between the laypersons' and experts' ratings.

Ford and Miura (1983) employed similar methods to determine people's implicit conceptions of "social competence." Using cluster analysis of categories provided by university students for descriptors of a prototypically socially competent adult, four facets of people's conceptions of social competence were identified: prosocial skills (e.g., responds to the need of others), social-instrumental skills (e.g., knows how to get things done), social ease (e.g., enjoys social activities and involvement), and self-efficacy (e.g., has a good self-concept).

Relationships between practical and other kinds of intelligence

The traditional psychometric approach to measuring intelligence has to be viewed as one of the largest, and many would argue, one of the most successful undertakings in American psychology. There can be no doubt that (1) individuals differ in their skill at solving academic-type problems, (2) these individual differences can be reliably measured, and (3) these individual differences are general to a wide variety of academic tasks. An imporant issue, then, for researchers in practical intelligence is to determine how practical intelligence is related to academic intelligence. Relations proposed between practical intelligence and academic intelligence can be classified as one of two types: hierarchical and nonhierarchical.

Hierarchical views. Willis and Schaie provide an example of a hierarchical view of the relations between practical and traditional kinds of intelligence. They consider *traditional intelligence* to be those genotypic ability factors that are identified with the psychometric approach. Examples of genotypic ability factors include verbal reasoning and spatial relations. *Practical intelligence* is "the phenotypic expression of that combination of genotypic factors which, given minimally acceptable levels of motivation, will permit adaptive behavior within a specific situation or class of situations" (p. 240). Thus, Willis and Schaie (this volume) view practical intelligence as an everyday manifestation of an individual's underlying cognitive abilities of the sort one might measure with a standard IQ test.

This view differs from that of other contributors in at least one important way. If we assume that a formal classroom setting meets the criteria of being "a specific situation or class of situations," then perfomance at the task of say, spelling, would count as a manifestation of an individual's practical intelligence. Few would deny that practical intelligence is useful in academic settings for such things as devising test-taking strategies and allocating one's study time (see, e.g., Ford, this volume; Wagner & Sternberg, in press), but by Willis and Schaie's criteria, the very essence of performance on a spelling test is as good an example of practical intelligence as is finding one's way out of a forest after being lost. In addition, one might question the extent to which the factors commonly identified with the psychometric approach are genotypic in nature.

Drawing on Hebb (1949) and Vernon (1969), Berry and Irvine provide a model of the relations between cognitive processes, cognitive competence, and cognitive performance that is similar in its hierarchical nature to the views of Willis and Schaie. For Berry and Irvine, *cognitive processes* are biologically rooted mechanisms that are universal across cultures. When nurtured and directed by a particular culture, cognitive processes develop into *cognitive competencies*. Finally, *cognitive performances* are the manifestations of cognitive competencies that we observe in everyday life and in testing situations. These cognitive performances occur at culturally appropriate times and in culturally appropriate ways.

Nonhierarchical views. Nonhierarchical views are characterized by positing two or more kinds of intelligence, which may or may not be mutually exclusive, but which are equal in stature. Consider two examples.

In their approach to understanding practical intelligence, Walters and Gardner adopt Gardner's (1983) *multiple intelligences* framework, which proposes seven kinds of intelligence: musical, bodily-kinesthetic, logical-mathematical, linguistic, spatial, interpersonal, and intrapersonal. The intelligences are viewed as being independent and of equal stature. Each individual has some of each of the seven intelligences. An individual's profile of intelligences is determined by his or her particular innate endowment and the history of training.

A potential problem of the Walters and Gardner approach is deciding whether to stop at one, seven, or seventy intelligences. Gardner (1983) has attempted to deal with this problem by carefully specifying criteria that must be met for an intelligence to be identified. One criterion, which reflects the biological roots of the framework, is that the skill must be found in all cultures, although its specific manifestation is allowed to vary as a function of culture. So, for example, language meets the criterion even though it may be expressed as writing in one culture and oratory in another.

Mercer, Gomez-Palacio, and Padilla divide intelligence into two mutually exclusive categories: academic intelligence, which refers to abilities characterizing the internal world of the individual, and practical intelligence, which refers to one's ability at dealing with the external world of social structures and social interactions (see Sternberg, 1985, for a related conceptualization of internal and external worlds). However, Ford (this volume) cautions not to make too much of the academic versus practical distinction, believing they represent overlapping rather than mutually exclusive aspects of intelligence.

What are viable approaches for understanding practical intelligence?

Having decided which aspects of practical intelligence one wishes to examine, one is faced with the nontrivial task of deciding how to set about doing so. The approaches to understanding practical intelligence represented by the contributors are of three basic types: the ethnographic, the simulation-based, and the psychometric. Each of these three approaches will be considered briefly. In doing so, it will become apparent that what these approaches have in common, when applied to practical intelligence, is a capitalization on group differences. Groups are variously identified across the approaches on the basis of on culture, age, or level of expertise.

Ethnographic approaches

A good example of the ethnographic approach is provided by Berry and Irvine. Their review of a number of studies in anthropology and psychology on cognitive competence in everyday life represents a useful compilation of examples of practically intelligent behavior. What is especially important about their contribution, however, is their consideration of how one might ever relate cross-cultural examples of practically intelligent behavior to a general theory of cognitive functioning.

Berry and Irvine distinguish three levels of generality for intellectual performance. The most general level is that of *general intelligence*, at which intellectual performance is viewed in terms of a single pattern of abilities that is invariant across ecological (cultural) contexts (see, e.g., Irvine, 1979; Vernon, 1969). The least general level is that of *specific abilities*, at which patterns of abilities are viewed as specific to ecological contexts (see, e.g., Berland, 1983; Cole, Gay, Glick, & Sharp, 1971; Serpell, 1979). In between is the level of *cognitive styles*, at which a limited number of patterns of abilities is presumed to characterize performance across ecological contexts (see, e.g., Annis, 1980; Berry, 1976; van de Koppel, 1983). Berry and Irvine suggest that each of these levels may hold for different aspects of intellectual functioning.

Berry and Irvine's framework for conceptualizing how to inform a general theory of cognitive competence from examples of practically intelligent performance consists of a 2×2 matrix, containing rows corresponding to areas of cognitive functioning (e.g., reasoning), and columns corresponding to societies (e.g., European). Determining *universals* for areas of cognitive functioning is to be accomplished by integrating across rows. Conversely, a *societal psychology* – a psychology of cognitive functioning for a given society – is accomplished by integrating down a column. Finally, integrating across both rows and columns yields a *universal cognitive psychology*.

The Berry and Irvine framework nicely captures the task at hand for those whose goal is a general theory of cognitive functioning. Of course, the real work begins when one attempts to fill in the cells, even forgetting for a moment the terribly difficult problem of extracting general aspects across rows (competencies) or columns (societies). Berry and Irvine suggest that we have achieved a societal psychology for a few, mainly Western, cultures, and that we have achieved universals for a few areas of cognitive functioning. Their appraisal may be overly optimistic, however, unless one is willing to identify Western Society exclusively in terms of the ecology of academic settings.

An approach that might be labeled "second-order ethnographic," because it attempts through interviews to obtain information that ordinarily would require countless hours of observation, is Klemp and McClelland's *job competence assessment*. Using peer nominations and other devices, outstanding individuals at a given job are identified to be compared with others working at the same job who are not identified as outstanding. Interviews are conducted in which individuals are asked to describe work-related situations they handled particularly successfully. Qualitative analysis of the transcripts of such interviews is the basis for identifying competencies associated with outstanding performance at the job. Across a number of job competence assessments, Klemp and McClelland extracted eight "generic" competencies for the role of senior executive: planning/causal thinking, diagnostic information seeking, conceptualization/synthetic thinking, concern for influence, directive influence, collaborative influence, symbolic influence, and self-confidence. Klemp and McClelland stress that what differentiates outstanding and average managers is their *disposition* to act in the most appropriate way in a problem situation, rather than in their capacity for such action. However, Wagner and Sternberg found relationships between managing success and practical knowledge useful for solving similar practical problems as well. One potentially important issue that appears to be neglected by the Klemp and McClelland formulation is some type of a feedback system that determines, among other things, how much one should engage in these various competencies in any given situation. For example, at what point is further diagnostic information seeking pointless? Can one exert a detrimental amount of directive influence on one's subordinates and a detrimental amount of collaborative influence on a group? When is the time for planning over and the time for acting on one's plans at hand?

Goodnow makes the case for combining ethnographic approaches, which stress observation of behavior in its everyday social context, and formal approaches, which stress more analytical analyses of behavior in laboratory settings, to obtain fresh perspectives and generate new questions about intelligence. Goodnow demonstrates this approach in an incisive analysis of two intelligent behaviors: *organizing*, or planning; and *reorganizing*, or regrouping when one's original plans go awry. She argues that organizing and reorganizing are relatively general across age and situation. From her perspective, practically intelligent individuals are good at devising plans that enable them to accomplish their tasks efficiently, and are good at revising their plans when the situation warrants it.

Goodnow's analysis of organizing and reorganizing derives in equal measure from naturalistic interviews with children about such tasks as getting ready for school in the morning and arriving on time, and from more formal studies of planning drawn from the problem-solving literature. Goodnow's exclusive focus on organization and reorganization as the targets of her investigation seems justifiable because there does appear to be a general quality about these two behaviors. What remains to be determined is whether these two behaviors largely constitute practical intelligence, or whether they represent but 2 of 200 practically intelligent behaviors one might examine.

Simulation-based approaches

The simulation-based approaches involve observation of individuals in situations that have been designed to simulate some aspect of their everyday environment.

Scribner's studies of "unskilled" milk-processing plant workers is an example of combining ethnographic and simulation-based approaches in the study of everyday intellectual skill. Scribner conducted observational studies of individuals working as product assemblers (i.e., individuals whose job is to assemble the correct quantity of different kinds of dairy products for delivery), wholesale delivery drivers, inventory persons, and office clerks. She then provided the workers with laboratory analogues of their work-related tasks that were observed previously. Her analysis reveals that workers evolve highly specialized procedures for mental computation that are more efficient in completing their tasks than the general-purpose algorithms taught in school.

What is not clear from Scribner's analysis is the nature of the relation between practical intelligence and the specialized procedures devised by the milk-processing plant workers. Scribner chooses not to place her work in the larger context of intelligence in the everyday world. Her goal is a functional account of practical modes of thought, and she prefers to make no claims about abilities of individuals or about the structure of intelligence. Her position on this matter is consistent with that of Olson. Olson rejects the view that intelligence is a quality of mind, the quantity of which varies from individual to individual, and which explains intelligent actions. Instead, he emphasizes competence in dealing with cultural artifacts and technologies, and sees the role of a theory of intelligence as limited to description of types and levels of intelligence that provide a general characterization of expected levels of performance in a domain, based on a sampling of tasks from that domain.

Another example of the simulation approach is provided by Ceci and Liker, who compared models of racehorse handicapping of expert and nonexpert (although still quite knowledgeable) handicappers. Using the factorial survey approach (Rossi & Nock, 1982), they asked their subjects to handicap simulated races in which variables believed to be related to estimating probable odds were systematically manipulated. They found differences between the expert and nonexpert groups in the extent to which they used a complex algorithm for weighting the variables. Furthermore, the use of this complex algorithm was unrelated to IQ.

Advantages of the simulation approach include the extent to which the assessment situation parallels criterion performance and that, compared to simple observation, the additional structure provided by the simulation lessens the problem of unreliable scoring. Nevertheless, it can be difficult to decide just what aspects of a situation to simulate, and it is not always clear just how performance should be evaluated. Further, simulation is costly in terms of time as well as money.

Psychometric approaches

The psychometric approaches involve applying traditional psychometric methods that have been used successfully to study academic intelligence to the domain of practical intelligence.

An example of the psychometric approach is provided by Willis and Schaie, who compared relationships between performance on the Basic Skills Test (Educational Testing Service, 1977), a test developed to assess real-life competencies achieved by high school seniors such as reading labels, filling out forms, comprehending newspaper text, and reading a street map, with performance on a battery of traditional tests, for a group of older adults (mean age = 68.6 years). They were surprised to find very high correlations (.7–.8) between performance on the Basic Skills Test and measures of fluid as well as crystallized intelligence. This important result, viewed in the context of other studies reported in this volume that examined relations between

IQ and practically intelligent performance, provides empirical support for the contention of Frederiksen and others that what a test measures may depend as much on the format as the content. Looking across the studies reported in this volume, the correlation between measures of practical and academic intelligence varies as a function of the format of the practical intelligence measure: Correlations are large when the practical intelligence measure is testlike, and virtually nonexistent when the practical intelligence measure is based on simulation.

How can practical intelligence be measured?

The previous section dealt with approaches to understanding practical intelligence. This section deals with the question, how might we measure the practical intelligence of an individual or groups of individuals? Three methods will be considered: traditional psychometric methods, methods based on expert-group comparisons, and qualitative methods.

Traditional psychometric methods

One approach to measuring practical intelligence is to apply traditional psychometric solutions. Examples of this approach include the Adaptive Behavior Inventory for Children (ABIC) used by Mercer, Gomez-Palacio, and Padilla, and the Basic Skills Test used by Willis and Schaie. Comparing the two instruments, it can be noted that whereas performance on the Basic Skills Test was highly related to performance on traditional IQ tests, performance on the ABIC was not. There are several probable explanations for this difference in results. First, the Basic Skills Test is a test in the sense that the examinee is presented with items in paper-and-pencil format, whereas the ABIC questions are to be answered not by the "examinee," but by a caretaker who knows the examinee. Second, the content of the Basic Skills Test, which includes reading newspaper passages, reading paragraphs for comprehension, and understanding technical documents, is more academic in character than the content of the ABIC. Third, the subjects given the Basic Skills Test were elderly, whereas the targets of the ABIC were children.

An advantage of the psychometric approach to measuring an individual's practical intelligence demonstrated by the work of Mercer et al. and Willis and Schaie is that it is possible to construct tests that are as reliable, and as easily administered and scored, as are traditional psychometric measures. But what remains to be determined is what proportion of real-world intellectual competence can suitably be measured with such tests.

Methods based on expert-group comparisons

A second approach to measuring an individual's practical intelligence involves comparing their performance to that of an expert group. Wagner and Sternberg presented business professionals and academic psychologists with descriptions of work-related situations, and then compared their responses to prototypes derived from the responses of expert groups of business professionals and academic psychologists. Similar approaches were taken by Ceci and Liker in their study of horse race handicapping, and by Klemp and McClelland in their study of business executives. And, although he does not specifically advocate such an approach, it should be possible following Ford's approach to measure an individual's everyday competence by quantifying the extent to which characteristics ascribed to an individual, based on ratings provided by others, the individual himself, or by both, match characteristics of the prototypically socially competent adult.

The legitimacy of methods for quantifying performance by comparison to the performance of an expert group depends on (1) whether it is possible unequivocally to identify individuals who qualify as experts, and (2) the interpretability of expert performance. It can be difficult objectively to select experts in aspects of everyday intelligent behavior because with the exception of some occupational settings, individuals rarely are ranked in terms of their practical abilities in like manner to the ranking of chess players or students in school.

The problem of the interpretability of expert performance arises because experts often differ from nonexperts in characteristics that are unrelated to their expertise (e.g., age). Thus, a score derived from similarity to expert performance can be contaminated by characteristics unrelated to criterion performance. An example of this problem arises in the case of interest inventories. Interest inventories are tools for providing career guidance that involve comparing an individual's interests to those of various occupational groups. Whereas firefighters may enjoy competitive sports such as bowling, just because an individual does not says nothing about how capable a firefighter the individual might make. Though it is possible in theory to restrict the items of an interest inventory to interests directly relevant to job performance (e.g., "enjoys solving abstract problems" for mathematicians), in practice, objective determination of the work-related relevance of an interest is problematic.

Qualitative methods

A third approach to measuring practical intelligence is qualitative analysis of the sort employed by Frederiksen to quantify performance on his in-basket test. A sample of protocols was evaluated to identify relevant categories of behavior (e.g., asks for further information, exhibits courtesy to subordinates). All the protocols were then rated for the (1) presence of each category of behavior, (2) total number of actions taken (an indicator of productivity), and (3) characteristics of the actions taken such as creativity. Each of these ratings was then compared with performance on psychometric tests and measures of criterion performance for validation. The adequacy of this approach depends on the ability of raters to make a reliable determination of differences in performance in the in-basket situation that ultimately affect job performance.

Some important questions for the future

Several questions will be mentioned in this section for which answers have yet to be sought in a serious way, largely because of uncertainty regarding the more basic questions discussed in previous sections.

What is the developmental course of practical intelligence?

The developmental course of academic intelligence, in the form of performance on IQ tests, has been charted at least in broad terms. In general, performance on early IQ tests, excluding tests for preschool children, is a good predictor of performance on later IQ tests, although some individuals are characterized by large changes in IQ. For most individuals, the point of maximum performance on IQ tests is reached before graduation from high school, although some people who remain in academic settings continue to increase in level of absolute performance. Finally, performance declines with aging, although the timing and extent of the decline are topics of hot debate.

What might we expect the developmental course to be for practical intelligence? Does practically intelligent performance depend largely on underlying abilities that develop over the course of childhood, or does most of the developmental "action" take place in adulthood? When does one reach asymptotic levels of intellectual performance in everyday settings, and what is the time course and extent of decline if indeed there is decline?

The work of Willis and Schaie and Dixon and Baltes represents promising approaches to answering developmental questions about practical intelligence, especially questions concerning the effects of aging. For example, the dual-process conception of Baltes, Dittmann-Kohli, and Dixon (1984) distinguishes two domains of intellectual functioning that appear to correspond roughly to fluid and crystallized intelligence. The first domain, termed the *mechanics of intelligence*, includes the content-free architecture of information processing and problem solving. Aging-related decline is expected for this domain. The second domain, termed the *pragmatics of intelligence*, includes specialized, accumulated systems of knowledge and skills, for which stability and perhaps even improvement are expected with aging. For Dixon and Baltes, successful aging involves selective optimization with compensation: selecting life goals and trajectories that take advantage of one's durable specialized intellectual skills and realms of expertise and that facilitate compensation in areas of competence that would otherwise show decline.

Can practical intelligence be increased?

Given the early stage of much of the work discussed and a desire to avoid some of the mistakes made in the academic intelligence area, it perhaps is not surprising that few contributors directly addressed the issue of the trainability of practical intelligence (see Detterman & Sternberg, 1982, for discussion of approaches for increasing academic intelligence). The views of the contributors do have implications about the ultimate feasibility of training practical intelligence, however, and it is these implications that will be considered briefly in this section.

Because of its biological roots, the multiple-intelligences framework of Walters and Gardner would appear to be more pessimistic about modifying practical intelligence than other views. Intelligences are viewed as the joint product of innate endowment and a particular history of training. Rather than emphasize a program of training to further develop one's intelligence, Walters and Gardner see the important task as helping individuals find vocational and avocational niches that take maximal advantage of their particular profile of abilities.

Wagner and Sternberg have little to say about improving practical intelligence, but their tacit-knowledge framework is potentially more optimistic regarding the training of practical intelligence than others. If it is possible to teach tacit knowledge that is of general use, or if it is possible to train strategies useful in the acquisition of tacit knowledge, meaningful increases in an individual's practical competence could be expected, at least for limited domains such as one's occupation. On the other hand, if differential acquisition of tacit knowledge reflects long-standing differences in underlying practical abilities that are similar in character to academic abilities, the task of improving one's practical intelligence may prove difficult.

Finally, an implication of the Dixon and Baltes model of selective optimization with compensation is that one might improve practical intelligence for the aged if it is possible to improve their aptitude for selecting life goals that maximally take advantage of their unique pattern of abilities and expertise.

How is expertise acquired and used in practically intelligent performance?

A theme for several of the contributors is that expertise plays an important role in adult intelligent behavior. Dixon and Baltes present the case for the view that intellectual development beyond adolescence is not related to further development in basic cognitive processes. Rather, the primary form of development through adult life involves the acquisition of procedural and declarative knowledge associated with education, occupational life, and everyday life. They argue for further study of the specialization of cognitive skills, the acquisition of professional knowledge, and the nature of wisdom. What is needed, in their opinion, is not just an elaboration of the concept of crystallized intelligence, but a cognitively grounded understanding of the acquisition and use of expertise.

Wagner and Sternberg are beginning work on understanding how tacit knowledge is acquired and actually put to use by professionals in making work-related judgments and decisions. Regarding the acquisition of tacit knowledge, they are attempting to determine whether the acquisition of tacit knowledge can be accelerated, and if so, for which kinds of tacit knowledge and through which methods of instruction. Regarding how tacit knowledge is put to use, their interest is determining whether the usefulness of tacit knowledge is limited to such things as deciding what one should be doing and the best strategy for doing it, or whether the usefulness of tacit knowledge extends to lower-level performance aspects of "real-time" judgment formation and decision making.

Some concluding remarks about the search for intraterrestrial intelligence

We have considered a number of basic questions about practical intelligence, including what it is, how best to study and understand it, how it might be measured, and some important issues for the future. The points of view expressed by the contributors represent a healthy degree of variability, yet most of the points of view were shared among more than one individual. Everyone agrees that IQ tests are measures of only limited aspects of intelligence in the everyday world, although there is little agreement about what should take their place. Everyone has wrestled with the issue of how to derive generalities from collections of practically intelligent performance, although some worry more about the issue than others.

In short, the search for intraterrestrial intelligence is on in earnest. Using devious and ingenious means, the contributors (the *bricoleurs* of contemporary psychology?) have broken new ground in their attempts to understand intelligence in the everyday world. Only time will tell the true importance of the exciting beginnings described in this volume, but I suspect that they represent the start of a truly important period for the field of intelligence, and for psychology more generally.

References

Annis, R. C. (1980). *Bantu and Pygmy perceptual patterns: An eco-cultural study*. Unpublished doctoral dissertation, University of Strathclyde, Glasgow.

Baltes, P. B., Dittmann-Kohli, F., & Dixon, R. A. (1984). New perspectives on the development of intelligence in adulthood: Toward a dual-process conception and a model of selective optimization with compensation. In P. B. Baltes & O. G. Brim, Jr. (Eds.), *Life-span development and behavior* (Vol. 6, pp. 33–76). New York: Academic.

Berland, J. (1983). Dress rehearsals for psychological performance. In S. H. Irvine & J. W. Berry (Eds.), *Human assessment and cultural factors* (pp. 139–154). New York: Plenum.

Berry, J. W. (1976). *Human ecology and cognitive style: Comparative studies in cultural and psychological adaptation*. New York: Sage–Halstead.

Binet, A., & Simon, T. (1905). Méthodes nouvelles pour le diagnostic du niveau intéllectuel des anormaux. *L'Année Psychologique, 11*, 191–244.

Cole, M., Gay, J. Glick, J., & Sharp, D. (1971). *The cultural context of learning and thinking*. New York: Basic.

Detterman, D. K., & Sternberg, R. J. (Eds.) (1982). *How and how much can intelligence be increased*. Norwood, NJ: Ablex.

Educational Testing Service (1977). *Basic Skills Assessment Test*. Princeton, NJ: Educational Testing Service.

Ford, M. E., & Miura, I. (1983). *Children's and adults' conceptions of social competence*. Paper presented at the meeting of the American Psychological Association, Anaheim, CA.

Gardner, H. (1983). *Frames of mind*. New York: Basic.

Hebb, D. O. (1949). *The organization of behavior*. New York: Wiley.

Irvine, S. H. (1979). The place of factor analysis in cross-cultural methodology and its contribution to cognitive theory. In L. Eckensberger, Y. Poortinga, & W. Lonner (Eds.), *Cross-cultural contributions to psychology* (pp. 300–341). Amsterdam: Swets and Zeitlinger.

Mercer, J. R. (1979). *System of multicultural pluralistic assessment: Technical manual*. New York: The Psychological Corporation.

Neisser, U. (1976). General, academic, and artificial intelligence. In L. Resnick (Ed.), *The nature of intelligence* (pp. 135–144). Hillsdale, NJ: Erlbaum.

Neisser, U. (1979). The concept of intelligence. In R. Sternberg & D. Detterman (Eds.), *Human intelligence: Perspectives on its theory and measurement* (pp. 179–189). Norwood, NJ: Ablex.

Rosch, E. R. (1978). Human categorization. In N. Warren (Ed.), *Studies in cross-cultural psychology* (pp. 1–47). London: Academic.

Rosch, E. R., & Mervis, C. B. (1975). Family resemblances: Studies in the internal structure of categories. *Cognitive Psychology, 7*, 573–605.

Rosch, E. R., Mervis, C. B., Gray, W., Johnson, D. M., & Boyes-Braem, P. (1976). Basic objects in natural categories. *Cognitive Psychology, 8*, 382–439.

Rossi, P. H., & Nock, S. L. (1982). *Measuring social judgments: A factorial survey approach*. Beverly Hills, CA: Sage.

Serpell, R. (1979). How specific are perceptual skills? A cross-cultural study of pattern reproduction. *British Journal of Psychology, 70*, 365–380.

Sternberg, R. J. (1985). *Beyond IQ: A triarchic theory of human intelligence*. New York: Cambridge University Press.

Sternberg, R. J., Conway, B. E., Ketron, J. L., & Bernstein, M. (1981). People's conceptions of intelligence. *Journal of Personality and Social Psychology, 41*, 37–55.

van de Koppel, J. (1983). *A developmental study of Biaka Pygmies and the Bangandu*. Lisse: Swets and Zeitlinger.

Vernon, P. E. (1969). *Intelligence and cultural environment*. London: Methuen.

Wagner, R. K. & Sternberg, R. J. (in press). Executive control of reading. In B. Britton (Ed.), *Executive control processes in reading*. Erlbaum.

Wagner, R. K., & Sternberg, R. J. (1985). Practical intelligence in real-world pursuits: the role of tacit knowledge. *Journal of Personality and Social Psychology*, *48*, 436–458.

Name Index

379

Subject Index

0